# PEDIATRIC COLORECTAL AND PELVIC RECONSTRUCTIVE SURGERY

# PEDIATRIC COLORECTAL AND PELVIC RECONSTRUCTIVE SURGERY

Edited by
**Alejandra Vilanova-Sánchez**
**Marc A. Levitt**

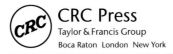

CRC Press
Taylor & Francis Group
Boca Raton London New York

CRC Press is an imprint of the
Taylor & Francis Group, an **informa** business

CRC Press
Taylor & Francis Group
6000 Broken Sound Parkway NW, Suite 300
Boca Raton, FL 33487-2742

© 2020 by Taylor & Francis Group, LLC
CRC Press is an imprint of Taylor & Francis Group, an Informa business

No claim to original U.S. Government works

Printed on acid-free paper

International Standard Book Number-13: 978-0-367-13651-2 (Hardback)
978-0-3671-3647-5 (Paperback)

---

**Library of Congress Cataloging-in-Publication Data**

---

Names: Levitt, Marc A. (Marc Aaron), 1967- editor. | Vilanova-Sanchez, Alejandra, editor.
Title: Pediatric colorectal and pelvic reconstructive surgery / [edited by] Marc A. Levitt, Alejandra Vilanova-Sanchez.
Description: Boca Raton : CRC Press, [2020] | Includes bibliographical references and index. | Summary: "This book provides comprehensive coverage of the anatomical and physiological aspects of complex colorectal and pelvic malformations. Also described are the surgical protocols for this specialized field within pediatric surgery. The benefits of high-level collaboration between surgical services when treating these anomalies are explained, as are treatment algorithms and care of complications. Includes evaluation and management of the newborn Describes surgical interventions of the newborn, and when a primary repair versus a staged approach is required Explains the value of laparoscopy and deciding in which cases to use it Looks at the importance of a transition program to adulthood Pediatric surgeons worldwide and the teams in which they work will benefit from this well illustrated and comprehensive work"-- Provided by publisher.
Identifiers: LCCN 2019042582 (print) | LCCN 2019042583 (ebook) | ISBN 9780367136475 (paperback ; alk. paper) | ISBN 9780367136512 (hardback ; alk. paper) | ISBN 9780429027789 (ebook)
Subjects: MESH: Colonic Diseases--surgery | Rectal Diseases--surgery | Pelvis--surgery | Reconstructive Surgical Procedures | Infant | Child
Classification: LCC RD544 (print) | LCC RD544 (ebook) | NLM WI 650 | DDC 617.5/55--dc23
LC record available at https://lccn.loc.gov/2019042582
LC ebook record available at https://lccn.loc.gov/2019042583

---

**Visit the Taylor & Francis Web site at**
**http://www.taylorandfrancis.com**

**and the CRC Press Web site at**
**http://www.crcpress.com**

# Contents

# Editors

**Dr. Alejandra Vilanova-Sánchez** is a pediatric surgeon who runs the Urogenital and Colorectal Unit at the University Hospital La Paz in Madrid.

Dr. Vilanova-Sánchez earned her medical degree at Universidad de Alcalá de Henares, Madrid and at Université de Montpellier, France. She completed her general pediatric surgical training at University Hospital La Paz, Madrid.

After finishing her training she completed a fellowship in Pelvic Reconstruction Surgery at the Center for Colorectal and Pelvic Reconstruction, Nationwide Children's Hospital, Columbus, Ohio. Her focus was on complex colorectal and pelvic surgery involving the gynecological and urological systems.

Dr. Vilanova-Sánchez is a member of the Spanish Association of Pediatric Surgeons, European Paediatric Surgeons' Association (EUPSA), and ARM-Net. She has written 35 peer-reviewed journal articles on colorectal and pelvic surgery, and has contributed to eight book chapters on the subject.

She is a frequent speaker at international meetings and has herself organized several national and international meetings on pediatric colorectal surgery.

She participates every year in surgical mission trips, collaborating with nonprofit organizations (Colorectal Team Overseas and Helping hands in Anorectal Malformations), where she helps patients with colorectal conditions around the world.

**Dr. Marc A. Levitt** has focused his clinical and academic career on helping patients with complex colorectal and pelvic problems. He received his undergraduate degree from the University of Pennsylvania, his medical degree from the Albert Einstein College of Medicine, and his surgical training at the Mount Sinai Medical Center in New York and the Children's Hospital of Buffalo. He is currently chief of Colorectal and Pelvic Reconstructive Surgery at Children's National Hospital in Washington, DC. Dr. Levitt has published over 300 articles, 80 book chapters, and three books. He has delivered more than 500 international, national, regional, and local presentations of his work and has been an invited visiting professor all over the world. He has trained dozens of clinical fellows, research fellows, nurses, and students in his career and has directed numerous colorectal training courses attended by established surgeons and surgical trainees from nearly every country. He is proud to have been a founding member of the Pediatric Colorectal and Pelvic Learning Consortium (www.pcplc.org). He dedicates much of his free time to mission trips around the world with an organization called Colorectal Team Overseas (www.ctoverseas.org) where he trains surgeons and nurses in complex colorectal surgical techniques.

# Contributors

**Marion Arnold**
Capetown, South Africa

**Mark Arnold**
Columbus, Ohio, USA

**Jeffrey Avansino**
Seattle, Washington, USA

**D. Gregory Bates**
Columbus, Ohio, USA

**Kristina Booth**
Columbus, Ohio, USA

**Giulia Brisighelli**
Johannesburg, South Africa

**Christina B. Ching**
Columbus, Ohio, USA

**Julie Choueiki**
Washington, DC, USA

**Daniel G. DaJusta**
Columbus, Ohio, USA

**Ivo de Blaauw**
Nijmegen, Netherlands

**Belinda Dickie**
Boston, Massachusetts, USA

**Karen A. Diefenbach**
Columbus, Ohio, USA

**Carlo Di Lorenzo**
Columbus, Ohio, USA

**Jennifer L. Dotson**
Columbus, Ohio, USA

**Sarah Driesbach**
Columbus, Ohio, USA

**Robert Dyckes**
Columbus, Ohio, USA

**Victor Etwire**
Accra, Ghana

**Meghan Fisher**
Columbus, Ohio, USA

**Molly E. Fuchs**
Columbus, Ohio, USA

**Alessandra C. Gasior**
Columbus, Ohio, USA

**Devin R. Halleran**
Columbus, Ohio, USA

**Geri Hewitt**
Columbus, Ohio, USA

**Stuart Hosie**
Munich, Germany

**Sebastian King**
Melbourne, Australia

**Wilfried Krois**
Vienna, Austria

**Martin Lacher**
Leipzig, Germany

**Victoria Lane**
Leeds, United Kingdom

**Jacob C. Langer**
Toronto, Canada

**Taiwo Lawal**
Ibadan, Nigeria

**Marc A. Levitt**
Washington, DC, USA

**Peter L. Lu**
Columbus, Ohio, USA

**Ross Maltz**
Columbus, Ohio, USA

**Kate McCracken**
Columbus, Ohio, USA

**Paola Midrio**
Treviso, Italy

**Dennis Minzler**
Columbus, Ohio, USA

**Onnalisa Nash**
Columbus, Ohio, USA

**Mikko Pakarinen**
Helsinki, Finland

**Lori Parker**
Normal, Illinois, USA

**Carlos A. Reck-Burneo**
Vienna, Austria

**Rebecca M. Rentea**
Kansas City, Missouri, USA

**Risto Rintala**
Helsinki, Finland

**Michael D. Rollins**
Salt Lake City, Utah, USA

**Brenda Ruth**
Columbus, Ohio, USA

**Greg Ryan**
Melbourne, Australia

**Sabine Sarnacki**
Paris, France

**Rita D. Shelby**
Columbus, Ohio, USA

**Caitlin A. Smith**
Seattle, Washington, USA

**Jonathan H. Sutcliffe**
Leeds, United Kingdom

**Duarte Vaz Pimentel**
Leipzig, Germany

**Alejandra Vilanova-Sánchez**
Madrid, Spain

**Stephanie Vyrostek**
Columbus, Ohio, USA

**Andrea S. Wagner**
Columbus, Ohio, USA

**Laura Weaver**
Columbus, Ohio, USA

**Tomas Wester**
Stockholm, Sweden

**Chris Westgarth-Taylor**
Johannesburg, South Africa

**Richard J. Wood**
Columbus, Ohio, USA

**Desalegn Yacob**
Columbus, Ohio, USA

# Where are we in pediatric colorectal and pelvic reconstructive surgery? New insights and the future

Marc A. Levitt

## Introduction

A popular children's book, *Everyone Poops*, by Tarō Gomi, demonstrates that the physiology of stooling is thought about, makes children and parents concerned, and is a focus of much of a child's early development. For those individuals currently delving into our book on colorectal and pelvic reconstruction, Gomi's children's book has deep meaning, particularly when one recognizes that there is a follow-up to this book—*Pooh Gets Stuck* about Winnie the Pooh, a beloved frictional character. References to pediatric colorectal problems go back many thousands of years. In fact, in the Babylonian Talmud written 2000 years ago, the following treatment is described: "An infant whose anus is not visible should be rubbed with oil and stood in the sun...where it shows transparent it should be torn crosswise with a barley grain." Our surgical techniques to manage such a patient have certainly evolved since that time, but the basic principles of care remain.

It was our desire to help children in whom "poo gets stuck" (in all of its forms) that motivated us to write about this physiologic problem in a very practical way, in the hope that ideas could be spread across the world, reach into remote clinics, wards, and operating rooms, and ultimately improve the lives of many children.

My personal journey in this field began when I was an eager medical student in 1992 and I signed up for an elective in pediatric surgery. I met Alberto Peña, one of the pioneers in the field of colorectal care (Figure I.1), and this changed my career trajectory in a very dramatic and positive way. I observed Dr. Peña providing all aspects of these patients' care, and was in awe, and inspired. However, as I advanced in my training I became more and more nervous that there was no way that I could provide this level of comprehensive care. I saw medicine becoming increasingly complex and knew I needed help from collaborators.

The modern pediatric colorectal story for the treatment of anorectal malformations began in Melbourne, Australia when Douglas Stephens (Figure I.2) worked on defining the

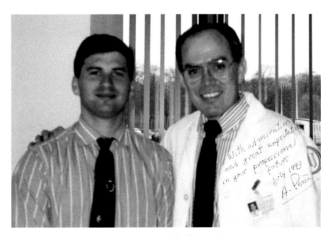

Figure I.1 Marc Levitt and Alberto Peña in 1993.

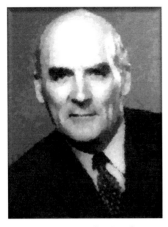

**Figure I.2** Douglas Stephens.

anatomy of children with these congenital defects. He did this by diligently performing autopsies on patients with these conditions. Prior to this, the anatomy of such patients was only a concept that existed in surgeons' minds, without anatomic precision, because no one had actually seen the anatomy. The anatomy was believed to look like the images shown in Figure I.3 from the bible of pediatric surgery in North America, the Gross textbook, which in retrospect was both oversimplified and inaccurate.

Dr. Stephens came to several anatomic conclusions during his autopsy dissections, most notably that a sphincter mechanism surrounded the rectum, the puborectalis sling. The surgery he proposed, the Stephens technique, as well as the Keiswetter technique, involved a perineal dissection to find a path for the distal rectum to be pulled through this sling (Figure I.4). Justin Kelly (Figure I.5), one of Stephen's trainees in Australia, learned

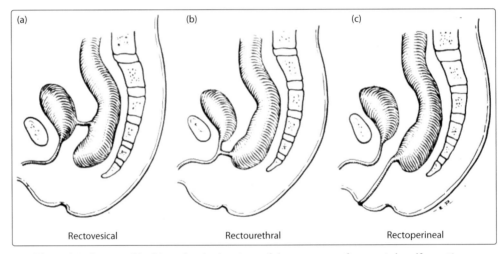

**Figure I.3** Gross and Ladd textbook, drawings of the anatomy of anorectal malformations.

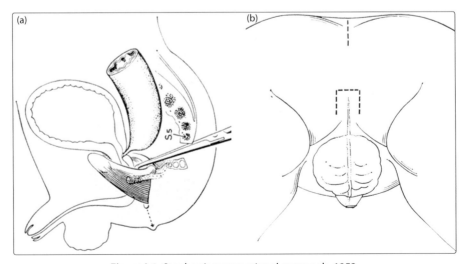

**Figure I.4** Stephen's sacroperineal approach, 1953.

how to do this and then traveled to Boston for further training. At Boston Children's Hospital he taught what he had learned from Stephens to the surgeons there, including another trainee, Alberto Peña (Figure I.6). At the same time Peña used to go across town to watch Hardy Hendren operate—Hendren was a master technician who was the first surgeon to successfully repair cloacal malformations. After completing his training in Boston, Peña went to Mexico City in 1972 to become the head of surgery at the National Pediatric Institute. When he asked his new partners to choose an area of specialization, no one chose colorectal, so he took on that group of patients and embarked on his revolutionary career. Peña at first applied the Stephens technique to children with anorectal malformations but he became increasingly frustrated by the procedure as it was blind and had very poor exposure. Over time his incision grew longer

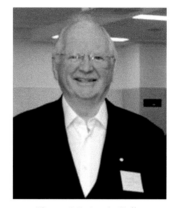

Figure I.5  Justin Kelly.

and longer. This culminated in 1980 thanks to a collaboration with Dr. Peter Devries (Figure I.7), who had come to Mexico City to work on these cases with Peña, with the first posterior sagittal anorectoplasty.

This posterior sagittal approach (Figure I.8) opened a Pandora's box. It allowed for a true understanding of the pelvic anatomy and led to the care of many conditions previously, to use Peña's description, very difficult to reach from above (via laparotomy) and very difficult to reach from below (perineally). The approach influenced the repair of cloacal malformations, urogenital sinus, pelvic tumors, urethral problems, reoperations for imperforate anus and for Hirschsprung disease, a transpubic approach (splitting the pubis for complex genitourinary problems inaccessible any other way), and a comprehensive strategy for the management of cloacal exstrophy. Perhaps the greatest contribution that came from a focused approach to these patients was nonsurgical, namely the development of the concept of bowel management for fecal incontinence. Thanks to such programs, thousands of children are no longer in diapers and have said goodbye to their stomas, an impact perhaps comparable to the use of intermittent catheterization for children with urinary incontinence.

During these years it was clear that myriad concerns related to patients' urologic, gynecologic, and GI/motility systems. It was at this point that I realized that a new paradigm of care was needed.

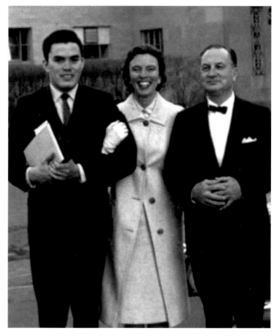

Figure I.6  Alberto Peña as a fellow at Boston Children's Hospital with his program director, Robert Gross.

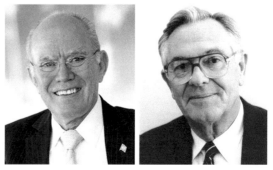

Figure I.7  Alberto Peña and Peter Devries.

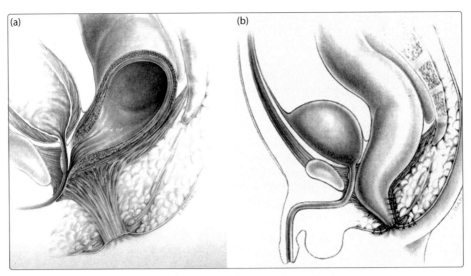

Figure I.8  The original diagrams of the posterior sagittal anorectoplasty.

I realized that much of the world works differently, and better, than medicine. For example, consider the project of creating a bridge. How does such a project start? I predict that the cement layers did not show up one day and lay cement prior to the steel team deciding where to place their beams. The project, I am certain, began with all parties sitting in a room and developing a comprehensive plan. Amazingly, that process does not happen often in the medical care of complex patients, but it most assuredly needs to.

I felt I had a unique perspective, having seen the care provided by a single individual needing to evolve into something more sophisticated. This idea of perspective is illustrated in Figure I.9, which shows what a little girl thought her mother did for work. One may assume they know the mother's occupation, but with perspective, and knowing that the mother worked for a hardware store, it was a snowy day, and there was only one shovel left to sell and many customers wanted it, you realize the importance of context. I saw the care of such children being done well by a single clinician, and simultaneously witnessed the complexity of medicine growing. I also realized that the care of children with colorectal problems is very difficult and harder than most realize (Figure I.10). It requires an integrated and collaborative approach because all the anatomic structures lie right next to each other (Figure I.11).

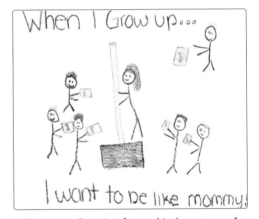

Figure I.9  Drawing from a kindergartner of what she thought her mother did for work.

To achieve success, patients with anorectal malformations (ARM), Hirschsprung disease (HD), fecal incontinence from a variety of conditions, and colonic motility disorders require care from specialists across a variety of fields throughout their lives. These include colorectal surgery, urology, gynecology, and GI motility, as well as orthopedics, neurosurgery, anesthesia, pathology, radiology, psychology, social work, and nutrition, amongst many others. Perhaps most important though, to their achievement of a good functional result, is their connection to superb nursing care.

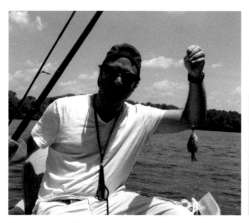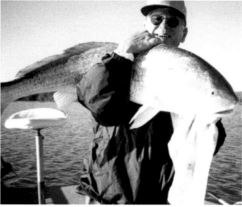

Figure I.10  What most people think it takes to do colorectal care compared to what it actually takes.

Having met many parents with newborns diagnosed with colorectal problems, I have made several observations. First, no parent seems to have ever thought that their child could have a problem with stooling—this is a physiologic ability that is taken for granted, and when told about this problem, they are usually shocked that something like this could happen. Second, when discussing with them that their child will need surgery to correct their colorectal anatomy, none focus on the surgical technique and elegance of the anal reconstruction, as I do. All instead focus on whether that technique will create an anatomy that will work, and will allow their child to stool without difficult, and become socially continent. Clinicians need to remember this—we always need to understand what it is that the family and patient wish for us to deliver to them. As proud of our skills as we are, it is the functional outcome that matters most.

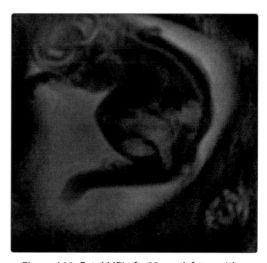

Figure I.11  Fetal MRI of a 22-week fetus with a cloaca. The bladder, vagina and rectum are all next to each other in the pelvis.

I like to say that a complex colorectal operation takes about four hours to perform, but in order to get a good result takes an additional 96 hours of work—the vast majority of which involves nursing care. From the very beginning of my journey in the field of pediatric colorectal surgery the value of a good nursing partner was clear. Their skills in identifying problems, solving them, being willing to get down in the weeds, and always striving to fill the gaps, are unique. I am so convinced, and often shout from the rooftops, that without my nursing partners I would have achieved very little as a surgeon.

With this collaboration we can achieve great things, and we need to always remember that "it is not the unanswered questions, but rather the unquestioned answers that one must pursue."

A few such advances achieved by a collaborative model, which will be discussed in the chapters of this book, include:

- Working in accurate prenatal diagnosis of anorectal and cloacal malformations (Figure I.11)
- Management of the complex newborn, particularly newborn radiology and neonatal care

- Recognizing and treating associated urologic anomalies
- Recognizing and treating associated gynecologic concerns
- Developing a protocol to predict continence, even in the newborn period
- Surgical interventions of the newborn and knowing when a primary repair versus a staged approach is appropriate
- Defining of anatomy so patients can be compared across centers, and treatment options and outcomes uniformly analyzed (Figure I.12)
- Recognizing the value of laparoscopy and knowing for which cases this approach should be applied
- Development of a treatment algorithm for management of cloacal malformations, taking into account the importance of their common channel and urethral lengths (Figure I.13)
- Recognizing key complications after ARM and Hirschsprung surgery, knowing when and how to do a reoperation, determining the outcomes of such reoperations, and ultimately figuring out how to avoid complications altogether
- Learning the physiology of fecal continence, which patients suffer from it, and the predictors of continence
- Development of a bowel management program and committing to following patients long term
- Recognizing the vital collaboration with GI/motility and offering surgical adjuncts to treatment, when appropriate, including colonic resection and antegrade options
- Collaborating with urology to render a patient clean and dry for both urine and stool and knowing when the colon could be used for a bladder augment, or if the appendix can

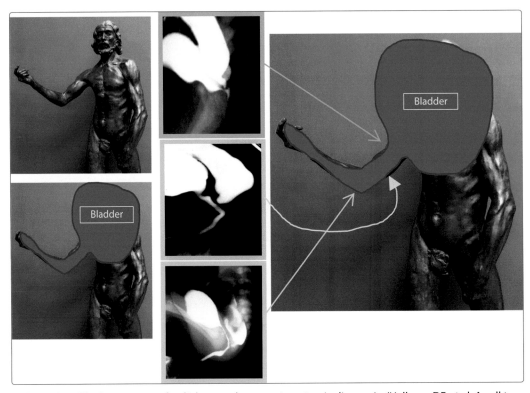

**Figure I.12** The importance of radiology and a correct anatomic diagnosis. (Halleran DR et al. A call to ARMs: *Accurate identification of the anatomy of the rectourethral fistula* in anorectal malformations. J Pediatr Surg. 2019, 54(8):1708–1710.)

be shared between Malone and Mitrofanoff

- Developing of new technologies, such as sacral nerve stimulation, and understanding for which patients they are appropriate
- Development of dedicated centers, that are integrated and collaborative and documenting that such centers provide better outcomes
- Recognizing the range of ages we need to care for and establishing transition program for adults
- Developing research protocols to define the genetics of these disorders and working toward tissue engineering of structures that congenitally have failed to correctly develop
- Using strategies to have real-time data, follow outcomes, and respond to changes
- Developing international consortiums that work well together to help patients in a way not achievable by a single institution
- Bringing complex care to all corners of the world including the developing world
- Learning the pathophysiology of motility disorders, and based on a better understanding of this, develop treatment protocols
- Reaffirming the key principles stated by Sir Dennis Browne to help set a standard of care rather than create a monopoly

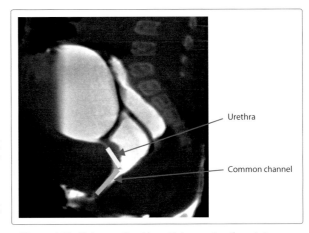

**Figure I.13** If the urethral length is greater than 1.5 cm, a total urogenital mobilization should be performed. If it is less than 1.5 cm, a urogenital separation is best.

We strove with this book to help other caregivers understand the daily struggle of improving a patient's quality of life, and to convey to the readers the skills and tricks to achieve good results. It was an honor to work on this book with colleagues who represent the authors, who have poured their heart and soul into their work and onto these pages, and to have my name appear as an author beside theirs. We hope you enjoy reading this book, and that it helps you help many children. If we have achieved that lofty goal, then we will feel very gratified.

# 1 Pediatric colorectal and reconstructive surgery: Fundamentals of surgical preparation

Rebecca M. Rentea and Andrea S. Wagner

## 1.1 Bowel preparation in pediatric colorectal surgery

### 1.1.1 Case 1

A 15-month-old female with history of constipation and weight loss presents for evaluation. Symptoms began at 4 months of age when she was transitioned from breast milk to formula. She had two previous hospitalizations for fecal impaction that required clean out and has tried multiple oral laxatives without improvement. Clinic examination reveals a funnel shaped anal opening admitting a 10 Hagar dilator. Abdominal radiograph reveals significant pancolonic stool burden.

The following should be considered:

- **A.** A diagnosis of anal stenosis
- **B.** A pelvic MRI to evaluate for a pre-sacral mass
- **C.** VACTERL workup should include spinal MRI, echocardiogram, and renal ultrasound
- **D.** Surgical plan includes posterior sagittal anorectoplasty with creation of diverting colostomy
- **E.** This child would benefit both from a mechanical bowel prep and oral antibiotics prior to surgery
- **F.** All the above are correct

*Answer:* F

### 1.1.1.1 Learning points

Any child presenting with anal stenosis should undergo full evaluation for VACTERL and Curarino syndrome. Although there is significant variation among surgeons regarding the use of bowel prep prior to surgery [1–4], we utilize it in our practice. The child has a significant pan colonic stool burden and is going to undergo a surgical anoplasty. Additionally, the colon is going to be diverted as an important surgical consideration when repairing nearly all cases of anal stenosis. Our current practice is to admit the patient a day prior to surgery for preparation with 25 mL/kg/hour of polyethylene glycol administered orally or via a nasogastric tube and clear liquid diet as tolerated. Oral antibiotics are also given preoperatively after the effluent is clear from the mechanical bowel prep. Mechanical cleansing of the colon decreases overall stool burden, but does not necessarily change the concentration of bacteria. For this reason, in addition to the intravenous antibiotics routinely given immediately prior to incision and re-dosed during surgery, oral antibiotics are given before colorectal surgery. A common oral antibiotic regimen includes neomycin and erythromycin which is given the day prior to surgery. Our current practice is to give Metronidazole instead of erythromycin because of its increased coverage of anaerobic organisms.

A specific group of patients who benefit from bowel preparation in the complex colorectal patient population include:

- Posterior sagittal anorectoplasty without ostomy creation
- Anticipated need for vaginal replacement
- Sigmoid resection
- Hirschsprung disease without ostomy creation, or with ostomy site serving as the pull-through
- Redo Hirschsprung disease or posterior sagittal anorectoplasty without ostomy creation
- Neo-malone appendicostomy creation

## 1.2 Rectal enemas and rectal irrigations

### 1.2.1 Case 2

A 5-year-old male with Hirschsprung disease who has previously undergone a laparoscopic-assisted Soave pull-through in infancy is scheduled for redo pull-through due to an obstructing Soave cuff.

Additional considerations while administering a bowel prep in children undergoing surgery for Hirschsprung disease include:

**A.** Rectal irrigations in the bowel prep
**B.** Do not administer a mechanical bowel prep, as it is not well tolerated in patients with Hirschsprung disease
**C.** Antibiotics are unnecessary in patients with Hirschsprung disease

*Answer:* A

### 1.2.1.1 Learning points

In addition to a mechanical bowel prep with polyethylene glycol and oral antibiotics, this child will benefit from rectal irrigations prior to surgery. Surgery for Hirschsprung disease involves a transanal dissection and an anastomosis above the dentate line. This is a good opportunity to teach caregivers how to successfully perform a rectal irrigation in case irrigations may be needed to treat distension after surgery. Postoperatively, there is a potential risk of anastomotic disruption with an irrigation. So the first few passages should be done by a trained clinician. The day prior to surgery when the child is already undergoing bowel preparation is an opportunity for rectal irrigation teaching and assists in emptying of the stool and decompressing the colon prior to surgery. Often due to the disease the patient has trouble emptying their colon, so irrigations from below are needed [5].

## 1.2.2  Case 3

A 3-month-old-male with Hirschsprung disease who underwent a transanal Swenson pull-through for rectosigmoid transition zone on the 8th day of life, is admitted for abdominal distension and bilious vomiting. He is diagnosed with Hirschsprung-associated enterocolitis (HAEC). The first step in treatment consists of

 **A.** Goltyely® (polyethylene glycol 3350 and electrolytes) clean out
 **B.** Rectal enema
 **C.** Rectal irrigations

*Answer:* C

### 1.2.2.1  Learning points

Hirschsprung-associated enterocolitis remains the greatest cause of morbidity and mortality in children with Hirschsprung disease [5]. Prompt rectal irrigations should be initiated immediately in the emergency department or clinic. Additionally, an examination of the anus with Hagar dilators and digitally to check for a stricture should be documented. A rectal irrigation is performed with a large bore soft silicone catheter, a 20-French for children less than 1 year of age, or a 24-French for children greater than 1 year of age. Using room temperature or warm saline, instill 10–20 mL of saline into the colon via the catheter and allow gas and stool to empty through the catheter. Repeat this process with aliquots of 10–20 mL of saline until the effluent runs clear. Saline instilled should be removed with the addition of gas and stool. If the saline is retained, the catheter is manipulated gently, and the abdomen massaged to allow "pockets" of gas and stool to empty during the irrigation. This process should be repeated at 6–8 hours intervals until the child's symptoms improve and they spontaneously stool between irrigations.

## 1.2.3  Case 4

An 11-year-old female with Hirschsprung disease presents to an outpatient clinic for evaluation of chronic fecal soiling. She had a pull-through in infancy for descending colonic transition zone and has struggled with constipation and soiling since being toilet trained. Her examination under anesthesia revealed she has patulous anal sphincters and partial loss of her dentate line.

**Treatment recommendations for this child?**

 **A.** Bowel management with rectal enemas
 **B.** Bowel management with oral laxatives
 **C.** Diverting ileostomy

*Answer:* A

To achieve fecal cleanliness, rectal enemas are used to mechanically empty the colon. It is important to distinguish between rectal irrigations and a retention enema, in which fluid is instilled and retained. Rectal irrigations use a small volume of saline flushed into and out of the colon to treat stasis. An enema is intended to instill a large volume of saline mixed with irritants like glycerin or castile soap that is used to mechanically clean the colon. The rectal enema is administered with a ballooned catheter and the solution is allowed to dwell for 5–10 minutes before removing the catheter and letting the stool pass. This solution cleans the colon of stool, then the colon remains "quiet" without any stool output until the enema is due the following day. A daily rectal enema will give this child periods of cleanliness and allow her to mechanically achieve social continence.

The infant in case 3, however, needs serial rectal irrigations as part of his treatment for HAEC. He could experience further bowel distention and bacterial translocation if given an enema rather than an irrigation.

## 1.3 OR setup for colorectal surgery: How to improve exposure?

### 1.3.1 Case 5

An adopted 2-year-old-female patient presents for surgical repair of long segment stricture of the recto-sigmoid pull-through for Hirschsprung disease. Diagnosis of her long segment stricture was made following admission for enterocolitis and difficulty performing home rectal irrigations.

**Operative considerations in this child include all of the following *except*?**

A. The family should be consented for both transanal and intra-abdominal dissection
B. Any style of anal canal retraction pins can be utilized
C. The patient should undergo a total body preparation
D. Possible diverting ileostomy may be needed if a tapering coloplasty is performed at the anastomosis

*Answer:* B

The case described above poses several important considerations. A full evaluation of the colon anatomy with contrast enema should be performed to assess the amount of colonic dilation. A dilated colon that fails to decompress with irrigations may require diversion. A tapering coloplasty for size mismatch at the anatomosis requires diversion. An ileostomy is a good temporary option in this setting as it does not disrupt the colonic marginal blood supply at the time of stoma creation and takedown [6]. The case described requires both trans-anal work of mobilizing the long stricture as well as potential intra-abdominal mobilization of the colon. Deep pelvic dissection can require the aid of a lighted retractor—such as a lighted St. Marks pelvic retractor (Figure 1.1). Lone star pins with silicone bungees and stainless-steel sharp hooks allow for several uses both during trans-anal dissection and for soft-tissue exposure during anorectal malformation surgery cases (Figure 1.2). A total body preparation should be performed to aid with rotating the patient for maximal visualization and exposure without having to re-prep the patient (Figures 1.3 through 1.7). While the steps of a total body preparation appear numerous, the resulting patient access by both the surgical and anesthetic team makes it very worthwhile.

The steps to total body preparation include

1. Cushion (we utilize Z-flos) to size under head
2. Chest roll under axilla to size available to anesthesia for prone position (placed by anesthesia on non-sterile side of drape)

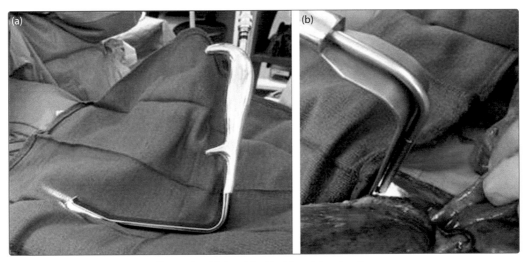

**Figure 1.1** Lighted St. Mark's pelvic retractor.

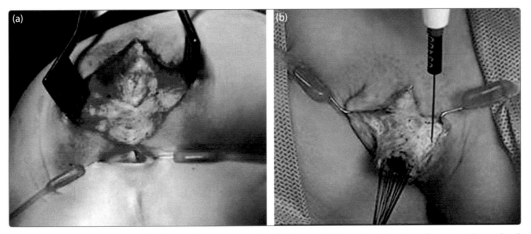

**Figure 1.2** Loan star pins with silicone bungees and stainless-steel sharp hooks allow for several uses both during trans-anal dissection and for soft-tissue exposure during surgery cases.

3. Two Z-flos available for arms in prone position (arms over the head) (Figure 1.3)
4. Anesthesia ether screen on bed and position small patients on bed so that feet can be lifted to the front of the anesthesia screen
5. Bovie pad placed high on back (between the shoulder blades) with 2–1000-drapes encircling the patient just below the bovie pad and around the chest (Figure 1.4)
6. 3/4 sheet placed under patient and over arms—before prep begins
7. Two people needed to prep—one person with prep sticks/one person who has sterile gloves on and lifts patient, 2 Chloraprep sticks
   a. One person preps anterior patient with 1st Chloraprep stick
      i. Make sure to get between toes, foot and ankle
   b. Second person puts on sterile gloves and lifts patient by prepped foot/ankle
      i. First person uses 2nd Chloraprep stick to prep posterior patient and sides
8. Prep person pulls the 3/4 sheet out from under patient and scrub nurse places sterile 3/4 sheet under patient and then legs are laid down

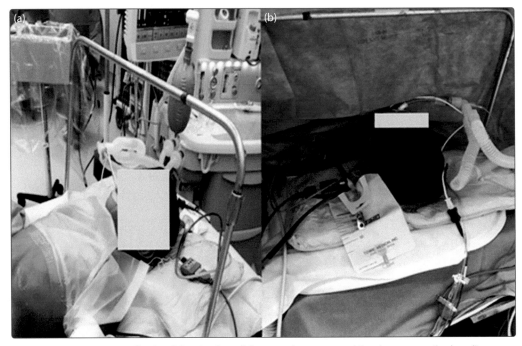

Figure 1.3 Two Z-flos (padding is placed) for arms in prone position (arms over the head).

9. Scrub nurse places second sheet across anterior abdomen covering the 1000 drape
   a. Two pieces of sterile tape are placed on each side of the patient in order to secure the drapes so that they are circumferentially around the patient (do not use hemostats or clips)
10. Large drape with circular hole is used to place the child through
    a. Do not stretch the hole in the drape until it rips—need intact sterile seal
    b. Place patients lower extremity through drape first and then up to mid-abdomen
11. Legs are wrapped—sterile, performed by scrub nurse (Figure 1.5)
    a. Soft sterile webril wrap and then Coban
    b. Need two rolls of each (sterile webril and Coban)
    c. Place all four rolls on operative field to facilitate case
    d. Start at toes first sterile webril and then Coban
    e. Coban should make a little extra "*toe flap*" (so that it can later have a clamp on it without crushing the toes or falling off)
    f. Make sure to go up high on upper thigh with the Coban
    g. Coban covers all of the sterile webril
12. Raytec (counted sponge) and large Tegaderm will be applied over stoma after prepping and draping
13. Foley catheter placed on sterile field (all children with anorectal malformation require Coude), for other children regular Foley would be okay, need 60 mL slip tip syringe for urine collection
14. Two people available to help anesthesia flip patient and pad arms
15. Arms need to be less than 90° at the shoulders
16. Surgeon/assistant will hold applied drapes under the circular drape in place as anesthesia flips
17. Have large sterile bump available for under patient's pelvis—small roll or blue towels to elevate feet (Figure 1.6)

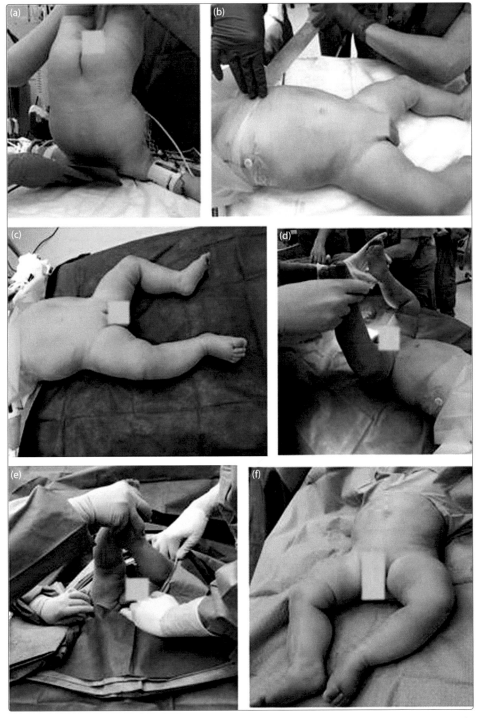

Figure 1.4  Bovie pad placed high on back, with 2–1000-drapes encircling the patient. Patient is placed following sterile prep through the opening of the surgical drape.

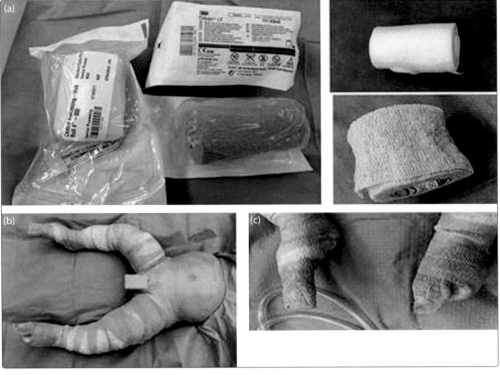

Figure 1.5  Supplies (soft sterile Webril wrap and then Coban) and technique to wrap the lower extremities.

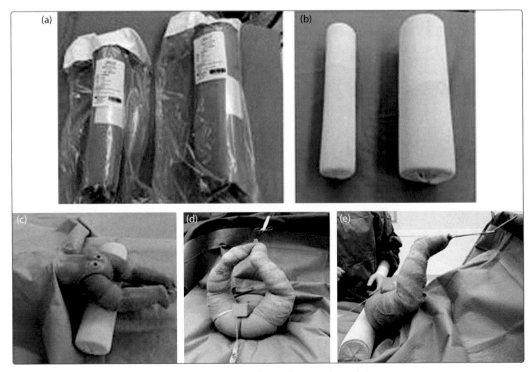

Figure 1.6  Sterile rolls to place under pelvis.

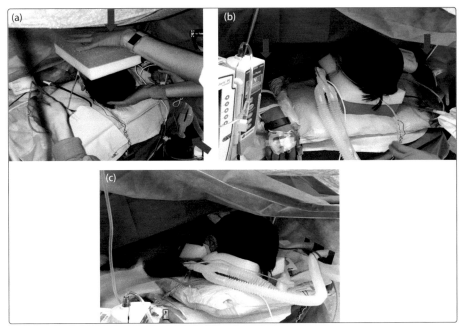

**Figure 1.7** Anesthetic prone position perspective. Arms are forward and padded.

# References

1. Anjali K.S., Kelleher D.C., Sigle G.W. Bowel preparation before elective surgery. *Clin Colon Rectal Surg.* 2013 Sep;26(3):146–52.
2. Bass L.M., Wershil B.K. Anatomy, histology, embryology, and developmental anomalies of the small and large intestine. In: Feldman M, Friedman LS, Brandt LJ, eds. *Sleisenger and Fordtran's Gastrointestinal and Liver Disease: Pathophysiology/Diagnosis/Management.* 10th ed. Elsevier Saunders, Philadelphia, PA, 2016: chap 98.
3. Feng C., Sidhwa F., Anandalwar S., Pennington EC. Contemporary practice among pediatric surgeons in the use of bowel preparation for elective colorectal surgery: A survey of the American Pediatric Surgical Association. *J Pediatr Surg.* May 2015;50(10).
4. Gosain A., Frykman P.K., Cowles R.A., Horton J., Levitt M.A., Rothstein D.H., Langer J.C., Goldstein A.M., American Pediatric Surgical Association Hirschsprung Disease Interest Group. Guidelines for the diagnosis and management of Hirschsprung-associated enterocolitis. *Pediatr Surg Int.* 2017 May;33(5):517–21.
5. Kiran RP, Murray AC, Chiuzan C, Estrada D, Forde K. Combined preoperative mechanical bowel preparation with oral antibiotics significantly reduces surgical site infection, anastomotic leak, and ileus after colorectal surgery. *Ann Surg.* 2015 Sep;262(3):416–25.
6. Soh H.J., Nataraja R.M., Racilli, M. Prevention and management of recurrent postoperative Hirschsprung's disease obstructive symptoms and enterocolitis: Systematic review and meta-analysis. *J Pediatr Surg.* 2018 Dec;53(12):2423–9.

# 2 Basic anatomic principles of pediatric colorectal and reconstructive surgery

Rebecca M. Rentea

## 2.1 Normal anatomy of the perineum in a newborn, toddler, and adolescent

### 2.1.1 Case 1

A 4-week-old full-term newborn female infant presents for surgical consultation with a history of constipation and concerns of an anterior location of the anus. Physical examination is performed in the clinic demonstrating the following perineal finding. Regarding this history and examination finding (Figure 2.1):

  A. Not enough information to decide if location of anus is correct
  B. Anterior anus may be normal variant and therefore does not require surgical correction
  C. Anal sphincter muscle complex stimulation will differentiate anterior anus vs. perineal fistula
  D. All the above

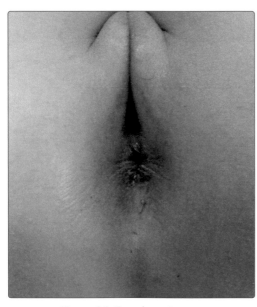

Figure 2.1 Female perineum.

**Does this young female who is examined in the clinic (with labia spread) need an examination under anesthesia or surgical intervention? (Figure 2.2)**

    **A.** Yes
    **B.** No

*Answers*: D,B

### 2.1.1.1 Learning points

Genital examination of the neonatal female is best conducted with the patient either in the frog-leg position, flexed and abducted at knees and hips or supine. Evaluation should include notation of the following anatomic structures. There are three qualities to anal location that should be noted—namely anal size, location (surrounded by sphincter muscle complex), as well as perineal body (separation from the introitus or urinary structures). Examination under anesthesia for the child in Figure 2.1 demonstrated normal anatomy with the anus surrounded by sphincter complex but anteriorly located. No surgery is indicated.

The child in Figure 2.2 has a congenital perineal groove. This anal opening is normal. This is a rare congenital malformation that is characterized by an exposed wet sulcus with non-keratinized mucous membrane that extends from the posterior vaginal fourchette to the anterior ridge of the anal orifice. The lesion can be misdiagnosed as contact dermatitis, trauma, or even sexual abuse. No surgery is indicated.

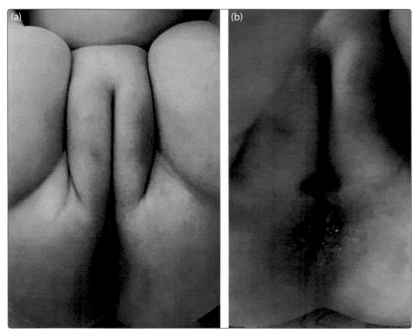

Figure 2.2 Congenital perineal groove.

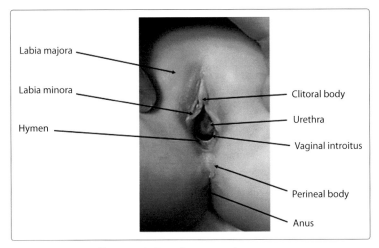

Figure 2.3 Female neonatal anatomy.

Examination in the clinic or operating room should include details regarding (Figure 2.3):

- Anus:
  - Size (Hegar dilator size)
  - Sphincter muscles (stimulation of the sphincter muscle complex takes places under anesthesia)
  - Strictures of the anus
  - Prolapse of anal mucosa
- Perineal body: Length in cm
- Hymen
- Labia minora and majora—normal or abnormal
- Clitoral body—normal or abnormal
- Vaginal introitus (Hegar dilator size of introitus, length of vagina to cervix [cm])
- Urethra: Length (cm) and location

## 2.2 Technical essentials of pelvic surgery

### 2.2.1 Case 2

A 2-year-old child with Hirschsprung disease is undergoing resection of a massively dilated Duhamel pouch with failure to empty stool and recurrent enterocolitis.

**While dissecting the intra-abdominal portion of the adherent pouch from surrounding structures, what are the key steps to reaching the pelvic inlet?**

    A. Taking down the bladder
    B. Carefully preserving the ureters and vas
    C. Avoiding gynecologic structures during dissection
    D. All the above

*Answer*: D

#### 2.2.1.1 Learning points

The relationship of the ureters relative to pelvic structures is of importance [3]: The ureter is close to numerous abdominal and pelvic structures, which puts it at risk during surgical procedures particularly in a reoperation. The ureters lie on the psoas muscle, passing medially to penetrate the base of the bladder. Descending into the pelvis the ureters course anterior to the iliac vessels and posterior to the gonadal vessels.

*Females*: The ureter runs posterior to the ovary and the broad ligament while coursing lateral to the uterus. The uterine arteries pass just anterior to the ureter at the ureterovesical junction.

*Males*: the ureter passes under the vas deferens before entering the bladder.

*Left ureter*: The uretero pelvic junction (UPJ) is just posterior to the pancreas and duodenal–jejunal junction and is crossed anteriorly by the inferior mesenteric artery and sigmoid vessels.

*Right ureter*: The right UPJ is posterior to the duodenum and lateral to the inferior vena cava, and is crossed by the right colic and ileocolic vessels.

### 2.2.2 Important points of the anatomy of the internal and external sphincter mechanism

#### 2.2.2.1 External sphincter

The external anal sphincter is under voluntary (CNS) control. It is a continuation of the funnel of pelvic muscles [3]. Innervation is via the inferior rectal (anal) branch of the internal pudendal nerve (sympathetic) and perineal branch of S4. The parasagittal fibers and muscle complex are part of the levator ani muscle group (striated muscle).

#### 2.2.2.2 Internal anal sphincter

The internal anal sphincter is under involuntary control. It is the continuation of the muscularis propria (colon circular layer, smooth muscle). Innervation is by pelvic splanchnics (S2–S4, parasympathetic, no voluntary control). There is no pudendal innervation. It is normally contracted, serving the role of a closed sphincter which can relax at the appropriate time.

### 2.2.3 In a Hirschsprung surgical procedure there are three different dissection planes that existing—defined by the Soave, Swenson, and Duhamel procedure

Three different dissection planes are utilized (Figure 2.4) [1]. *Swenson*: full thickness rectosigmoid dissection with an end-to-end anastomosis. *Soave*: performed as a way to

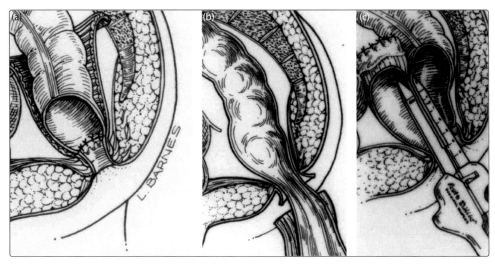

Figure 2.4 Three dissection planes. (a) Soave, (b) Swenson, (c) Duhamel.

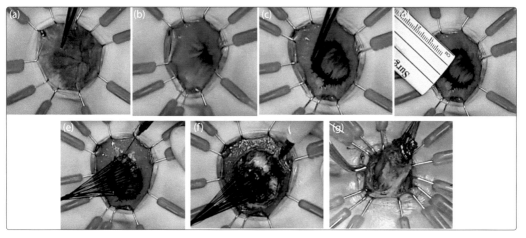

**Figure 2.5** (a) Exposure of the dentate line. (b) Followed by covering the dentate line. (c,d) The *purple line of Lee* (C) is drawn, 1 cm proximal to the dentate line. (e,f) Full thickness rectal dissection are performed, and (g) the hooks are moved for a third time covering the cuff.

avoid the risks of injury to pelvic structures inherent to the external rectal wall dissection. The *Swenson* procedure consists of removing the mucosa and submucosa of the rectum and placing the pull-through bowel within a "cuff" of aganglionic bowel (the external wall of the rectum). *Duhamel*: The aganglionic colon is resected to the rectum and the normal proximal bowel is brought retrorectally. The ganglionated colon and rectum are brought together in an end-to-side anastomosis. Understanding these key differences between procedures is vital to understanding potential complications related to HD surgery.

### 2.2.4 Anal canal exposure during Swenson pull-through

When performing a Swenson full thickness dissection, hooks to expose the dentate line are moved three times. Lone star retractor hooks are placed (Figure 2.5) initially inside the anal canal at the level of the mucocutaneous junction. Then just proximal to the dentate line so that it is no longer visible; assuring that it will be protected during the dissection. Finally, 0.5 cm of anal canal is preserved proximal to the dentate line (also referred to as the *Purple Line of Lee*) [1]. Electrocautery is used to perform *full-thickness* dissection along the traction line of silk sutures that were placed above the preserved anal canal. The pins are then placed into this cut edge to facilitate the full thickness dissection.

## 2.3 Colonic vascularization and its importance in pediatric colorectal surgery

### 2.3.1 Case 3

A 6-month-old male with an anorectal malformation and a history of a divided sigmoid colostomy presents for reconstruction. Prior to reconstruction, a high-pressure distal colostogram is performed demonstrating a recto-bladderneck fistula. In a patient with recto-bladderneck fistula, mobilization of a very high rectum requires:

   A. Ligation of the IMA
   B. Dissection of the distal IMA branches preserving the intramural rectal blood supply to the distal rectum, preserving the IMA branches and thus the intramural blood supply

    **C.** Ligation of the superior epigastric arcade

    **D.** Ligation of the middle colic artery

**In the previous question, what is the reason for avoiding ligation of the IMA?**

    **A.** IMA does not perfuse the rectosigmoid

    **B.** Previously done colostomy may have ligated the marginal branches

    **C.** IMA is not readily visible with laparoscopy

    **D.** The hemorroidal vessels depend on IMA blood flow

*Answers*: B, B

### 2.3.1.1 Learning points

Understanding the vascular supply to the colon (Figure 2.6) is essential for the technical success of any colorectal surgery. There are several considerations unique to children who require surgical intervention for Hirschsprung disease, ARM, or require re-operative interventions in the setting of past colorectal surgery. The three main vessels supplying the colon include the

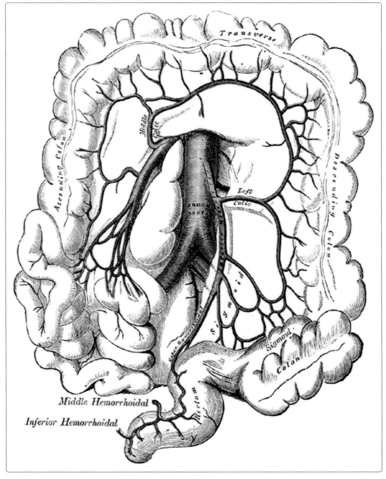

**Figure 2.6** Colonic arterial blood supply—note the marginal supply between the ileocolic and middle colic as well as middle colic and inferior mesenteric artery blood supply.

ileocolic, middle, and the left colic vessels. The rectum is mainly supplied by the hemorrhoidals which come from the internal iliacs.

*Right colon*: Is supplied by the ileocolic trunk and the middle colic artery. The middle colic artery generally divides early in its course into right and left branches. The left branch usually forms a well-developed *marginal artery* that connects with the left colic artery at the splenic flexure. The origin of the middle colic artery is from the superior mesentery in most cases and is absent in 5%–8% of the population. The marginal blood supply at the splenic flexure is poor in 32% of the population and absent in 7%. The marginal anastomosis between the right colic and ileocolic arteries is absent in 5% of subjects [4,5].

*Left colon*: The left colon is supplied by the inferior mesenteric artery (IMA) which arises from the aorta. Branches of the IMA are the left (ascending) colic artery (contributing to the marginal artery), one to nine sigmoid arteries, and the superior rectal (hemorrhoidal) artery.

*Rectum*: Vascularization of the rectum is through the superior hemorrhoidal (branch of the IMA and middle and inferior hemorrhoidal (branches of internal iliacs).

*Special considerations in Hirschsprung disease*: There is usually marginal supply between the ileocolic and middle colic as well as middle colic and left colic vessels. However, in a portion of the population (20%–40%) the marginal artery is absent [4,5]. This anatomic variation impacts pull-through operations that are dependent on marginal blood supply. A classic example is a transition zone at the splenic flexure in Hirschsprung disease that requires ligation of the middle colic artery. If there is no marginal supply to the ileocolic system, this pull-through will not survive.

*Special considerations for patients with a history of ARM*: Children with ARM who have undergone previous descending or sigmoid colostomy may have an interruption in the colonic vascular arcade. This means that the most distal portion of the rectosigmoid receives all of its blood supply from IMA. Therefore, the IMA cannot be ligated to bring down the rectosigmoid as it may result in loss of the rectum.

*Mobilizing the rectum*: During reconstruction surgery, operative length and mobilization of a high rectum is gained by ligating peripheral branches of the IMA vessels close to the rectal wall, being sure to preserve at least one or two proximal branches. The rectum thus relies on the intramural blood supply. Damaging the rectal wall results in interruption of the intramural distal blood supply.

## 2.4 Sensation of the anal canal

### 2.4.1 Case 4

A 4-year-old male presents for evaluation following a posterior sagittal anorectoplasty performed in the neonatal period for a recto-perineal fistula. He suffers from constipation, daily fecal smearing, and inpatient bowel cleanouts requiring GoLytle via nasogastric tube. He is not on any medication or enemas at home. Elements of bowel control consist of:

  A. Sensation
  B. Sphincter and rectosigmoid motility
  C. Reservoir function
  D. All the above

*Answer*: D

#### 2.4.1.1 Learning points

Bowel control requires sensation, sphincter, and rectosigmoid motility and reservoir function. The three parts of the bowel—anal canal, rectosigmoid, and colon perform different functions that are important to understanding bowel function and control.

The anal canal is capable of discriminating gas from liquid and from solid fecal matter. The muscle tone of the sphincter mechanism maintains the anal canal in a collapsed configuration. When gas, liquid, or stool reaches the anal canal, the voluntary sphincter mechanism can occlude the lumen of the anal canal to avoid a bowel movement. The rectum has the capacity for proprioception, or the ability to feel fullness, and acts a fecal reservoir as it remains in a relaxed state. Rectosigmoid motility and reservoir function are additional elements of bowel control. A colonic pull-through removes this rectal reservoir and may result in stooling.

Preservation of the anal canal in operations of patients born with normal anal canals assist with continence (e.g., Hirschsprung disease, severe constipation, inflammatory bowel disease, familial polyposis). Patients with ARM are born without an anal canal (exception is rectal atresia).

## 2.5 Ostomy creation

### 2.5.1 Case 5

An ex-34-week newborn male presents as a transfer at 30 hours of life with prenatal diagnosis of trisomy 21 and a cardiac defect. On examination, his abdomen is distended, and he does not have an anus.

**Given the anorectal malformation, he requires a colostomy; which type of colostomy is ideal?**

    A. Transverse loop
    B. Hartman's
    C. Divided proximal sigmoid colostomy
    D. Loop ileostomy
    E. Cecostomy

**What are potential disadvantages of a transverse colostomy?**

    A. Likelihood of prolapse
    B. Difficult to perform a distal colostogram
    C. Possibility of absorption of urine into the colon via a rectourethral fistula
    D. Distal fecal impactions
    E. All the above

In a male patient with an anorectal malformation, the distal colostogram demonstrates a rectoprostatic fistula, with the distal rectum just under the coccyx. During the dissection of the distal rectum, special care needs to be taken to avoid injury to:

    A. The vas deferens
    B. An ectopic ureter
    C. The seminal vesicles
    D. The bladder neck
    E. All the above

*Answers*: C, E, E

#### 2.5.1.1 Learning points

In anorectal malformation, separate stomas should be created ideally in the proximal sigmoid colon (a diverting loop is acceptible as well) (Figure 2.7). The mucous fistula can be tiny as its only purpose is to be used for the distal celestogram. To avoid stomal prolapse, the stoma is placed at the first mobile portion of the sigmoid colon after the descending colon, which is normally fixed.

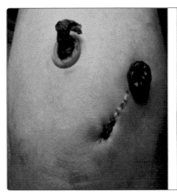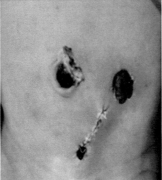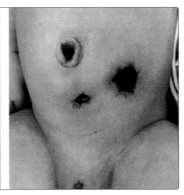

Figure 2.7 Forms of acceptable divided sigmoid colostomy with mucous fistula.

Why perform a separated divided colostomy? There are several pitfalls that exist with regard to the creation of transverse or some loop colostomies [2]. We recommend a divided sigmoid colostomy with mucous fistula and intact skin bridge or a diverting loop (Turnbull type stoma). Issues encountered include:

*Inadequately placed stomas*: If the colostomy is opened too distal in the sigmoid, it will interfere with the pull-through and not leave enough length of the bowel. During attempts to perform a transverse colostomy, cases of inadvertent sigmoid colostomy placed in the right upper quadrant have occurred. Anchoring of the sigmoid in the right upper quadrant can interfere with the pull-through of the bowel during reconstructive surgery.

*Transverse colostomy*: A transverse colostomy also allows for accumulation of mucous in the distal segment, distal stool is hard to clean out, makes a distal colostogram difficult, and potentially allows for colonic absorption of urine via the rectourethral fistula if present.

*Loop colostomies may cause*: Severe stomal prolapse. A loop colostomy does not completely divert the stool and may allow for distal stool impaction (occasionally requiring operative disimpactions) and urinary tract infections.

Patients with a cloaca pose unique considerations when forming a colostomy with mucous fistula as a hydrocolpos may be present which may operative drainage (30% of patients) if perineal decompression is inadequate. Drain age of the hydrocolpos at the time of colostomy may require a midline sub-umbilical incision, and then creating two separate orifices for the colostomy/mucous fistula (medial mucous fistula, lateral colostomy) and placement of the vaginostomy in the tube right lower quadrant. A majority of patients have two hemivaginas with both sides requiring adequate drainage. When the hydrocolpos is not large enough to reach anterior abdominal wall, pigtail catheter is best.

## 2.5.2 Technique for creation of laparoscopic divided sigmoid colostomy with mucous fistula

- Needs to be created prior to massive abdominal distension caused by the distal obstruction, between 24 and 48 hours of life.
- Camera access via 5 mm port at umbilicus.
- 5 mm port at colostomy site.
- 3 mm stab incisions for additional graspers if needed (suprapubic or right lower quadrant)
- When sigmoid loop is chosen near the retroperitoneal proximal attachment, enough to just get it out of the abdomen, enlarge the stoma site at the 5 mm port site.
- A small enterotomy can be created to wash out the distal bowel stool contents.
- Bowel is then divided using a staple load across it.

- The corner of the distal divided end is brought out through a separate incision medially, under visualization, only a corner of the staple line is removed (it is only required for a distal high-pressure colostogram in the future) and should not be matured like the functional end (this also makes bagging the functional colostomy easier).
- The functional proximal sigmoid colon staple line is resected, and the ostomy is matured in the lateral abdomen.

### 2.5.3  Hirschsprung disease and type of stoma: Leveling colostomy, loop colostomy, or ileostomy?

A stoma may be indicated for children with severe enterocolitis, perforation, malnutrition, or massively dilated proximal bowel, as well as in situations where there is inadequate pathology to support reliable identification of the transition zone on frozen section. So, if colonic anatomy is unclear, especially proximal to the splenic flexure, children under 6-months of age who would require division of the middle colic artery and may not have a right marginal present should be given an ileostomy. A leveling colostomy is a good option if pathology is available or the stoma can be opened in the dilated colon if a surgeon does not have a pathologist as a guide. An ileostomy is a good option if colonic mapping has not been completed or is pending. An ileostomy is a good option if the middle colic needs to be divided and a right marginal branch may not be present. If a loop is created, the distal end should be closed (can be performed with a circular suture placed in a purse string fashion closing the lumen of the distal bowel) to prevent stool from entering the diverted bowel.

## References

1. Levitt MA, Hamrick MC, Eradi B, Bischoff A, Hall J, Pena A. Transanal, full-thickness, Swenson-like approach for Hirschsprung disease. *J Ped Surg.* 2013;48(11):2289–95.
2. Levitt MA, Pena A. Operative management of anomalies in male. In *Anorectal Malformations in Children* Edited by: Holschneider AM, Hutson J. Heidelberg: Springer; 2006:295–302.
3. Skandalakis JE et al. *Skandalakis' Surgical Anatomy: The Embryologic and Anatomic Basis of Modern Surgery.* eds. Skandalakis JE, Colborn GL. Paschalidis Medical Publications; 2004:861–1002.
4. Gust L, Outarra M, Coosemans W et al. European perspective in Thoracic surgery-eso-coloplasty: When and how? *J Thorc Dis.* 2016 Apr; 8(Suppl 4):S387–98.
5. Meyers MA. Griffiths' point: critical anastomosis at the splenic flexure. Significance in ischemia of the colon. *AJR Am J Roentgenol.* 1976 Jan;126(1):77–94.

# 3 Anorectal malformations: The newborn period

Sabine Sarnacki, Sebastian King, and Wilfried Krois

## 3.1 VACTERL association (and syndromes) screening

### 3.1.1 Case 1

Prenatal diagnosis was made in a male fetus with a duodenal atresia associated with tetrology of fallot, a right renal multicystic kidney, with a polyhydramnios in the second semester of gestation who was then born at 33rd week gestation, with a birth weight of 1450 g. At birth, confirmation of the malformations suspected on prenatal US and MRI and a diagnosis of an esophageal atresia type III and of an imperforate anus was made.

**What is your work-up?**

A. Chest x-ray
B. Abdominal x-ray
C. Spinal cord US
D. Abdominal US
E. Echocardiogram
F. All of the above

*Answer:* F

### 3.1.1.1 Learning points

- The presence of these congenital malformations indicates a VACTERL/VACTER association which is defined by the presence of at least three of the following congenital malformations: vertebral defects (V), anorectal malformation (A), cardiac defects (C), trachea-esophageal fistula with or without esophageal atresia (TE), renal anomalies (R), and limb abnormalities (L). The incidence is estimated at approximately 1 in 10,000 to 1 in 40,000 live-born infants [1].
- A chest x-ray is mandatory not only to evaluate for the length of the upper esophageal pouch but also to detect costal and/or spinal anomalies which are present in about 60%–80% of patients with VACTERL association. Vertebral anomalies typically include segmentation defects, such as hemivertebrae, "butterfly vertebrae," "wedge vertebrae," and vertebral fusions, supernumerary or absent vertebrae, and other forms of vertebral dysplasia. Of note, the sacral abnormalities frequently associated with ARM are usually not included as true vertebral malformations for the diagnosis of VACTERL association, if isolated.
- An abdominal x-ray was done to confirm the diagnosis of duodenal atresia and also to show the level of the upper esophageal pouch. In VACTERL association, a number of subtypes of tracheo-esophageal fistula (TEF) may occur and may present with or without esophageal atresia. Overall, TEF occurs in approximately 5%–9% of patients. Abdominal x-ray is also useful to identify spine anomalies.
- *Sacral x-ray*: Sacral anomalies may be linked to the ARM, independent of the VACTERL association and consisting in sacral abnormalities ranging from a missing coccyx, a few sacral vertebrae, or hemi-sacrum, to complete absence with fused iliac bones. Sacral x-ray allow also to calculate the sacral ratio, which correlates with a continence prognosis and as well as to associated urological malformations [2].
- *Spinal cord US*: The presence of sacral anomalies is associated frequently with spinal anomalies. This exam should be done before 3 months of age prior to ossification of the sacral units. The most frequent anomaly is tethered cord but other dysraphisms can be identified such as filum lipoma, transitional lipoma, low conus medullaris, and short spinal cord (or caudal regression). It is of great interest to know if there is a spinal anomaly before surgery of the anorectal malformation because these patients are at high risk of post-operative urinary retention that could thus be anticipated.
- *Abdominal US*: This exam is mainly intended to identify renal or urological malformations whose presence should lead to measures to prevent renal infection and dysfunction, especially before and during ARM repair. It is thus better to perform this exam as soon as possible and before surgery. In this case the patient has only the left kidney and renal function should be carefully preserved. Vesicoureteral reflux must be diagnosed and proactively managed.
- *Echocardiogram*: Cardiac malformations have been reported in approximately 40%–80% of patients with VACTERL association. They can range from mild-to-severe congenital cardiac leisions requiring multiple step surgery. Patent ductus arteriosus or patent foramen ovale are not considered component features of the VACTERL association.

**What is your next step in management?**

Esophageal atresia should be repaired as a first step after birth along with a duodenal atresia repair and colostomy.

- If the patient is too fragile, the duodenal atresia repair could be done as a second step but then a gastrostomy is mandatory.
- If the esophageal atresia is a long gap type, the procedure is limited to the ligature of the fistula, gastrostomy, and colostomy plus duodenal atresia repair.

Later, when the esophageal atresia repair is planned, esophageal replacement with gastric tube or pull-up should be preferred to colonic replacement because of the associated anorectal malformation. The presence in this case of an associated duodenal atresia ensures a good volume to the stomach and allowed the creation of a gastric tube without compromising the volume of the stomach.

## 3.1.2 Case 2

Prenatal diagnosis is made of sacral anomalies in a female fetus. The baby is born at the 37th week of gestation, with a birth weight of 3150 g. Meconium was passed within the first 24 hours but progressive appearance of constipation developed. The anus is normally placed but has an infundibular aspect ("funnel anus") and high ano-cutaneous junction.

**What is your diagnostic hypothesis?**

    **A.** Anorectal malformation with sacral anomalies
    **B.** VACTERL association
    **C.** Currarino syndrome

**What is your work-up?**

    **A.** Spinal cord US
    **B.** Pelvic and abdominal US
    **C.** Sacral x-ray
    **D.** Spinal cord MRI
    **E.** All of the above

*Answers:* E

### 3.1.2.1 Learning points

Currarino syndrome (CS) is a rare cause of constipation. It was described in 1981 as a triad consisting of a sickle-shaped sacrum, a hindgut anomaly, and a presacral mass. In 1998, heterozygous point mutations in the *MNX1* (*HLXB9*) homeobox gene were identified in some CS cases with an autosomal dominant transmission, in half of patients, and in 90% of familial cases. Screening for sacral and spinal cord anomalies should be proposed to the parents as well as genetic analysis of the child and the parents. Beside the typical sickle-shaped sacrum (Figure 3.1), sacral anomalies may be less typical with total sacral agenesis or sacral unit anomalies below S2 or bifid sacrum. Although sacral anomalies are found in more than 95% of cases, a normal sacrum has been reported in genetically proved CS. Hindgut anomalies are found in 100% of cases as a typical infundibular anus with high ano-cutaneous junction in most of the cases associated with a more or less severe anorectal stenosis (Figure 3.2). A presacral mass, cystic, solid, or mixed is observed in 90% of cases and consist of a teratoma or anterior meningocele. A spinal cord anomaly is the 4th major sign identified in 70% of cases and consists of tethered cord, short filum, low-lying conus, lipoma of the filum or of the conus, or syringomyelia. Finally, a Müllerian duplication is diagnosed in 70% of CS females [3].

Spinal cord US should be done before 3 months of age to identify a spinal cord anomaly, which should confirm the diagnosis by showing any of the previously described anomalies. In cases of highly suspicious CS, spinal cord MRI is recommended because of its higher accuracy.

Sacral x-ray should confirm the prenatally diagnosed sacral anomalies that could also be analyzed on the spinal cord MRI or even better on pelvic MRI. This latter exam has the advantage

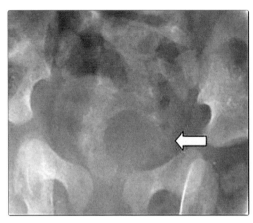

Figure 3.1 Typical sickle-shaped sacrum in CS.

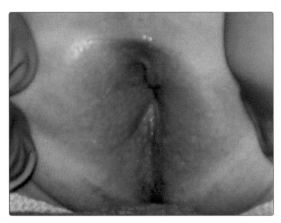

Figure 3.2 Typical infundibular anus in CS.

of identifying the presacral mass (Figure 3.3). A Müllerian duplication is difficult to identify in the neonatal period and pelvic US and/or MRI should be repeated at the beginning of puberty.

**What is your next step in the management?**

   **A.** Dilatation
   **B.** Surgery of the anorectal stenosis

*Answers:* A and B can both be correct

### 3.1.2.2 Learning points

Dilation of the anorectal stenosis may be sufficient to relieve obstruction when it is incomplete. This is of course if a presacral mass has been ruled out or resected. Dilations have been done in such cases without diagnosing a presacral mass which could have serious consequences in that a teratoma

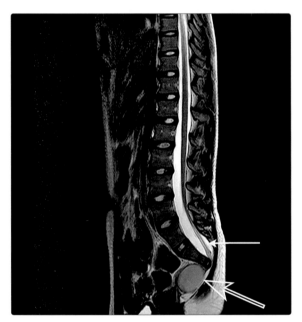

Figure 3.3 Typical presacral mass in CS (thick arrow) with tethered cord (thin arrow).

could be missed and undergo malignant transformation [4]. Special attention should be paid to a potential hidden communication between a presacral mass and the medullary conus, which is frequent and not always clearly identified on spinal MRI. Cases of meningitis has yet been reported which were linked to bacterial translocation induced by iterative anorectal dilatation [5]. When the stenosis is not manageable with dilatation, surgery should be done. The resection of the presacral mass during the same operation is recommended [6]. Unless a spinal correction is needed which may require separating the mass resection from the anal repair. A protective colostomy is not required but is a safe approach.

### 3.1.3 Case 3

A female neonate is born at term, at the 38th week gestation, with a birth weight of 2990 g. A diagnosis of an imperforate anus is made. There is meconium in the urine suggesting a high

ARM type. A colostomy is performed. Two weeks later a perineal hemangioma appears (Figure 3.4).

**What is your work-up**

   A. Pelvic and abdominal US
   B. Spinal cord US
   C. Spinal cord MRI
   D. Distal colostogram
   E. All of the above

*Answer:* E

### 3.1.3.1  Learning points

Pelvic hemangioma and ARM may be associated with LUMBAR syndrome: lower body hemangioma (LBH), urogenital anomalies, myelopathy, bony deformities, ARM, arterial anomalies, and renal anomalies [7]. The natural history of LBH is often associated with an initial phase characterized by unrecognized telangiectatic lesions and a second phase of rapid growth. Some hemangiomas extend deeply into the perineal region or may ulcerate and bleed. In the presence of an associated ARM, hemangiomas are typically located in the perineum.

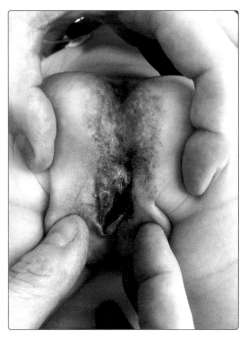

Figure 3.4 Female patient with perineal fistula and a perineal hemangioma in PELVIS-syndrome (patient in a prone position).

The work-up should screen all the potential associated anomalies and thus comprises at least pelvic and abdominal US, spinal cord US, and spinal cord MRI.

**What is your next step in the management?**

   A. Delayed ARM repair after disappearance of hemangioma
   B. Medical treatment
   C. ARM repair at 3 months of age

*Answers:* A and B

### 3.1.3.2  Learning points

Hemangiomas may regress spontaneously but generally do so very slowly. Treatment with nonselective β-adrenergic receptor-blocking agent (e.g., Propanol®) is currently the rule (after appropriate work-up) which allows for rapid involution within a few months [6]. ARM repair is performed when complete regression is achieved.

## 3.2  Key anatomical findings in the newborn to identify the different types of anorectal malformations

A careful clinical perineal inspection in the newborn is essential and provides important clues about the type of malformation. It is important to assess the perineum and the anal opening carefully because the passage of meconium does not necessarily indicate normal anatomy. In most of the cases with anorectal malformations, the clinical examination will suggest the correct diagnosis with more complex malformations needing additional studies and imaging.

The examination of the newborn is done in a supine position and with the legs relaxed and bent upwards. The form and shape of the bottom cheeks (i.e., "flat bottom" as a sign for more complex malformation) is evaluated and the area of the assumed muscle complex ellipse can be identified by a more pinkish color than the surrounding skin. Other than in perineal or vestibular fistula, it is impossible to identify the type of anorectal malformations by clinical examination alone. Some findings like meconium in the urinary stream can give hints about the existence of a fistula to the urinary tract, but it is impossible to tell the exact type of malformation without further studies. In female patients, you need to look for three orifices—the urethra, the vagina, and the rectum.

Practical tips for clinical evaluation in anorectal malformations

1. Hold the baby in a comfortable supine position with upward bend and relaxed legs.
2. Inspect the form and shape of the buttocks gluteal groove ("flat bottom").
3. Identify the assumed muscle complex as an area with a pinkish color.
4. Spread the perineal body to identify the anatomy and look for a fistula, meconium, or mucous beads or a "bucket handle" in the male.
5. The clinical examination of the female patient starts with the inspection and determination of the three perineal openings (urethra, vagina, anus/fistula).
6. Spread the perineal body by applying gentle traction to the labia outwards and laterally to identify the length and configuration of the perineum.
7. Lift the labia in cases where you cannot identify the three openings to get a better view of the vestibule to identify a vestibular fistula.

## 3.2.1  Perineal fistula in male

In this malformation, the rectum is seen to form a fistulous tract to the perineum anterior to the anal dimple (Figure 3.5), in some cases meconium or mucous beads can be seen on the perineum and may run along a fistulous tract along the midline raphe of the scrotum (Figure 3.6). The fistulous tract starts anterior to the correct location of the anus and there is no communication with the urinary tract. A "bucket-handle" deformity is associated with a perineal fistula (Figure 3.7). In cases without a clear visible fistula, mucous beads, or meconium, it is important to wait at least 20–24 hours after birth and repeat the clinical examination, because a significant intraluminal pressure is required for meconium to be forced through a fistula in order for it to be seen. A cross-fire film can show the rectal air column very close (within 1–2 cm to the perineal skin).

## 3.2.2  Perineal fistula in female

In females with perineal fistula, the fistula is separated from the vagina and the urethra with a small perineal body (Figure 3.8). In some cases, the perineal body seems short, but the anus may lie within the muscular complex. It is important to spread the perineum to identify the anatomy. In unclear cases, the patient may need an examination under anesthesia and electric stimulation to rule in or out a perineal fistula and/or confirm regular anatomy and muscular contraction within a centered anus.

## 3.2.3  Vestibular fistula

In patients with vestibular fistula, the fistula appears directly posterior to the vagina, but still, three openings can be seen (Figure 3.9). In some cases it can help to lift the labia on both sides to have a better view of the posterior part of the vestibule to visualize the fistula.

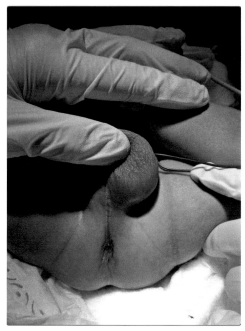

Figure 3.5  Perineal fistula with meconium indicating the orifice 24 hours after birth.

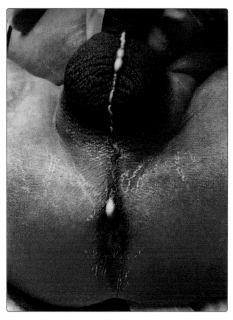

Figure 3.6  Perineal fistula with mucus beads along the midline raphe of the scrotum.

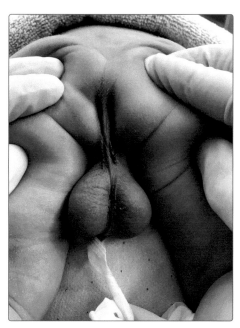

Figure 3.7  "Bucket handle" deformity as seen in male patients with perineal fistula (patient in a prone position).

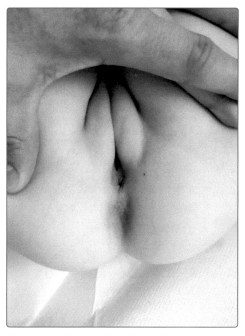

Figure 3.8  Perineal fistula in a female patient. The fistula is posterior to the vaginal vestibule and the muscle complex can be assumed in the pinkish area posterior to the fistula.

### 3.2.4  Recto-vaginal fistula

In this rare type of anorectal malformation, there are two openings. There is no visible anus and the fistula opens into the posterior aspect of the vagina. The urethra and vagina can be identified separately, the fistula can be hard to see by visual inspection only but can be assumed by vaginal meconium.

### 3.2.5  Cloaca

In cases of a cloaca, there is no anal opening and only one orifice in the perineum just under the distance in the majority of cases (Figure 3.10). It is impossible to assess the length of the common channel without further imaging studies.

### 3.2.6  Posterior cloaca

In a posterior cloaca, the urethra and vagina are fused, forming a urogenital sinus that deviates posteriorly to open in the anterior rectal wall or immediately anterior to the anus. The posterior location of the single perineal opening differentiates this malformation from the classic cloaca [8] (Figure 3.11).

### 3.2.7  Urogenital sinus

In a urogenital sinus, the urethra and vagina open in one single common channel. The anus is in normal position and centered within the muscle complex (Figure 3.12).

### 3.2.8  Additional perineal findings in patients with anorectal malformations

#### 3.2.8.1  Perineal masses

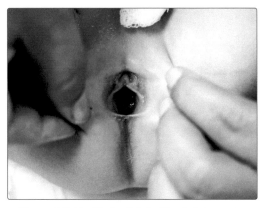

Figure 3.9 Vestibular fistula. The fistula can be identified with mildly elevated labia directly posterior to the vaginal introitus.

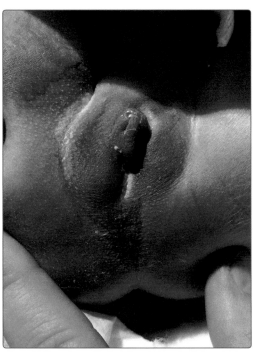

Figure 3.10 Cloaca. Only one opening can be identified by clinical examination.

Some cases of anorectal malformations present with a perineal mass. Usually, there are congenital isolated perineal lipomas and can be present in patients with or without an anorectal malformation (Figure 3.13). They result from a failure of caudal regression of the fetus and can contain skin, soft tissues, glia, osteoid, nephrogenic rests, and endocervical-type mucosa. MRI imaging is recommended to rule out a sacrococcygeal teratoma or spinal cord defect prior operative repair, although these rare vestigial appendages usually are not associated with anomalies of the spinal canal [9,10]. However, most of the lesions can be excised with preservation of the muscle complex during operative repair of an underlying ARM.

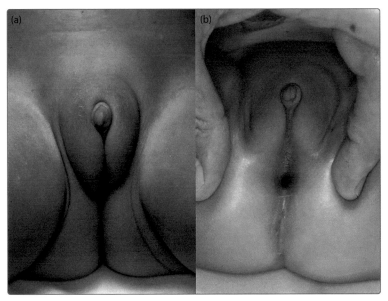

Figure 3.11 Perineum of a posterior cloaca without spreading the labia. (a) and after spreading the labia. (b) showing the single orifice. (From Peña A et al. *J Pediatr Surg* 2010;45:1234–40.)

### 3.2.9  Clinical scenario 1

You are asked to see a male newborn in the neonatal unit without an anus. During the clinical examination you cannot find a fistula in the perineal or scrotal region. Your impression of the bottom cheeks is that they are very flat.

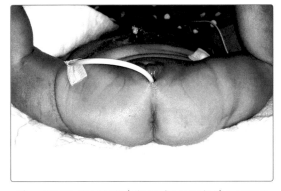

Figure 3.12 Urogenital sinus. An anus in the correct position and a long perineal body lead to one orifice for vagina and urethra.

**What is your diagnosis?**

A.  ARM without fistula
B.  Rectobulbar fistula
C.  At this time, the exact type of ARM cannot be specified

*Answer:* C

**How would you proceed in this case?**

A.  Go straight to the OR to perform a posterior sagittal anorectoplasty
B.  Wait for another 24–48 hours to see if you find a perineal fistula
C.  Opt for a diverting sigmoid colostomy and subsequent colostogram to specify the correct type of ARM and proceed with a repair in 2–3 months

*Answer:* C

### 3.2.10  Clinical scenario 2

You see a 4-year-old female with constipation and episodes of soiling in your clinic. During the clinical examination, you inspect the perineal area and find the anal orifice anterior to

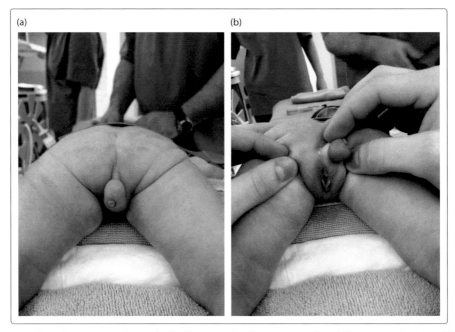

(a)     (b)

**Figure 3.13** Female patient with vestibular fistula and a "human pseudo-tail" congenital perineal lipoma (patient in prone position).

the pinkish area where you would suspect the muscle complex.

**How do you proceed in this case? (Figure 3.14)**

A. You suspect a perineal fistula and schedule an examination under anesthesia for electric stimulation to confirm your suspicion

B. You treat the patient with laxatives, because this looks like a normal anus

*Answer:* A

## 3.3 How to talk with the family—Potential for bowel control: Type of malformation, sacral ratio, and spine status (the ARM continence index)

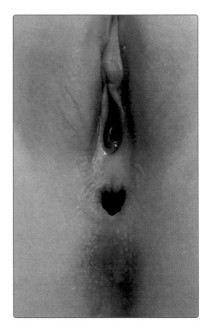

**Figure 3.14** Normal urethra, normal introitus and anal opening anterior to the pink ellipse of the sphincter mechanism.

### 3.3.1 Clinical scenario

The parents of new baby girl with a rectovestibular fistula have come to you to discuss her chances of long-term fecal continence. Her spinal ultrasound demonstrates no evidence of spinal cord tethering, nor associated fatty changes. Her sacral ratio, as calculated from her lateral sacral radiograph, is 0.78.

Pediatric surgeons are the most privileged of surgical specialists as we have the potential to impact upon the entire lives of patients. With this privilege comes great responsibility, as the impact of fecal incontinence upon children and their families is profound.

The ARM continence index is a newly developed tool that aids in prognosticating the likelihood of the patient being able to establish long-term fecal continence. The three main components are:

1. ARM type
2. Spine
3. Sacrum

The ARM type ranges from the simple (rectoperineal fistula) to the most complex (cloacal exstrophy). Assessment of the spine entails two components, namely the termination of the conus (normal, tethered, myelomeningocele) and the appearance of the filum (normal, thickened, myelomeningocele). The sacral ratio is calculated, preferably using a lateral sacral radiograph, to determine the tip of coccyx (C), the inferior point of the sacroiliac joints (B), and the iliac crests (A). The sacral ratio is then determined as the ratio of BC:AB. A normal sacral ratio is greater than 0.7, while the presence of a hemi-sacrum, presacral mass, or sacral hemivetebra is a poor prognostic sign.

According to these assessments, the patient described previously has an excellent opportunity to establish fecal continence. She has one of the milder types of ARM, has a normal spine, and a sacral ratio that lies within the normal range.

## 3.4 How to proceed when there are major co-morbidities—What should the surgeon do first?

### 3.4.1 Clinical Scenario

You are asked to see a new baby boy in the Neonatal Intensive Care Unit with a suspected esophageal atresia (EA) and an associated anorectal malformation (Figure 3.15a). Twelve hours following the initial radiograph, the baby has developed increasing abdominal distension

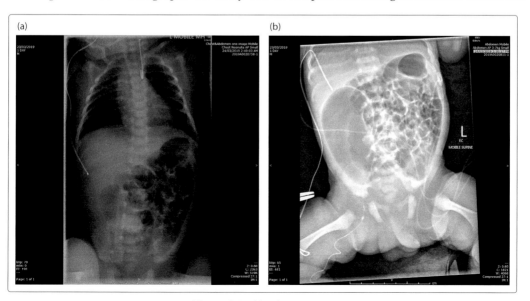

Figure 3.15  Newborn x-rays.

and the Neonatal team have requested an urgent review (Figure 3.15b). The baby is taken immediately to the theater for repair of the EA and formation of a divided sigmoid colostomy.

A significant proportion of children born with an anorectal malformation (ARM) will demonstrate at least one associated anomaly. In many children, these anomalies may represent a major co-morbidity that impacts upon their immediate prognosis, as well as their short- and long-term outcomes. Mortality related directly to the ARM is extremely rare, and is most likely the result of a complex associated anomaly.

Esophageal atresia (EA), though a relatively uncommon finding in children with an ARM, has significant implications for their immediate clinical management. In the majority of published series, EA occurs in 5%–9% of ARM patients, and often impacts upon the timing of operative intervention. As the majority of EA patients will have an associated tracheo-esophageal fistula (TEF), the passage of air through to the rectum may be expedited by preferential passage of air through the fistula. In these patients, the requirement for earlier formation of colostomy must be considered.

The presence of duodenal atresia (DA) in a child with an ARM, though less frequent than EA, does impact upon the operative approach to the ARM. As the flow of enteric content has been minimized during the fetal period, there is limited meconium in the rectum and the distal colon is typically less dilated. While this may facilitate an easier formation of a divided colostomy, the surgeon must be mindful of selecting the correct section of bowel and appropriately orientating the divided sigmoid colostomy. A potential operative trick that may facilitate choosing the correct section of bowel is to use the vision afforded by the transverse laparotomy incision for the duodeno-duodenostomy to mark the proximal and distal sigmoid colon with sutures. This will then hasten the delivery of the correct bowel loops through a limited left lower quadrant incision.

In ARM patients with associated EA/TEF and DA, it is recommended that a "top-down" approach to operative repair is taken. Division of the TEF, esophageal anastomosis, formation of a duodeno-duodenostomy, and then colostomy formation may be undertaken in one procedure, as long as the patient remains hemodynamically stable.

The most common major co-morbidities found in ARM patients are cardiac lesions. The cardiac lesion most commonly requiring operative repair is a ventricular septal defect (VSD), and this will rarely impact physiologically upon the patient undergoing formation of a colostomy. All patients with an ARM should undergo a thorough VACTERL screen, though in many patients the cardiac echocardiogram may be delayed until after colostomy formation, unless the patient demonstrates signs of cyanosis.

Abdominal wall defects are rarely associated with an ARM, except in the setting of exstrophy. The omphalocele-exstrophy-imperforate anus-spinal defects (OEIS) complex, first described in 1978, includes cloacal extrophy [13]. Improvements in prenatal ultrasonography have led to increased fetal diagnosis, and suggestions of a greater incidence of the complex than previously thought. In addition, the association between prune belly syndrome and congenital pouch colon has been described by a number of authors, but appears largely limited to the Indian populations [14].

The co-existence of colonic atresia and an ARM is exceedingly rare, and is limited to very small series in the literature [15]. The key clinical findings that may aid in the diagnosis include the small calibre of the distal rectum and the character of its contents, namely white mucus rather than normal meconium. The relationship between colonic atresia and Hirschsprung disease must also be borne in mind, though it is a rare finding.

## 3.5  Who needs a colostomy?

The decision about performing a colostomy or a primary operation must be made after 20–24 hours. As the meconium needs a significant intraluminal pressure to be forced through a fistula, and the rectum is still collapsed and not filled with gas directly after birth, the radiologic evaluations will not show the real anatomy before that time.

If the newborn with perineal or vestibular fistula is ill from associated anomalies, or is premature, the fistula can be gently dilated and the repair should be delayed. In patients with perineal or vestibular fistulas who are in good clinical condition without associated anomalies a primary anoplasty can be performed without a protective colostomy. Studies have shown that in cases with perineal and vestibular fistulas within a proper setting and careful surgical technique, the outcome in terms of continence seems similar in primary repair or multi-level approach with protective colostomy [16]. Although, this procedure strongly depends on the surgeon's experience and the potential advantages of an early repair must be weighed against the possible disadvantages of an inexperienced surgeon unfamiliar with the posterior sagittal operation and anatomic structures and the risk of perineal dehiscence.

In male patients where no meconium is seen at the perineum or urinary stream after 24 hours, a cross table lateral x-ray (cross-fire) in a prone position should be obtained. If the gas in the rectum is below the coccyx and the baby is in good condition, a primary posterior sagittal operation without colostomy is feasible. But it should be kept in mind that a repair without a colostomy is done without precise anatomic information about the patient's specific type of anorectal malformation. Horrible complications with injuries of the urethra, ectopic ureter, or bladder neck occurred in patients without a preoperative distal colostogram. In all cases where rectal gas is seen above the coccyx or the patient has meconium in the urine, significant associated defects or complex malformation with flat bottom or abnormal sacrum, a colostomy is recommended and the repair should be delayed for 2–3 months. Particularly in regions with insufficient medical supply and limited expertise in posterior sagittal operations, it is advisable to perform a colostomy and plan the definitive repair within an optimized setting.

In female patients without a visible fistula or a cloaca, a colostomy is indicated. In patients with a cloaca it is mandatory to perform an urologic evaluation prior the colostomy and drain a hydrocolpos if present. In rare cases, where the patient is unable to empty the bladder, a vesicostomy may be required [17].

# References

1. Salomon BD. VACTERL/VATER association. *Orphanet J Rare Dis*. 2011;6:56.
2. Vilanova-Sanchez A, Reck CA, Sebastião YV et al. Can sacral development as a marker for caudal regression help identify associated urologic anomalies in patients with anorectal malformation? *J Pediatr Surg*. 2018;53:2178–82.
3. Crétolle C, Pelet A, Sanlaville D et al. Spectrum of HLXB9 gene mutations in Currarino syndrome and genotype-phenotype correlation. *Hum Mutat*. 2008;297:903–10.
4. Rod J, Cretolle C, Faivre L, Jacquot C, Yacoub O, Ravasse P, Cheynel N, Sarnacki S. Malignant transformation of presacral mass in Currarino syndrome. *Pediatr Blood Cancer*. 2019 Feb 10:e27659.
5. Jeltema HR, Broens PMA, Brouwer OF, Groen RJM. Severe bacterial meningitis due to an enterothecal fistula in a 6-year-old child with Currarino syndrome: Evaluation of surgical strategy with review of the literature. *Childs Nerv Syst*. 2019;35:1129–36.
6. Baselga E, Dembowska-Baginska B, Przewratil P et al. Efficacy of propranolol between 6 and 12 months of age in high-risk infantile hemangioma. *Pediatrics*. 2018;142(3).
7. Iacobas I, Burrows PE, Frieden IJ et al. LUMBAR: Association between cutaneous infantile hemangiomas of the lower body and regional congenital anomalies. *J Pediatr*. 2010;157:795–801.e1–7.
8. Peña A, Bischoff A, Breech L, Louden E, Levitt MA. Posterior cloaca – further experience and guidelines for the treatment of an unusual anorectal malformation. *J Pediatr Surg*. 2010;45:1234–40.
9. Shaul DB, Monforte HL, Levitt MA, Hong AR, Peña A. Surgical management of perineal masses in patients with anorectal malformations. *J Pediatr Surg*. 2005;40:188–91.
10. Wester T, Rintala RJ. Perineal lipomas associated with anorectal malformations. *Pediatr Surg Int*. 2006;22:979–81.
11. Frade F, Kadlub N, Soupre V et al. PELVIS or LUMBAR syndrome: The same entity. Two case reports. *Arch Pediatr*. 2012;19:55–8.

12. Girard C, Bigorre M, Guillot B, Bessis D. PELVIS Syndrome. *Arch Dermatol.* 2006;142:884–8.
13. Carey JC, Greenbaum B, Hall BD. The OEIS complex (Omphalocele, exstrophy, imperforate anus, spinal defects). *Birth Defects Orig Artic Ser.* 1978;XIV:253–63.
14. Bangroo AK, Tiwari S, Khetri R, Sahni M. Congenital pouch colon with prune belly syndrome and megalourethra. *Pediatr Surg Int.* 2005;21(6):474–7.
15. Goodwin S, Schlatter M, Connors R. Imperforate anus and colonic atresia in a newborn. *J Pediatr Surg.* 2006:41(3):583–5.
16. Short SS, Bucher BT, Barnhart DC et al. Single-stage repair of rectoperineal and rectovestibular fistulae can be safely delayed beyond the neonatal period. *J Pediatr Surg.* 2018;53:2174–7.
17. Timothy BL, Ankur M, Jayant R. VACTERL associations in children undergoing surgery for esophageal atresia and anorectal malformations: Implications for pediatric surgeons. *J Pediatr Surg* 2015;50:1245–50.

# 4 Anorectal malformation: Definitive repair and surgical protocol

Belinda Dickie, Taiwo Lawal, and Paola Midrio

## 4.1 Preoperative considerations

### 4.1.1 Case 1

A newborn female with an anorectal malformation (vestibular fistula) is seen in the neonatal intensive care unit. On initial workup what imaging is required?

What if it were a male? Does it change the initial imaging if there is a perineal fistula opening?

What if the newborn male does not have any obvious perineal opening?

The importance of preoperative imaging to plan for a successful surgery cannot be stressed enough. Knowing the location of the fistula and associated anomalies can prevent potential surgical misadventures and provide an accurate guide for surgical planning.

At birth, a child should be screened for renal and bladder anomalies, the presence or absence of a tethered cord, and sacral abnormalities. If there is significant urologic issues, a voiding cystouretherogram should be obtained. This may reveal ectopic insertions of the ureters that may need to be addressed at the time of surgery, vesicoureteral reflux, and bladder emptying.

Sometimes overlooked in initial screening is the ruling out of a presacral mass. This can be done during the initial screening spinal ultrasound, and if present, the child may have Currarino's triad. If there is a presacral mass, a dedicated spinal and pelvic MRI should be done prior to surgery. This will determine if there is an intraspinal component to the presacral mass and whether neurosurgery needs to be involved prior to or coordinated with the procedure.

In both male and females, if the child has a perineal opening, often no further imaging is required prior to surgery to determine the location of the fistula.

If there is no obvious fistula site, cross-table lateral image (cross-fire) is sometimes done in the newborn period to see the location of the rectal gas. A bump is placed under the hips to place pressure on the abdomen and force the air distally into the rectum. Unless the gas is able to pass the levators/pelvic floor, this may not be accurate in the determination of the potential distance of the fistula/rectum to the perineum.

In males, a distal colostogram is currently the most widely accepted way to determine the location of the fistula. In collaboration with radiology, a balloon catheter is inserted into the distal mucus fistula. With the balloon inflated in the mucus fistula and below the level of the fasica, injection of the contrast can be instilled with enough pressure to allow the contrast to flow distal to the levator complex and outline the most distal aspect of the rectum and subsequent rectourethral fistula. A true lateral is needed to determine the location of the fistula to the tip of the coccyx to plan for a posterior sagittal approach only or if an abdominal approach is also required. A line drawn from the pubic bone to the coccyx (PC line) is helpful—if the rectum lies below this line a posterior sagittal approach can be done; if the rectum lies above this line a trans abdominal approach (laparotomy or laparoscopy) is needed. Enough contrast needs to be instilled into the rectum until the connection to the urologic system is delineated—usually apparent once the child starts to pass urine. An anteroposterior view is also needed to show the length and redundancy of the rectum. Ultrasound is emerging as a useful modality to provide the same information without ionizing radiation (Figure 4.1).

In females, rectoperineal and rectovestibular fistulas do not require imaging prior to surgery to delineate the fistula. However, if there is no noted normal vaginal introitus, a pelvic ultrasound may be needed to determine the presence or absence of internal Müllerian structures.

### 4.1.1.1 Imaging of the cloaca

Cloacal imaging is more complicated, as there are a number of anatomical issues that need to be addressed. Both contrast studies and endoscopic evaluation are required in order to plan appropriately for the reconstruction.

Initially, the standard imaging was two-dimensional fluoroscopy with a catheter at the common channel opening. This has subsequently evolved to catheterization of each structure (uretheral catheter, vaginal catheter, and injection via the mucus fistula) and 3D cloacagrams with computerized reconstruction.

Important landmarks during the study to note are the length of the common channel, length of the urethra off the common channel, location of the rectum, and take-off. These measurements determine the type of reconstruction and approach.

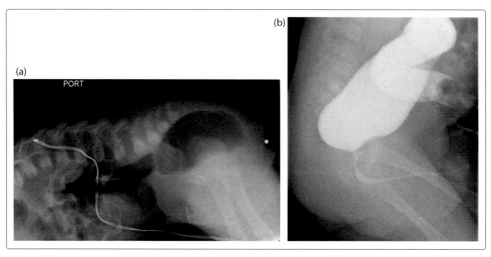

**Figure 4.1** (a) Cross table lateral with hips elevated to push air column in rectum distally past the levators. (b) Distal colostogram demonstrating rectourethral fistula.

### 4.1.1.2 Bowel preparation

The literature regarding bowel preparation in children is lacking, but it appears recently that the use of mechanical bowel preparations and preoperative oral antibiotics in elective adult colorectal procedures reduces surgical site infections.

Although the literature is lacking in the pediatric population, there are single center papers that have compared mechanical bowel preparations to no preparations and have found no difference in elective colorectal procedures.

The difference in anorectal malformation cases is the mucosa to skin anastamosis, which is likely a higher risk for healing. Postoperatively, it is important to avoid any impaction or hard stools, as this may cause undue stress on the coloanal anastamosis.

Because of this, children who are not diverted should undergo a mechanical bowel preparation. Patients who are diverted with a mucus fistula do not require a mechanical bowel preparation. In diverted patients with a mucus fistula or loop ostomy, irrigation of the distal limb bowel to be pulled through will help evacuate any impacted stool prior to surgery. Any child with a short distal limb, and cloaca patients with the potential need for vaginal replacement, should undergo a mechanical bowel preparation due to the potential need for proximal colon needed for the reconstruction.

### 4.1.1.3 Preoperative antibiotics

Preoperative antibiotics should be administered within 1 hour of making the incision for surgery to reduce the risk for surgical site infections. Antibiotic choice should cover lower gut flora, and consensus guidelines suggest cefoxitin, cefazolin plus metronidazole, or enhanced ampicillin with sulbactam. If penicillin allergy is present, a combination of clindamycin and gentamicin or ciprofloxacin is suggested.

In patients with risk of urinary contamination, a history of recurrent urinary tract infections, or known urologic issues with risk of infection, preoperative urine cultures are obtained and if bacteria are present, treatment and clearance of any bacterial presence should be considered.

## 4.2  Intraoperative considerations

### 4.2.1  Case 2

A 3-month-old male, with anorectal malformation and a colostomy performed at birth, is scheduled for PSARP, after execution of the distal colostogram that shows the level of recto-urinary fistula (rectobulbar fistula).

**What is your plan for him in the O.R.?**

  A.  Place the Foley catheter before PSARP
  B.  Place the Foley catheter if urethral damage occurs during PSARP
  C.  Place the Foley catheter at the end of PSARP

### 4.2.1.1  Learning points

- Male ARM patients undergoing PSARP, with or without a demonstrated rectourinary fistula, must have a Foley placed before surgery begins. During the posterior sagittal dissection, indeed, the bulbar urethra, especially in an infant, is quickly encountered and may be accidentally injured. The Foley helps to detect the urinary tract during surgery and will keep the urethra dry after closure of the fistula.

- In a male with rectourinary fistula, the Foley should stay at least 7 days postoperatively if no injuries occurred during surgery. In case of additional urethral repair or extensive dissection of the lower urinary tract, it may be required for longer. In a female with recto-vestibular or perineal fistula the catheter is left from 24 to 48 hours. In case of cloaca, it should stay 2–4 weeks.

### 4.2.1.2 Foley

Every patient submitted to an anorectal reconstruction must have a Foley catheter placed into the bladder per *urethra* before surgery. Due to the high prevalence of latex allergy observed in these patients and the possible need for urinary catheterization or bowel management with rectal probes in their future, it is recommended to use silicon catheters.

Placement of a Foley catheter in females with perineal or vestibular/vaginal fistula and males with perineal fistula is generally straightforward and should be performed before turning the infant prone and prepping the surgical field.

Placement of the catheter in males with rectobulbar prostatic fistula or bladder neck fistula is also performed before turning the infant prone and prepping the surgical field. However, in rare cases the Foley may proceed only a few centimeters from the meatus as it hits the fistula dimple and does not reach the bladder. In these cases, the catheter should be guided into the bladder by means of cystoscopy (cystoscope 8—9,5 Fr. with an operative channel to introduce the wire and the catheter with open tip over it).

The correct placement of a urinary catheter in case of cloaca, instead, is quite difficult or impossible as, most of the time, it goes into the vagina. In these complex cases the patient is prepped and the correction starts in prone position. By the time the common channel is isolated and opened, the urinary meatus becomes visible and it is possible, at this time, to insert a silicone catheter into the bladder.

### 4.2.1.3 Electrical stimulation

The use of electrical stimulation is very important to identify and correctly place the neo-anus within the muscle complex.

In the past the "Pena stimulator" was the only available device, but nowadays other instruments are present on the market, including a muscle-nerve stimulator commonly used by the anesthesiologists [1,2].

To obtain the best contraction no muscle relaxant should be infused at the time of initial stimulation and a continuous current should be used. When the tip of the stimulator is placed on the perineal skin, the best contraction is expected to be where the anal dimple is visible and/or where the skin has a different color, generally pinker and darker than the rest of the intergluteal fold. The stimulator is moved along the midline until no contractions are visible. The muscle complex of an infant is usually 2–3 cm long and it is not uncommon to observe right and left asymmetry. The sphincter should be marked prior to starting the operation.

### 4.2.1.4 Key steps

The PSARP (posterior sagittal ano-rectoplasty) is performed, in prone position with an indwelling urinary catheter placed before turning the patient and a roller pad underneath the pelvis (Figure 4.2). This approach is recommended for the majority of anorectal malformations and, as opposed to in the past, it is now best performed with surgeons standing on both sides of the patient. For those rarer forms of malformations for which a combined perineal-abdominal approach is foreseen, it is recommended to prep the patient from nipples to toes in order to be able to flip during the operation.

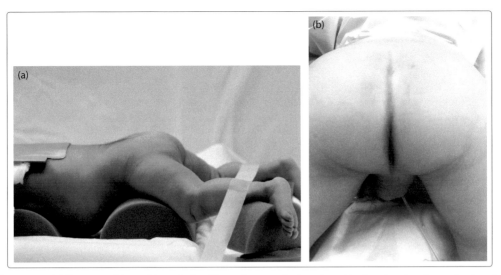

Figure 4.2 (a) Prone position with an indwelling urinary catheter placed before turning the patient and a roller pad underneath the pelvis. (b) This allows the perineum to be elevated and visible to the surgeon.

In the case of a classical PSARP (i.e., a male with rectourethral fistula), the incision must be kept in the midline from skin to deeper dissection. The use of retractors that help to maintain the exposure are also vital (i.e., two adjustable Weitlander or disposable hooks (Figure 4.3).

Once the dissection is deepened, the first encountered structure is, usually, the posterior rectal wall. This fact should be known and anticipated based on the distal colostogram. A couple of traction sutures are then placed on both sides of the midline and the rectum opened longitudinally in the midline. As long as the dissection proceeds more distally, more traction sutures are symmetrically placed on both sides until the fistula is encountered at the end of the rectum, on the anterior wall. At this point, a fine traction suture is placed in the midline on the fistula to better expose it. A series of fine traction sutures are placed across midline right above the fistula and the rectum cut between the fistula and the suture line. All traction sutures are put together by means of a mosquito clamp and by constant

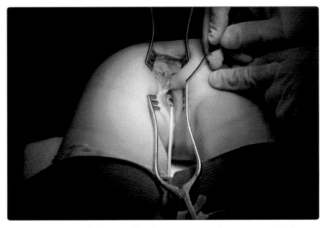

Figure 4.3 Position of the Weitlander retractors for symmetrical exposure.

traction. First the lateral walls are defined and then a plane between the anterior rectal wall and the urinary tract is developed, with great attention not to cause injury to the urethra. During this dissection the presence of the Foley catheter can be easily palpated and it helps to localize the urethra.

To gain enough length to reach the perineum, the rectum has to be dissected along both sides, posteriorly under the sacrum and anteriorly up to the peritoneal reflection.

Before pulling through the rectum, a meticulous reconstruction of the posterior urethra has to be performed. The rectum is then pulled to the perineum. The space anterior to the sphincter is cleaned, then the *levator ani* approximated behind it with absorbable sutures that include the posterior rectal wall (rectopexy). Finally, a neo-anus is fashioned within the muscle complex identified at the beginning of surgery with the muscle stimulator and rechecked at this time. Four absorbable sutures, including full thickness rectum and skin, are first placed at the four cardinal points and three stitches per quadrant (total of 16 stitches) complete the anoplasty. These are placed at slight tension and clipped to the draper. After cutting these stitches the anoplasty retracts in slightly.

### 4.2.1.5 Laparoscopic key points

Anorectal malformations with rectobladder fistula, some cases of rectoprostatic fistula, and cloacas may require an abdominal approach to mobilize the rectum and close the fistula. In these selected cases, laparoscopy can be very useful [3]. The patient is total body prepped and a Foley catheter inserted on the surgical field.

A 3 or 5 mm 30° camera and two 3 mm ports are used (Figure 4.3) and 6–8 mmHg pneumoperitoneum created. In some cases, a fourth 3 mm trocar is required to pull the bladder against the anterior rectal wall and facilitate the dissection of distal colon. The dissection is kept close to the rectal wall and continued distally until the caliber of the rectum becomes as thin as the dissector. The rectourinary fistula is closed with either a transfixed nonabsorbable stitch or an endoloop. The use of metallic clips is not recommended.

The patient's legs are lifted in order to expose the perineum. The patient remains supine. A midline incision is performed where the muscle complex is identified by the muscle stimulator. The dissection is deepened and by means of Hegars (size 8–15) a sort of "anal canal" is created that reaches the pouch of Douglas. Under laparoscopic vision a clamp is inserted through the neo-anal canal, and the dissected rectum is grasped and pulled out straight from the abdomen. Experience is required to understand how tense the rectum is in order to avoid postoperative retraction and stricture. The anoplasty is fashioned, in supine position, as previously described.

## 4.3 Follow-up Long term (anal dilations)

*Postoperative considerations*: At 2 weeks after PSARP or LAARP anal calibrations are started with Hegars dilatators or any other available tools that have a smooth surface and adequate increasing sizes (i.e., very thin candles or pipettes).

The most common schedule of calibrations is: bi-daily calibration (30–60 seconds each calibration) with weekly increases in size until 13–14 mm is reached (Table 4.1). Once the adequate anal size is reached, the colostomy can be closed, but calibrations are recommended, daily, for a couple of more months. Calibrations should not be painful, except for the first few days, nor should blood be noted. There is some speculation as to whether dilators are needed at all and this is currently being prospectively studied. If a good anoplasty is done and a patient does not dilate, a skin level stricture many result, which can be easily solved using a Heineke–Mikulicz plasty in four quadrants.

*Table 4.1*  Target anal dilator size for different ages

| Age | Size |
| --- | --- |
| 1–4 months | 12 |
| 4–8 months | 13 |
| 8–12 months | 14 |
| 1–3 years | 15 |
| 3–12 years | 16 |
| >12 years | 17 |

*Source:*  Elizabeth Speck K et al. Pediatric Surgery NaT
online resource, Anorectal Malformations.

## 4.3.1  Case 3

A 6-week-old female with an anorectal malformation (vestibular fistula) has two normal kidneys and normal sacrum, and cystoscopy and vaginoscopy showed a vaginal septum. She had a primary PSARP done a few hours ago.

**What is your plan for her to recommence feeding?**

   **A.**  NPO for 24 hours, then feed
   **B.**  NPO for 7 days, keep the patient on hyperalimentation, then feed
   **C.**  Feed immediately after recovery from anesthesia
   **D.**  Clear liquids or breast milk for 5 days, then feed

*Answer*: D is acceptable, and once adequate perineal body healing is confirmed a normal diet can start.

### 4.3.1.1  Learning points

- It is important to note differences in the postoperative care of patients with ARM based on the specific type of malformation.
- A primary PSARP for a patient with vestibular fistula places the additional challenge of preventing wound dehiscence on the surgeon and this has to be meticulously prevented.
- The period of NPO is shorter in patients who have a protective colostomy and discharge from the hospital is also earlier than in those repaired without a colostomy.
- In some circumstances an colostomy is appropriate to reduce the risk of perineal body dehiscence.

## 4.3.2  Case 4

A 4-month-old male with a anorectal malformation (rectoprostatic urethral fistula) was referred to you after a divided colostomy was done on the second day of life. He was scheduled for a PSARP, which was completed a few hours ago.

**How will you manage the Foley catheter left in place?**

   **A.**  Leave the Foley catheter for 5 to 7 days
   **B.**  Remove the Foley catheter after 48 hours
   **C.**  Leave the Foley catheter for 3 weeks

*Answer*: A

### 4.3.2.1 Learning points

- The Foley catheter placed in the urethra helps in its identification during surgery and prevention of urethral injury. The catheter serves to divert urine from soiling the wound in the postoperative period.
- The Foley catheter is kept for longer periods in boys; the higher the malformation, the longer the duration of catheterization.
- If the urethral catheter falls off, it should not be repassed through the urethra, as this may lead to disruption of the wound if urethral repair was done; it is not necessary to repass if it falls off in a patient who had an uncomplicated repair, as they usually void without difficulty.
- If the patient has an associated spiral anomaly such as a tethered cord, the surgeon needs to be more worried about urinary retention and may leave the catheter longer, and the surgeon also needs to be prepared for the possible need for intermittent catheterization.

### 4.3.2.2 Foley catheter

The Foley catheter can be removed in girls with vestibular fistula, as well as in boys with perineal fistula, within 24 hours of surgery but can be left longer to keep the perineal incisions dry. A similar measure is done for patients with ARM without fistula. In boys with rectourethral fistula, the Foley catheter is left in place in the urethra for 5 to 7 days. The catheter is retained for longer in those who had rectovesical fistula or in whom urethral repair was done, in which case the Foley is kept for 10–14 days, or in patients with spinal anomalies who may need to do intermittent catheterization. Another option is to pass a suprapubic catheter or perform a vesicostomy in boys with rectovesical fistula or following urethral repair, especially with a laparotomy or laparoscopy-assisted anorectoplasty. A transurethral silicon stent can also be used. This stent exits the lower abdomen at one end and the urethral meatus at the other end. The two ends are tied together to prevent the stent from being dislodged (circle stent) and the stent is removed after cystoscopy confirms healing of the urethra at 6–8 weeks.

### 4.3.2.3 Antibiotics

Patients continue on broad-spectrum antibiotics given at induction of anesthesia for another 24 hours. Antibiotic ointment can be applied to the sutures on the perineum for 7 days, or the wound can be left dry.

### 4.3.2.4 NPO

The patient can be fed on the same day of surgery, once fully recovered from the anesthesia, if there is a protective colostomy. Neonates who undergo surgery for perineal fistula are commenced on oral intake within 48–72 hours of surgery. In patients with vestibular fistula who undergo primary repair without a colostomy, the period of NPO is extended to 5 to 7 days. Older patients with perineal fistula who have surgery outside the neonatal period are treated similarly and placed NPO for 5 to 7 days. Clear liquid or breast milk may be given as those keep the stools liquid.

### 4.3.2.5 NG tube

The nasogastric tube is generally removed after the surgery unless an ileus is expected.

### 4.3.2.6 Diet in the long term

Patients usually have multiple bowel movements after colostomy closure. This may lead to perineal skin excoriation. A constipating diet is commenced to slow down the bowel. After several weeks, constipation ensues and the patient is commenced on dietary modification, fiber, and a senna-based laxative. Small volume enemas may be necessary to clean the rectum. The bowel movement becomes more regular at about 3–6 months postoperatively. The diet is tailored to ensure one to three bowel movements each day. A patient is likely to be toilet trained if he/she has one to three bowel movements each day, is clean in between bowel movements, and feels the urge to push or there is evidence of pushing during bowel movements. Dairy products are added to the diet to meet the calcium requirement.

### 4.3.2.7  Special considerations

Urologic evaluation through USS of the kidneys, ureters, and bladder is done at 3 months postoperatively. A voiding cystourethrogram (VCUG) is indicated if there is hydronephrosis, reflux, or urinary tract infection. The urinary tract is evaluated yearly and multidisciplinary management with a urologist is recommended. Urodynamic study is required to evaluate for the presence of neurogenic bladder.

## Selected references

1. Levitt MA, Peña A. Imperforate anus and cloacal malformations. In: Holcomb III GW, Murphy PJ, Ostlie DJ, eds. *Ashcraft's Pediatric Surgery*. Elsevier-Saunders, New York, 2014, pp. 492–514.
2. Kapuller V, Arbell D, Udassin R et al. A new job for an old device: A novel use for nerve stimulators in anorectal malformations. *J Pediatr Surg*. 2014;49(3):495–6.
3. Short S, Kimble K, Zhai S et al. A low-cost improvised nerve stimulator is equivalent to high-cost stimulator for anorectal malformation surgery. *Eur J Pediatr Surg*. 2013;23(1):25–8.
4. Georgeson KE, Inge TH, Albanese CT. Laparoscopic assisted anorectal pull-through for high imperforate anus – A new technique. *J Pediatr Surg*. 2000;35(6):927–30.
5. Bischoff A, Levitt MA, Lawal TA, Peña A. Colostomy closure: How to avoid complications. *Pediatr Surg Int*. 2010;26(11):1087–92.
6. Wood, RJ, Levitt MA. Anorectal malformations. *Clin Colon Rectal Surg*. 2018;31(2):61–70.
7. Levitt MA, Peña A. Anorectal malformations. *Orphanet J Rare Dis*. 2007;2:33.
8. Levitt MA, Peña A. Operative management of anomalies in male. In: Holschneider AM, Hutson J, eds. *Anorectal Malformations in Children*. Springer, Berlin, 2006, pp. 295–302.
9. Levitt MA, Peña A. Operative management of anomalies in female. In: Holschneider, AM, Hutson J, eds. *Anorectal Malformations in Children*. Springer, Berlin, 2006, pp. 303–6.
10. Elizabeth SK, Avansino J, Lane V, Reck C, Asokan I, Levitt MA. Operative management of anomalies in female. In: Holschneider, AM, Hutson J. Pediatric Surgery NaT (online resource), *Anorectal Malformations*.

# 5 Cloaca: Important steps and decision-making for pre- and post-definitive repair

Richard J. Wood, Ivo de Blaauw, and D. Gregory Bates

## 5.1 Introduction

Cloacal malformations are characterized by a single perineal orifice and confluence of the distal ends of the urological, genital, and gastrointestinal tracts. This represents the most complex end of the spectrum of female anorectal malformations. These rare malformations occur 1 in 25–50,000 live births. Due to this very low incidence, the majority of pediatric general surgeons and urologists will be exposed to only a few cases throughout their careers, even in a busy practice. This has led to the need to create protocols to allow for improved management. The work of Pena and Hendren to establish treatment guidelines was an essential basis for the modern understanding of these malformations [1,2]. Separating the genital tract from urethra and emphasizing the urologic component of this surgery during cloacal repair were key foundational works [3]. Measurement of the common channel, defining the posterior sagittal anorecto-vaginourethoplasty (PSARVUP), and the total urogenital mobilization (TUM) procedure were all significant contributions to the field [4]. Recently, as technology has allowed for more complex and accurate imaging techniques, it has become clear that other aspects in the anatomical assessment are important for predicting complexity and surgical planning [5–7]. The goal of preoperative assessment is to predict in an accurate manner which cases of cloaca can be repaired with a reproducible operation, the TUM, and which cases require a more complex repair (urogenital separation) with or without the added complexity of vaginal replacement [8].

## 5.2  Case study

A 1-day-old full-term female infant is examined in the neonatal ICU. She is found to have a single perineal orifice on clinical examination.

**What are the key components to this examination and what are the key components of care in the next 24–48 hours?**

The most important aspect in the care of a patient with a cloacal malformation is making an accurate initial diagnosis. This can be made clinically with good lighting and an effective physical examination technique. Initially the perineum is spread to identify the absence of an anal opening. Then the labia are lifted up and out to reveal a single perineal orifice. After confirming the diagnosis of cloacal malformation by physical exam, the presence of hydrocolpos and associated hydronephrosis should be assessed by pelvic and renal ultrasound. Imaging will assist in determining the approach for perineal drainage if amenable.

This decision-making can be challenging for several reasons. First, at this early stage patients may be in the physiologic oliguric stage and may therefore not produce enough urine to cause significant hydronephrosis despite it being present in utero. Second, almost all patients with a cloacal malformation require a colostomy as part of their initial treatment. The ideal time to drain the hydrocolpos would be at the time of the colostomy formation. However, it may not yet be apparent whether intermittent perineal catheterization (a viable option to manage hydrocolpos) is working by the time the patient undergoes colostomy formation. In the past this has led surgeons to drain the hydrocolpos formally with a vaginostomy; however, there is no good evidence that drainage with a vaginostomy is superior to intermittent catheterization [9–11] and therefore there has been a shift in practice in many centers away from default vaginostomy formation. Whichever drainage method is chosen, there needs to be a commitment to ongoing care. Regular ultrasound investigations to confirm decompression of the hydrocolpos and improvement of the hydronephrosis are essential to prove that the method chosen is working.

Much speculation exists about the ideal diversion site for the colon in cloaca patients. There are variations in practice, but the main principles are to create a completely diverting stoma, which can be successfully bagged and is created in an adequate position in the bowel, which does not interfere with the future rectal pull-through and the arcades, which may be needed for a future vaginal replacement [12]. We have formed end stomas in the descending and sigmoid colon junction with a mucus fistula at a separate site and have found these to be successful; however, other options do exist. The disadvantages of transverse colostomies are well documented; increased urine absorption leading to acidosis, increased rates of prolapse, and difficulty in distending the rectum for imaging of the distal colon for surgical planning. Several authors have proposed the use of loop stomas in the literature, and if these can be completely diverting, which requires a refined technique, then the evidence would suggest they are a reasonable alternative [13].

**After initial care of the infant, she is thriving with her colostomy and intermittent catheterization of her vagina/s. The patients family was taught how to do this cathing and successful decompression of the hydrocolpos and hydronephrosis were confirmed by ultrasound. At what point should she be imaged prior to her definitive repair, and what are the options available?**

A detailed understanding of the anatomy of a cloacal malformation is critical to the successful repair of these challenging surgical patients. There are multiple components to consider and having an organized approach is beneficial. The use of multimodal and multidisciplinary input has been found to provide all the necessary information to make good decisions [6]. All patients should undergo an endoscopic examination just prior to reconstruction. We do not advocate endoscopy in the neonatal period as this can cause trauma to delicate structures, and the images provided by small endoscopes are often suboptimal.

Endoscopy should be performed with all surgical teams (colorectal, urology, and gynecology as available) and radiology present. A detailed understanding of the anatomy of the urogenital tracts and the location of the rectal fistula can be obtained. The bladder and ureteric anatomy can be reviewed as well as the anatomic characteristics of the bladder neck and the urethra above the common channel. Measurements of the length of the urethra and the length of the common channel can be taken; however, the measurements taken with 3D reconstructed imaging are more accurate than those taken with endoscopy (Figure 5.1). This relates to the angle change of the common channel and urethra as they traverse the area posterior to the pubic symphysis and is therefore more dramatic in longer common channel malformations. In addition, endoscopy is able to delineate the anatomy of the female genital tract if it is connected to the common channel. The presence of a longitudinal vaginal septum and uterine didelphys can be diagnosed as well as the number of cervices and their patency. The presence of a didelphys configuration is the most definitive from a diagnostic point of view; the presence of a single cervix could mean either normal uterine anatomy or perhaps a bicornuate uterus, which may not be obvious on imaging. Multimodal imaging and longitudinal follow-up is required, especially around puberty, to fully define the uterine anatomy in many cases [14]. The location of the rectal fistula can be assessed during endoscopy; however, the location is only part of the story. It is important to not only know the location of the fistula's entry into the vagina or common channel but also the location of the true rectum in the pelvis (Figure 5.2). Spatial understanding of the relationships between all structures requiring reconstruction and the pelvis is vital.

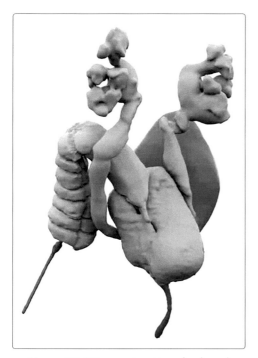

Figure 5.1 3D reconstruction of a cloacal malformation.

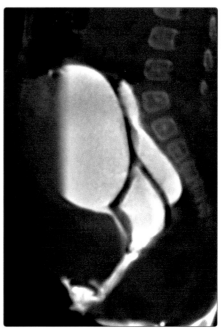

Figure 5.2 2D view of cloaca in the sagittal plane illustrating a cloacal malformation with a 2.8 cm common channel and an adequate 1.8 cm urethra with a very high rectum.

**What imaging techniques are available and how should they be used?**

The options for cloacal assessment are 2D fluoroscopy, 3D reconstructed fluoroscopy with or without the ability to manipulate the imaging, 3D printed images, and pelvic MRI with or without MR urography. When analyzing imaging options it is important to assess what information the different modalities are able to provide and additionally how easily this can be interpreted by surgical teams. The necessary measurements would appear to be obtainable from any of these modalities; however, their interpretation differs between the different modalities. The levels of experience definitely affect the ability to understand these images, with less experienced surgeons faring better on more complex imaging, approaching the abilities of experienced surgeons [15]. The fact that cloacal malformations are rare further emphasizes the need to use more complex imaging modalities. While 3D printing may be beneficial for the purposes of explanation to families [16] it adds significant cost and does not add significantly to the understanding of the anatomy by the surgical team [15]. MRI is able show great soft tissue definition, which may further aid the spatial understanding of the anatomy of pelvic musculature and hollow visceral structures [17]. There may be questions about the ability of MR to define fine structures like the common channel and urethral length accurately due to a lack of distension and at this time should probably be used in conjunction with fluoroscopy. Other modalities like contrast-enhanced ultrasound are currently under investigation and may hold future promise. At the conclusion of the endoscopy and review of the imaging, the surgical team should know: (1) the length of the common channel, (2) the length of the urethra, (3) the anatomy of the vagina or vaginas, and sometimes the anatomy of the upper genital tract, and (4) the location of the rectal fistula and the true rectum and its position in the pelvis, notably the pubococcygeal (PC) line. This information will allow the surgical team to decide on a surgical strategy, which we have found consistently predict the correct surgical plan [8].

**Do you have a specific protocol for how you might perform a 3D cloacagram on this 6-month-old child prior to her definitive reconstruction?**

At our institution, rotational fluoroscopy and 3D reconstruction are performed after initial examination under anesthesia (EUA) in the operating room (1). During the EUA, an 8-French end-hole Foley catheter (Folysil Pediatric Foley; Coloplast, Minneapolis, MN) is placed into the bladder under cystoscopy guidance and the balloon inflated. If you have to catheterize the bladder, I recommend attempts with a 6 or 8 Fr Coude catheter (Coloplast Self-Cath; Coloplast, Minneapolis, MN, USA) with the tip directed anteriorly. A similar 8-French end-hole Foley catheter may or may not be placed through the child's mucous fistula and the balloon inflated (this can be performed in radiology). Following completion of the EUA, the patient is immediately transported to the interventional radiology (IR) suite, under general anesthesia, where the 3D cloacagram is performed.

After positioning the patient on the IR table, metallic BBs are taped in place on the perineum at the expected location of the anus and at the single perineal opening. Radiopaque rulers can be placed beneath the patient for accurate adjusted magnification measurements from 2D images. Frontal and lateral fluoroscopic images of the sacrum are initially obtained to calculate the sacral ratio [2]. A voiding cystourethrogram (VCUG) is initially performed in the supine position. The bladder is distended with water-soluble contrast (Cysto-Conray; Mallinckrodt Inc., St. Louis, MO) to expected bladder capacity ([age in years $+ 2$] $\times$ 30) under gravity until maximum capacity is reached and/or spontaneous voiding occurs (the Foley catheter is manipulated under real-time fluoroscopy to allow spontaneous voiding as needed to opacify common channel). Bladder size, position, and morphology, as well as any vesicoureteral reflux (VUR), are documented. Oblique views of the bladder are obtained to document distal ureteral insertion sites (occasionally one/both ureters may arise from vagina/vaginas). The Foley catheter is repositioned at the bladder base under minor tension to maintain bladder

*Table 5.1*  Key measurements to be taken during cloacagram

Sacral ratios (AP and lateral)—x-ray images

Urethral length—oblique sagittal reconstructions CT

Common channel length—oblique sagittal reconstructions CT

Colonic length (to include rectum)—CT images

Rectal fistula length and position in relation to the vagina/vaginas—CT images

Distance from rectum to expected position of anus (marked by metallic BB)—CT images

Number and dimensions of vagina/vaginas—CT images

Presence of presacral mass

Position of rectal fistula above or below pubococcygeal line (PC line)—Lateral x-ray or CT images

distention, while colostogram and vaginagrams are performed. Leave contrast is connected to the Foley catheter, but the flow of contrast is turned off for now.

Next, a high-pressure distal colostogram is performed via the Foley catheter in the mucous fistula to fully distend the colon and document total length of distal colon, length, and location of rectal fistula, and the distance from the rectum to the expected position of the anus on the perineum (marked by external BB). This can performed in either supine or lateral position under fluoroscopy. The vagina/vaginas and common channel are typically opacified from this injection. If there is insufficient opacification, a third 8-French end-hole Foley catheter can be placed through the perineal opening and the balloon inflated to opacify these structures with hand injection of contrast.

Once all cavities have been opacified and the technologists have verified appropriate patient position and function of the rotational fluoroscopic C-arm, the patient is positioned in either supine or lateral position. Just prior to the start of the acquisition, the balloon in the bladder is deflated to allow voiding and reinjection of the colostomy Foley and perineal Foley catheters (if present) are undertaken to ensure maximum distention. Ensure that the external BBs at the perineum will be covered on the CT reconstructions. Rotational fluoroscopy is performed on a Siemens Artis Q angio/interventional System by selecting an image acquisition protocol originally developed for 3D rotational angiography. During rotational fluoroscopy, 120 images are acquired as the C-arm rotates 180° around the child; this takes 8 seconds. A 3D reconstruction is immediately available on a dedicated 3D workstation. Images can be evaluated both in a 3D rendering mode and as "CT like" slices in any obliquity (3). Key imaging involves reconstructed oblique sagittal imaging along the long axis of the native urethra and common channel on one image if possible (1 mm reconstructions). Each is measured directly from this image. Axial and coronal images are also utilized to document other required anatomy (see Table 5.1). Following imaging acquisition, the residual contrast is drained and catheter(s) are removed.

At the conclusion of this study and on review of the endoscopic exam the surgical team should have all the data necessary to formulate their reconstructive plan for the repair of the patient's cloacal malformation. The definitive care of these patients is discussed in detail in Chapter 6.

## 5.3  Postoperative care and follow-up

What is your postoperative follow-up plan for an 8-month-old patient who underwent urogenital separation and circle stent placement in her vesicostomy, for a 4 cm common channel and 1 cm urethra cloacal malformation repair? Her native vaginas were mobilized to the perineum and the septum was divided.

Patients who undergo urogenital separation require a formal review of the reconstructed urethra and vagina/s in the postoperative period. In addition the anoplasty needs to be assessed and postoperative anal dilations need to be started. The timing of such an assessment is somewhat controversial. We would suggest waiting until 6 weeks to assess the urethra to ensure ample healing has taken place. A cystoscopy can then be performed to look for a urethra-vaginal fistula, and the urethra can also be catheterized to ensure that it will be catheterizable by the family if required to empty urine after the vesicostomy has been closed. A vaginoscopy can be performed to review healing of the introitus and the site from where the vaginal septum was removed. The anoplasty can be sized and dilations started to ensure an adequate-sized anoplasty at the conclusion of the healing process. Dilations are advanced by one size per week in the usual fashion.

In the future, once the patient is able to pass urine successfully and urodynamics have been shown to be safe, the vesicostomy can be closed. This usually cannot done at the time of the colostomy closure.

### How would your management change in a patient who undergoes a total urogenital mobilization (TUM)?

In patients with a TUM there is no risk of urethra–vaginal fistula formation and the urethra itself has not been reconstructed; therefore the repair can be assessed once the postoperative swelling has subsided enough so that the urethra can be catheterized, if required. In most instances this can be reviewed without difficulty in a clinic setting and a catheter can be passed to ensure that it goes easily. Dilations can then be started if the anoplasty and perineal body have healed adequately and advanced in the standard fashion. An examination under anesthetic is only required if this review cannot be performed effectively in clinic.

### What is the long-term care and follow-up of cloaca patients?

Cloaca patients require longitudinal follow-up for multiple reasons. Notably they have a lifetime risk of up to 50% of developing renal impairment and this needs to be aggressively and proactively managed to keep the risks as low as possible. Ensuring good bladder emptying can be a key component to protecting the kidneys as the patient grows. The kidneys can be assessed on an ongoing basis with renal ultrasounds. Effective management of constipation and fecal incontinence will form a key component of care as the patient grows and can usually be performed between 4 and 5 years of age. Some patients may require further surgery in order to get dry for urine. In two large series [2,18] more than 50% of long common channel cloaca patients needed further surgery or ongoing clean intermittent catheterization (CIC) in order to get dry for urine and protect their kidneys. Reconstructive surgery, either bladder neck reconstruction or Mitrofanoff formation, which leads to continence, needs to be done very thoughtfully, as it can place the patient's kidneys at risk. Some patients may be more safely managed with incontinent diversions due to various circumstances. Renal and bladder care should be continued on a long-term basis. Another concern in postoperative cloaca patients is the quality of their gynecological repair and the ability to pass menstrual blood effectively. Six months after telarche, a pelvic ultrasound can be performed to start assessing for obstructive menstruation. In many cloaca patients the gynecological anatomy may not be completely clear and longitudinal care is important. Some patients may exhibit signs of obstruction with cyclical abdominal and pelvic pain and may need to have surgery to manage obstructed uterine structures. In addition an assessment of the introitus is required prior to sexual debut. Some patients may require an introitoplasty or vaginoplasty in order to accommodate penetrative intercourse. We generally suggest waiting until after puberty to ensure the tissue is estrogenized prior to surgery. Like all ARM patients ongoing bowel management is required to treat constipation and fecal incontinence. Many patients may benefit from antegrade enemas to achieve social continence; however, no patient should be offered a Malone appendicostomy until a decision has been made on the patient's need for Mitrofanoff to empty the bladder effectively.

# References

1. Hendren WH. Cloaca, the most severe degree of imperforate anus: Experience with 195 cases. *Ann Surg.* 1998;228(3):331–46.
2. Levitt MA, Peña A. Cloacal malformations: Lessons learned from 490 cases. *Semin Pediatr Surg.* 2010;19(2):128–38.
3. Hendren WH. Urogenital sinus and cloacal malformations. *Semin Pediatr Surg.* 1996;5(1):72–9.
4. Peña A. Total urogenital mobilization—An easier way to repair cloacas. *J Pediatr Surg.* 1997;32(2):263–7.
5. Patel MN, Racadio JM, Levitt MA, Bischoff A, Racadio JM, Peña A. Complex cloacal malformations: Use of rotational fluoroscopy and 3-D reconstruction in diagnosis and surgical planning. *Pediatr Radiol.* 2012;42(3):355–63.
6. Reck-Burneo CA, Vilanova-Sanchez A, Wood RJ, Levitt MA, Bates DG. Imaging in anorectal and cloacal malformations. *Pediatr Radiol.* 2018;48(3):443–4.
7. Riccabona M, Lobo ML, Ording-Muller LS et al. European Society of Paediatric Radiology Abdominal Imaging Task Force recommendations in paediatric uroradiology, part IX: Imaging in anorectal and cloacal malformation, imaging in childhood ovarian torsion, and efforts in standardising paediatric uroradiology terminology. *Pediatr Radiol.* 2017;47(10):1369–80.
8. Wood RJ, Reck-Burneo CA, Dajusta D, Ching C, Jayanthi R, Bates DG, Fuchs ME, McCracken K, Hewitt G, Levitt MA. Cloaca reconstruction: A new algorithm which considers the role of urethral length in determining surgical planning. *J Pediatr Surg.* October 2017. https://doi.org/10.1016/j.jpedsurg.2017.10.022
9. Bischoff A, Levitt MA, Breech L, Louden E, Peña A. Hydrocolpos in cloacal malformations. *J Pediatr Surg.* 2010;45(6):1241–5.
10. Chalmers DJ, Rove KO, Wiedel CA, Tong S, Siparsky GL, Wilcox DT. Clean intermittent catheterization as an initial management strategy provides for adequate preservation of renal function in newborns with persistent cloaca. *J Pediatr Urol.* 2015;11(4):211.e1–4.
11. Speck KE, Arnold MA, Ivancic V, Teitelbaum DH. Cloaca and hydrocolpos: Laparoscopic-, cystoscopic- and colposcopic-assisted vaginostomy tube placement. *J Pediatr Surg.* 2014;49(12):1867–9.
12. Levitt MA, Bischoff A, Peña A. Pitfalls and challenges of cloaca repair: How to reduce the need for reoperations. *J Pediatr Surg.* 2011;46(6):1250–5.
13. Liechty ST, Barnhart DC, Huber JT, Zobell S, Rollins MD. The morbidity of a divided stoma compared to a loop colostomy in patients with anorectal malformation. *J Pediatr Surg.* 2016;51(1):107–10.
14. Pradhan S, Vilanova-Sanchez A, McCracken KA, Reck CA, Halleran DR, Wood RJ, Levitt M, Hewitt GD. The müllerian black box: Predicting and defining müllerian anatomy in patients with cloacal abnormalities and the need for longitudinal assessment. *J Pediatr Surg.* 2018;53(11):2164–9.
15. Gasior AC, Reck C, Lane V, Wood RJ, Patterson J, Strouse R, Lin S, Cooper J, Gregory Bates D, Levitt MA. Transcending dimensions: A comparative analysis of cloaca imaging in advancing the surgeon's understanding of complex anatomy. *J Digit Imaging.* October 2018. https://doi.org/10.1007/s10278-018-0139-y
16. Ahn JJ, Shnorhavorian M, Amies Oelschlager AE, Ripley B, Shivaram GM, Avansino JR, Merguerian PA. Use of 3D reconstruction cloacagrams and 3D printing in cloacal malformations. *J Pediatr Urol.* 2017;13(4):395.e1–395.e6.
17. Jarboe MD, Teitelbaum DH, Dillman JR. Combined 3D rotational fluoroscopic-MRI cloacagram procedure defines luminal and extraluminal pelvic anatomy prior to surgical reconstruction of cloacal and other complex pelvic malformations. *Pediatr Surg Int.* 2012;28(8):757–63.
18. Warne SA, Wilcox DT, Ransley PG. Long-term urological outcome of patients presenting with persistent cloaca. *J Urol.* 2002;168(4 Pt 2):1859–62.

# 6 Cloaca: Definitive repair and surgical protocol

Richard J. Wood, Carlos A. Reck-Burneo, and Marc A. Levitt

## 6.1 Introduction

Cloacal malformations are a rare and complex spectrum of congenital defects affecting the development of the urological, gynecological, and colorectal systems. The challenges in the reconstruction of these patients are multi-faceted. The goal of their work-up is to allow the surgical team to effectively plan and execute a strategically sound reconstruction. The main components of this plan involve accurately predicting which techniques will allow for the reconstruction of the urethra, vagina/s, and rectum in the most functional way possible. Avoiding changing the plan during surgery is very important and is now possible with proper imaging. For example, if one technique is chosen, a total urogenital mobilization, and the surgeon is then unable to mobilize the urethra to reach the perineum, the plan would then need to change, which may have significant consequences. In such a case the urethra would need to be fully mobilized and separated from the vagina, which may lead to ischemia and urethral loss. Prior to embarking on a repair the surgical team needs a clear picture of the length of the common channel, the length of the urethra, the length and position of the vagina/s, and the position of the rectum in relation to the pubococcygeal (PC) line. This information will allow the team to make sound choices prior to starting the surgery. This knowledge will also help the surgeon know whether they have the experience to do such a case or if the patient should be referred.

## 6.2 Case study

A 9-month-old female presents to you with a classic cloacal malformation with a single perineal orifice. An initial colostomy was performed in the newborn period. Your evaluation after endoscopy and cloacagram notes the following findings: the common channel is 4 cm long with a 1 cm long urethra and the rectum lies just at the level of the PC line. There is a longitudinal vaginal septum and uterus didelphys, with two normal cervices seen on vaginoscopy. The vaginas are symmetrical each with a length of 4 cm.

Patients requiring a urogenital separation, as this patient does due to the very short urethra, require more challenging reconstructive techniques. Identifying these patients up front may facilitate referral to high volume centers as required. Except in cases of very long common channels (with all three structures above the PC line), we would advocate starting with a posterior sagittal approach. The incision runs from the coccyx to just posterior to the common channel. Where possible the common channel should be left intact at the perineal level (Figure 6.1). The wound is widely opened and the surgeon's preoperative understanding of whether the rectum and vagina/s lie above or below the levators (PC line) is important at this point in the operation. If present in the posterior sagittal field the rectum should be identified and mobilized as described for the rectal mobilization in any PSARP. The rectal attachment to the vagina/s or common channel needs to be identified, confirming what was seen on preoperative imaging, and divided. If the connection is to the common channel, care must be taken not to injure or narrow the common channel. At this stage, the posterior vagina is opened close to where it joins the common channel (urethrovaginal fistula). Sutures are placed on the edges of the vagina/s and the surgeon is able to look inside and identify the connection between the vagina/s and the common channel and urethra (Figure 6.2). The next stage is to start the separation of the vagina/s from the common channel, urethra, and bladder neck. This is done in the same way as is performed in a male undergoing a PSARP for a rectourethral fistula, with lateral dissection done first, then anterior (Figure 6.3). The lateral dissection is particularly vital as this plane, once the surgen enters the abdomen, is greatly facilitated by having started the dissection posterior sagittaly.

Once the bladder neck is reached or the dissection becomes too high, the surgery should be continued in a transabdominal fashion. This will prevent placing the ureters in danger of being injured. If the ureters are ectopic they can be stented cystoscopically at the start of the procedure.

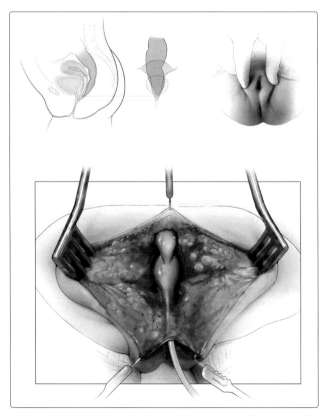

**Figure 6.1** Posterior sagittal incision with the rectum vagina and common channel displayed.

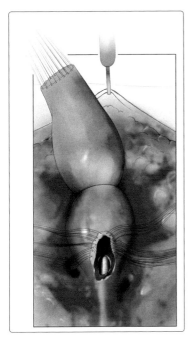

Figure 6.2 Rectum mobilized and vagina opened with view of Foley catheter in urethra through urethra-vaginal fistula (congenital).

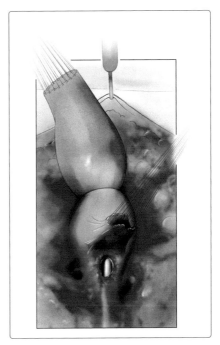

Figure 6.3 Careful mobilization of the vagina off the urethra and bladder neck.

The common channel needs to be meticulously repaired in order to leave the patient with a catheterizable channel. Urologic involvement can be advantageous and a repair in multiple layers with 5-0 PDS is our preference (Figure 6.4). A meticulous technique is essential and on table flexible cystoscopy can be helpful in some cases to identify precisely where the repair of the common channel is needed, particularly if it is close to the bladder neck. Thereafter,

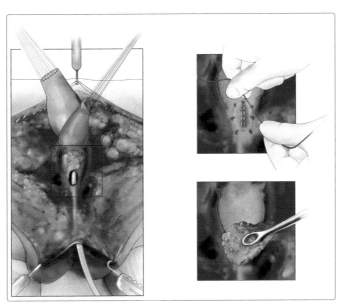

Figure 6.4 Repair of the common channel (urethra) with 5-0 PDS, covered by SIS and then and Ischiorectal fat pad.

the repair is covered with a single layer of SIS and the previously described ischiorectal fat pad [1]. This repair is vital to the successful reconstruction of these patients [2], in an attempt to avoid a vaginourethral fistula. Using this technique and adequate bladder drainage for at least 1 month has led to a fistula rate of less than 5% (2/41) in patients requiring urogenital separation. This is less than reported but still challenging to manage, if it does occur. Bladder drainage can be accomplished with a transurethral Foley catheter or circle stent if the patient has a vesicostomy. The advantage of the circle stent is that there is no balloon in the bladder, which may help to prevent bladder spasms in the postoperative period.

The abdominal portion of the procedure can be accomplished with open or MIS techniques. From a transabdominal approach, the ureters are carefully identified and protected and the separation of the vagina from the urinary tract is continued in the midline until the structures are fully separated. The vagina/s are then mobilized off the retroperitoneum until they reach the perineum, preserving both round ligaments and thus their main blood supply. Advanced technology like fluorescein dye can be used to assess blood supply during this process. At this stage either the vagina/s are able to reach the perineum or a tissue replacement will be required to bridge the gap. We hope one day that tissue engineered vagina could be used, perhaps avoiding this difficult dissection altogether.

If vaginal replacement is required, rectum, colon, and ileum are available. The rectum should only be considered in cases where the likelihood of fecal continence is low due to a sacral ratio of less than 0.4 or very abnormal spinal development. After the tissue for replacement has been prepared and is determined to reach the perineum with adequate blood supply, and no tension, it can be anastomosed to the distal native vagina/s. On occasion, the blood supply dictates that the neo-vagina be placed in an anti-peristaltic direction. If there is a longitudinal vaginal septum this may be divided to allow for future menstrual egress. The neo-vagina is then carefully pulled through to the perineum and reconstructed posterior to the common channel opening, which has become the urethra following its repair as already described.

The posterior extent of the labia majora is often a helpful guide for the location of the posterior limit of the introitus. As before, the location of the rectum and perineal body should be planned prior to beginning the introitoplasty.

**If the common channel was 2.3 cm long with a 1.8 cm urethra, and the rectum lies below the PC line, with a single vagina 6 cm long, and a single cervix is seen on vaginoscopy, how would the operative plan change?**

The description of the technique of the TUM has been previously reported and the technique we employ does not differ from this approach [3]. The surgery is started with mapping of the anal sphincter. In this instance, a full posterior sagittal incision will be required. The incision is carried from the coccyx to the common channel and the common channel is opened posteriorly until the rectum and vagina/s are visible. The rectum is then mobilized in the same usual manner. Thereafter, sutures are placed in the edge of the urogenital complex and the entire structure is mobilized in a full thickness fashion without compromising the integrity of the wall. The tissue is divided 5 mm posterior to the clitoris to allow for the urethroplasty (after incising up the center of the mobilized common channel) to be placed directly posterior to the clitoris in a visible position in case intermittent catheterization is required and to avoid vaginal voiding. The posterior lateral blood supply of the vagina needs to be dissected to allow the vagina to be adequately mobilized. The careful division of the suspensory ligaments of the urethra will be needed to allow for mobilization of the urethra into the position posterior to the clitoris. Full mobilization is realized once these ligaments are incised and the recto pubic fat below is visualized. There is much discussion in the literature regarding partial and complete TUM. The reality is that only those fibers needed to adequately mobilize the urogenital complex should be divided and this may vary from case to case. Once all three structures (rectum, vagina, and urethra) are adequately mobilized to reach the perineum, the reconstruction proceeds in the standard fashion. After the anterior common channel has been divided in its midline and the urethra has been adequately reconstructed, the sphincter complex and perineal body are planned and the remaining incision is used to create the introitus. The split common channel can be used to form the labia minora on each side. As mentioned previously, a longitudinal vaginal septum, if present, can be divided at the time of the introitoplasty.

**If, however, the common channel was 0.8 cm long with a 2 cm urethra and a single 6 cm vagina and a rectum well below the PC line, how would the plan change then?**

In a type 1 cloaca, this description represents that the patient is placed in a prone position and the anal sphincter complex is marked with an electrical stimulator. An incision is then carried from the posterior extent of the muscle complex (sphincter) through to the common channel, opening the common channel to reveal the urethral take-off, rectum, and vagina/s. The rectum is then mobilized, taking care to protect both the intramural blood supply of the rectum and the posterior vaginal wall. Once the rectum is separated, the vagina is opened to facilitate the formation of an adequate introitus. No urethral dissection is required. An electrical stimulator is employed to mark the anterior and posterior extent of the muscle complex. The length of the perineal body, between 1 and 2 cm depending on the age and size of the patient, is then selected. The remainder of the incision is left for the introitus. It is important that the repair be planned in this manner to allow the rectum to be placed in the muscle complex and to create an adequate perineal body. The perineal body is repaired in layers with 3-0 long-term absorbable interrupted sutures and the skin of the perineal body is repaired with vertical mattress sutures to take tension off the skin edge. The PSARP and posterior sagittal incision are repaired in the standard fashion and a vaginal septum, if present, is divided at the time of the introitoplasty.

The three most likely scenarios in these cases are the following:

1. *Type 1 cloaca:* Common channel less than 1 cm in length: The urethra is left untouched and the surgical team performs an introitoplasty and a posterior sagittal anorectoplasty (PSARP).
2. *Common channel less than 3 cm in length and a urethral length of at least 1.5 cm:* Total urogenital mobilization (TUM) and PSARP, which may require laparoscopy or open approach if the rectum is high.
3. *Common channel greater than 3 cm or urethra less than 1.5 cm:* Urogenital separation with common channel kept as urethra and PSARP. A proportion of these patients require vaginal replacement with colon, rectum, or small bowel. Open or MIS techniques may be required in these cases, especially where rectum or urogenital confluence lies above the PC line.

## 6.3 Conclusion

The definitive repair of cloaca malformations presents challenges to the surgical team on various levels. To obtain reproducible excellent results, accurate prediction of the technical complexity of the surgery and the correct strategic plan for each patient greatly facilitate this process. While anatomic repair is obviously very important, long-term functional outcomes need to be a key consideration.

# References

1. Levitt MA, King SK, Bischoff A, Alam S, Gonzalez G, Pena A. The Gonzalez hernia revisited: Use of the ischiorectal fat pad to aid in the repair of rectovaginal and rectourethral fistulae. *J Pediatr Surg.* 2014;49:1308–10.
2. Wood RJ, Reck-Burneo CA, Dajusta D et al. Cloaca reconstruction: A new algorithm which considers the role of urethral length in determining surgical planning. *J Pediatr Surg.* 2017. doi: 10.1016/j.jpedsurg.2017.10.022
3. Peña A. Total urogenital mobilization—An easier way to repair cloacas. *J Pediatr Surg.* 1997;32:263–7; discussion 267–8.

# Long-term urologic and gynecologic follow-up in anorectal anomalies: The keys to success

Geri Hewitt, Daniel G. DaJusta, and Christina B. Ching

## 7.1 Urologic long-term follow-up

### 7.1.1 Case 1

A 5-year-old female with a history of cloaca consisting of a 2 cm common channel and 1 cm urethra presents for evaluation of urinary incontinence. As an infant she underwent posterior sagittal anorectovaginourethroplasty (PSARVUP) with separation of her vagina from her urethra (urogenital separation) and interposition of bowel (left colon) from her native vagina to her perineum. She is interested in toilet training and shows the ability to generate a stream and urinate on command. She will, however, have dribbling between volitional voiding. She has not had any urinary tract infections. A renal ultrasound is normal. An MRI of her spine is normal. She underwent video urodynamics that show a large capacity, compliant bladder without overactivity. The video portion, however, shows significant pooling of urine in the vagina with voiding (Figure 7.1). Cystoscopy shows an urethrovaginal fistula in her mid-urethra distal to her bladder neck.

**What is your next step in management?**

  A. Refer her to neurosurgery for reevaluation of a possible tethered cord
  B. Close her bladder neck and create a continent catheterizable channel
  C. Advise spread leg voiding with timed and double voiding

*Answer:* C

### 7.1.1.1 Learning points

- As a child ages, the ability for continence after cloacal surgery becomes apparent. Urinary incontinence can be divided into dysfunction of bladder urine storage and abnormalities of the bladder outlet. It is important to evaluate for each of these causes in isolation or together as potential etiologies for urinary incontinence. In particular, spinal cord malformations can affect how either of these function and are vital to consider as underlying etiologies for urinary incontinence in children with cloacal malformation due to their increased risk of having spinal cord abnormalities [1,2]. It is important to be sure that there is not a neurogenic etiology for their inability to store urine. In addition, one has to consider the inherent length of the urethra in children with cloacas to determine if the proper operation was performed to facilitate continence [3–5]. Furthermore, one has to consider the possible complications from surgery such as a stricture or fistula. An important consideration is that the patient be able to empty their bladder completely and that their incontinence is not a sign of persistent high residual urine volumes. Such residual volumes and/or a high pressure bladder can lead to renal injury.

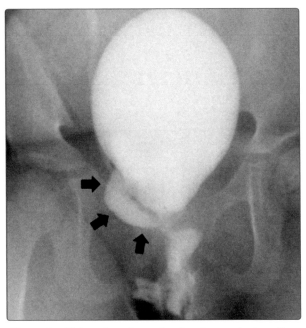

**Figure 7.1** Video of urodynamics showing vaginal pooling (black arrows) during urination due to urethrovaginal fistula.

- Behavioral changes are an important first step in managing many forms of urinary incontinence. These include having the child regularly void in timed intervals (referred to as "timed voiding") and to have them try to void multiple times in one sitting (referred to as "double voiding"). For this patient, also ensuring good positioning (they can sit backward on the toilet) to help empty the vagina during voiding is important and could be all that is needed to solve her problem of incontinence.
- Surgical repair may be necessary for postoperative urethrovaginal fistulas; however, the location of the fistula plays an important role in the timing of this decision. If the fistula is distal to the bladder neck and external urinary sphincter, the patient may be able to be dry without requiring surgery. While ultimately the fistula may need to be closed to protect against infection during sexual intercourse, delaying surgery until after puberty may enable a transvaginal approach for closure.

## 7.1.2 Case 2

A 6-year-old male with a history of ARM (rectoprostatic fistula) has a status of post-primary posterior sagittal anorectoplasty (PSARP) as an infant and posttethered cord detethering at 14 months and presents with urinary incontinence. The patient has been on clean intermittent catheterization (CIC) every 3 hours for poor bladder emptying and recurrent urinary tract infections. Despite being on CIC, however, he is wet between catheterization intervals.

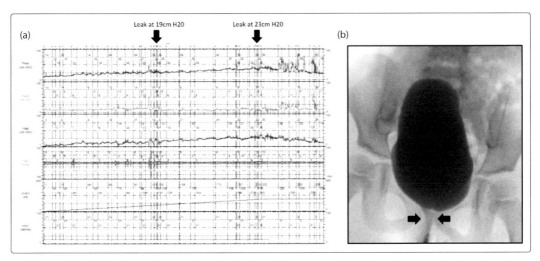

**Figure 7.2** (a) Urodynamics showing low leak point pressure with otherwise compliant and good bladder capacity bladder without overactivity. Video of urodynamics. (b) Open bladder neck (black arrows) during video.

He underwent urodynamic testing that showed bladder overactivity with a small capacity bladder. An MRI of his spine showed concern for retethering, so the patient was reevaluated by neurologists and underwent redo-detethering of his spinal cord. With no improvement in his incontinence, he was put on anticholinergics with some improvement in wetting between CIC but he was still not completely dry. He requires pull-ups and would like to be in regular underwear. Repeat urodynamics shows improved bladder capacity and resolution of his overactivity but leakage per urethra at low detrusor pressures of only 19–23 cm $H_2O$. A voiding cystourethrogram shows an open bladder neck with leakage (Figure 7.2).

**What is your next step in management?**

A. Proceed with bladder neck reconstruction with the creation of continent catheterizable channel
B. Increase CIC to every hour
C. Increase anticholinergic dosage and schedule patient for cystoscopy with Botox injection in his detrusor muscle

*Answer:* A

### 7.1.2.1 Learning points

- It is always important in a pediatric patient with a history of neurogenic bladder to reevaluate for spinal cord issues such as cord tethering or retethering when there is concern for urinary symptoms. Children grow and manifestations from a tethered cord can become apparent with time. In this patient, the urodynamics confirm that the bladder overactivity is well controlled and that the bladder capacity is adequate. Any additional measure to decrease bladder overactivity and increase compliance such as Botox detrusor injection or bladder augmentation would not render this patient dry.
- Methods to control urinary continence have to be practical for the family. Clean intermittent catheterization more than every 2–3 hours is difficult for patients and their families to maintain.

- When performing procedures at the bladder outlet, it is important to consider alternative methods of draining the bladder such as simultaneously creating a continent catheterizable channel (mitrofanoff). Additionally, it will be important to follow this patient closely postoperatively given 30%–50% of these patients will have bladder decompensation following an outlet procedure alone and require subsequent delayed augmentation [6,7]. Without close monitoring and appropriate changes in intervention, elevated bladder pressures could lead to renal damage and loss of renal function [8].

### 7.1.3 Case 3

A 13-year-old male with a history of ARM (rectobladder neck) status post-PSARP as an infant and normal spine imaging is found by his pediatrician to have a systolic blood pressure of 145 mm Hg at his annual well child checkup. 24-hour blood pressure monitoring confirms elevated systolic blood pressures. A renal ultrasound shows bilateral global cortical renal scarring. Upon further questioning, the father does remember the patient having frequent urinary tract infections as a toddler. His serum creatinine is 1.1 mg/dl. A voiding cystourethrogram shows bilateral grade 4 vesicoureteral reflux. A DMSA scan confirms bilateral renal scarring (Figure 7.3). Urodynamics shows a compliant bladder with no detrusor overactivity.

**What is your next step in management?**

- **A.** Consult nephrology for control of blood pressure and renoprotective management
- **B.** Avoid nephrotoxins such as NSAIDs and high protein and salt diets
- **C.** Surgical management of his vesicoureteral reflux with a bilateral reimplant
- **D.** All of the above

*Answer:* D

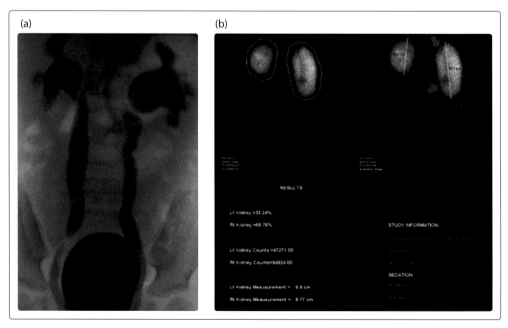

(a) (b)

**Figure 7.3** (a) Voiding cystourethrogram shows bilateral grade 4 vesicoureteral reflux. (b) A DMSA scan confirms bilateral scarring (globally of the left kidney, which only functions at 33%, and of the upper and mid/lower pole of the right kidney [red arrows]).

### 7.1.3.1 Learning points

- There is a high incidence of urologic abnormalities in patients with ARMs [1]. In particular, the higher the level of the ARM, the more likely the patient is to have an associated urologic abnormality [9]. Concomitant vesicoureteral reflux can be seen in up to 35% of patients with ARM [9,10].
- Patients with a history of ARM are at high risk for renal dysfunction [8,11,12]. Patients with a history of ARM require periodic monitoring of their renal function via imaging, blood work, and blood pressure measurements given the association of urologic abnormalities in this patient population. It is especially important if a patient has had a history of febrile urinary tract infections to understand what may be predisposing them particularly to pyelonephritis and the subsequent sequela of having had these infections (i.e., renal cortical damage).
- Follow-up is even more important in patients who require complex urological reconstruction to achieve continence, such as bladder neck procedures and catheterizable channels. Lack of symptoms or complaints should not preclude regular follow-up as early changes on renal ultrasound and renal function laboratory work could identify at-risk patients [8]. In addition, patient adherence to advised bladder care is of great importance as lack of adherence could lead to devastating and irreversible renal damage.

## 7.1.4 Case 4

An 8-month-old male with a history of imperforate anus and colostomy awaiting his primary repair has a history of recurrent left epididymitis requiring hospitalization and IV antibiotics. He has been put on antibiotic prophylaxis but has had persistent issues with recurrent left epididymitis despite this. A voiding cystourethrogram shows a likely rectobulbar fistula with right grade 2 vesicoureteral reflux and left-sided reflux of contrast into the left vas deferens and seminal vesicle during voiding (Figure 7.4). A renal ultrasound is normal. His serum creatinine is 0.32 mg/dl. Urodynamics shows bladder overactivity of a normal-sized bladder. An MRI of his spine shows sacral bone anomalies but no signs of tethering.

**What is your next step in management?**

- **A.** Vesicostomy creation
- **B.** L orchiectomy
- **C.** R ureteral reimplant

*Answer:* A

### 7.1.4.1 Learning points

- An easy and safe form of bladder management is to promote drainage through a vesicostomy. When there are concerns about bladder function and recurrent infections, a vesicostomy is a safe form of temporizing these medical issues. A vesicostomy is an especially nice option in infant patients who are not otherwise toilet trained and already in diapers. Once the patient reaches an age appropriate for toilet training, further work-up can be performed in order to evaluate for the best surgical management to enable continence and to safely address infections.

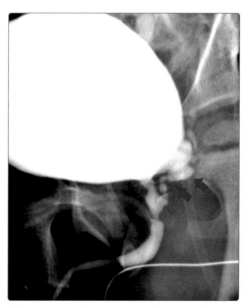

Figure 7.4 Voiding cystourethrogram showing reflux into the left vas deferens and seminal vesicle (red arrows) during voiding.

- Epididymitis may be a sign of other abnormalities of the urinary tract, especially when seen in young prepubescent males, and should necessitate evaluation of the urinary tract anatomy including the genitourinary tract and the kidneys [13,14]. This patient may require more definitive surgery to prevent recurrent epididymitis. At the time closure of his vesicostomy he may need further urologic reconstruction, but temporizing vesicostomy is an important first step and enables the patient time to be infection free.

### 7.1.5 Case 5

An 8-year-old male with a history of ARM (rectoprostatic fistula) has a status of post-primary laparoscopic PSARP and presents with dysuria. In addition, he complains of intermittent gross hematuria. His urinalyses have shown microscopic hematuria and leukocyturia but his urine cultures have been negative for bacteria. He is continent of urine. A renal ultrasound is normal without hydronephrosis. He has no postvoid residual. Cystoscopy demonstrates a large remnant of the original fistula (ROOF) off of the prostatic urethra with a stone in the lumen (Figure 7.5a,b). His bladder is otherwise normal without signs of inflammation or stone. An MRI of the pelvis also shows a remnant of an original fistula (Figure 7.5c).

**What is your next step in management?**

- **A.** Laser lithotripsy of the stone
- **B.** Remove the remnant of the original fistula (ROOF) through a redo PSARP
- **C.** Refer to nephrology for medical management of the stone

*Answer:* B

#### 7.1.5.1 *Learning points*

- There are several reasons to remove a remnant of the original fistula (ROOF). These include preventing difficulties with catheterization, removal of potential nidus for urinary stones and/or urinary tract infections, prevention of a place where urine can accumulate

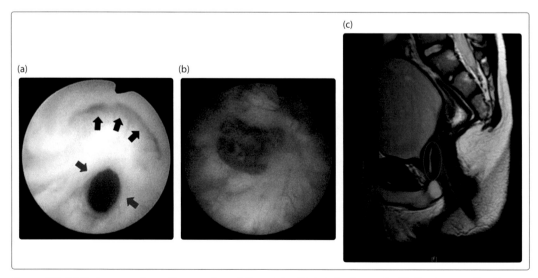

Figure 7.5 (a) Cystoscopy shows the opening of the original fistula (red arrow) with the true urethral lumen to the bladder marked by a black arrow. (b) Inside the opening to the original fistula there is a stone. (c) MRI of the pelvis showing the remnant of original fistula off of the posterior urethra (red circle).

and lead to urinary dribbling, and prevention of the possibility of adenocarcinoma developing in the remnant bowel mucosa interposed in the urinary tract.

- An MRI of the pelvis can be used to evaluate for a ROOF along with cystoscopy. We recommend both as we have found a ROOF can be missed on either. As a result, MRI scan and direct cystoscopic visualization are used together to evaluate for a ROOF.
- An asymptomatic small (1 × 1 cm) ROOF can be left alone with removal only performed in cases in which another operation such as a redo PSARP for mislocated anus is required. The rectum must be fully mobilized to visualize the urethra up to the bladder neck in order to safety remove the ROOF and repair the urethra.

### 7.1.5.2 Preoperative considerations

- Baseline evaluation of the spine
- Baseline evaluation of bladder function with video urodynamics
- Baseline evaluation of renal function including serum creatinine and cystatin C, and in selected cases a DMSA scan
- Baseline evaluation of anatomy to determine appropriate reconstruction (i.e., for cloaca repair to decide if the urethral length is appropriate for total urogenital mobilization vs. urogenital separation) and to take into account the high risk of associated urologic abnormalities in ARM

### 7.1.5.3 Postoperative considerations

- Ensuring and reinforcing good urologic follow-up due to the risk of silent renal injury
- Reinforcing close patient adherence to prescribed bladder management
- Evaluating the spine for the possible impact of neurologic pathology on urinary status
- Reevaluation of the anatomy to be sure of appropriate postoperative healing and bladder function

### 7.1.5.4 Follow-up protocol

- There are no universal protocols that have been outlined and/or adopted by Pediatric Surgery or Pediatric Urology Associations for these patients.
- Our practice has been at a minimum to obtain annual renal imaging, serum creatinine and cystatin C, and blood pressure measurements.
- Urodynamics can be done annually for patients with a known neurologic lesion causing a neurogenic bladder and/or when there is a change in urinary status such as new or persistent urinary incontinence or new urinary tract infections. We perform urodynamic evaluation before and after tethered cord surgery as well as before and after major reconstruction surgeries such as a cloacal repair. It should also be used to closely monitor patients after reconstruction with an isolated bladder neck reconstruction.

## 7.2 Gynecologic long-term follow-up

### 7.2.1 Case 1

A 15-year-old girl with a previously repaired rectovestibular fistula presents for follow-up. She has excellent bowel control and is otherwise healthy. Thelarche was at age 11 and she experienced menarche 18 months ago. She reports her periods are now monthly, lasting up to 7 days, with menstrual cramps relieved by ibuprofen. She changes her pads every 3–4 hours and has no menstrual accidents overnight. The patient recently began using tampons and reports that they "don't work" for her. She reports she is able to insert and remove the tampon without difficulty, but experiences menstrual accidents every time she uses them. This causes her distress because she is an elite swimmer and the inability to successfully use tampons has disrupted both training and competitions.

**What is your next step in management?**

    **A.** Perform a pelvic exam
    **B.** Order a pelvic ultrasound
    **C.** Order a pelvic MRI

*Answer:* A

### 7.2.1.1 Learning points

- Patients with anorectal malformations (ARM), who are otherwise healthy, undergo a normal pubertal process, both in timing and tempo. The menstrual pattern reported here is normal. Menses should occur every 21–35 days and last up to 7 days. The normal interval for pad changes (3–4 hours) and lack of overnight accidents are very reassuring and eliminate heavy menstrual bleeding (due to hormonal or bleeding abnormalities) as a likely cause of the tampon failure. Teens, unlike adult women, rarely have structural causes of heavy menstrual bleeding.
- Patients with ARM are at increased risk of Müllerian anomalies Figure 7.6. The normally timed menarche rules out vaginal and uterine atresia. The lack of significant dysmenorrhea makes an obstructive anomaly unlikely. Ovarian estrogen production during puberty promotes increased linear growth as well as breast and Müllerian development. While pelvic imaging has limited usefulness prior to puberty in the evaluation of Müllerian structures, after thelarche pelvic ultrasound is an excellent screening tool. Pelvic MRI is useful to further define suspected Müllerian abnormalities identified on ultrasound. Pelvic imaging is not, however, the next best step to identify this patient's underlying problem.
- Patients who struggle with tampon use require a pelvic examination. Patients who report difficulty in inserting or removing a tampon often have hymenal abnormalities. This patient, however, reports the classic symptoms of a nonobstructive longitudinal vaginal septum. The

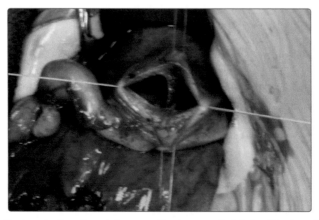

**Figure 7.6** Longitudinal vaginal septum. Intraoperative image of a bilateral hydrocolpos, with the dome of the vagina opened to remove part of the septum to allow for vaginostomy drainage of both sides with a single tube.

tampon is being placed on only one side of the septum and menstrual egress is persisting out the other side. Examination of the vaginal introitus and/or digital vaginal exam identifies the septum (see Figure 7.7). If a patient has been using tampons, she can tolerate a pelvic exam in the office with education and support. Neither pelvic ultrasound nor MRI would identify the septum.

- Approximately 5% of girls with rectovestibular fistula will have a longitudinal vaginal septum. If the septum was not removed at the initial repair, it should subsequently be removed to allow for successful tampon use, decrease the likelihood of pain with intercourse, and avoid obstetrical trauma during vaginal delivery (see Figure 7.7). If the septum is identified prepubertally and no other surgery is planned, delaying septum removal until puberty, allowing for an estrogenized vagina, may enhance postoperative healing, and, the longer introitus allows for better operative exposure.

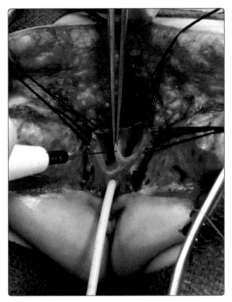

Figure 7.7 Intraoperative pictures of a longitudinal vaginal septum.

## 7.2.2 Case 2

A 16-year-old patient with previously repaired imperforate anus with rectovestibular fistula presents to the emergency department with abdominal pain. She has not yet had her first period and has never been sexually active. She denies any urinary or GI symptoms. She has regular bowel movements without soiling. The patient underwent thelarche and adrenarche approximately 3 years ago. Her mother notes increasing lower abdominal pain over the past couple of months that appears to be cyclic in nature. She is afebrile and has normal vital signs. Her abdomen is soft, with normal bowel sounds, with fullness and tenderness in the lower abdomen.

**Which of the following is the best imaging study to order?**

- **A.** Acute abdominal series
- **B.** Pelvic ultrasound
- **C.** Abdominal-pelvic CT scan

*Answer:* B

### 7.2.2.1 Learning points

Given her age and history of thelarche 3 years prior, this patient should have experienced menarche. This finding, coupled with her cyclic abdominal pain, raises the suspicion of an anatomic, obstructive cause of her amenorrhea. She needs an investigation of her reproductive anatomy to understand her Müllerian anatomy and confirm a patient outflow tract.

The next best steps in her management would include an external genital examination and pelvic imaging. The goal of the external genital exam is to evaluate the vaginal introitus

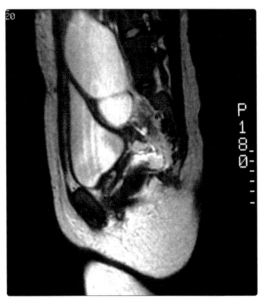

Figure 7.8 MRI of an obstructed Müllerian horn.

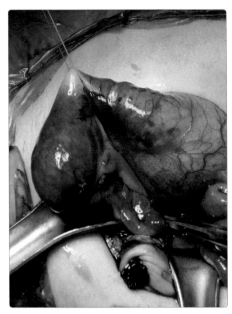

Figure 7.9 Intraoperative images of an obstructed uterine horn.

as well as the length of the vagina by inserting a small, cotton swab. This can be accomplished in the office setting with patient education and support. A pelvic ultrasound is the best initial screening tool to evaluate Müllerian anatomy and ascertain if there is blood in the vagina (hematocolpos) and/or uterus (hematometria). If either the exam or the ultrasound is abnormal, the patient may need a pelvic MRI to further delineate reproductive anatomy (see Figure 7.8).

Patients with ARM are at increased risk of congenital reproductive track anomalies. Ideally, families should be counseled about this risk at the time of the initial ARM diagnosis. This patient population requires close surveillance as they move through puberty. If the patient is normal weight and generally healthy, pubertal timing and tempo is normal. Best screening tools include the combination of an external genital examination, a pelvic ultrasound after thelarche, and a careful menstrual history. Lack of menses raises concern for either atresia (vaginal and/ or Müllerian) or obstruction. Dysmenorrhea (painful menses) could indicate an obstruction (obstructed Müllerian horn) as well.

This patient's presentation suggests an outflow tract obstruction. All functional endometrial tissue responds to estrogen stimulation by proliferating and eventually creating menstrual blood. Vaginal causes of obstruction include imperforate hymen, vaginal atresia, transverse vaginal septum, OHVIRA (obstructed hemivagina and ipsilateral renal agenesis), and vaginal–cervical atresia. Uterine causes of obstruction include bicornuate uterus with an obstructed horn (see Figure 7.9) and obstructed uterine remnants associated with Müllerian agenesis.

### 7.2.3  Case 3

A 20-year-old woman with a previously repaired cloacal malformation has recently attempted penetrative sexual activity. Her primary reconstruction was with a posterior sagittal anorectoplasty and total urogenital mobilization. She has a native vagina with normal Müllerian structures. She reports pain with penetration and during intercourse despite positional changes and use of vaginal lubricant. She has also experienced bright red bleeding after intercourse. She reports she has been with her partner for 2 years and they have a healthy, loving relationship with good communication. She reports normal monthly cycles with minimal pain prior to using progestin-only hormonal contraception. She is worried about her inability to enjoy sexual intimacy with her boyfriend and what that may mean for her relationship.

**What is the next best step in her evaluation?**

    **A.** Pelvic examination in the office
    **B.** Examination under anesthesia
    **C.** Pelvic ultrasound

*Answer:* A

### 7.2.3.1 Learning points

This patient reports both postcoital bleeding and dyspareunia, or painful intercourse, which occurs both at penetration and throughout intercourse. Both of these complaints require investigation, which should begin with a pelvic exam in the office. Examining the patient under anesthesia would eliminate the ability to reproduce her symptoms. Since the patient has known normal Müllerian structures, a pelvic ultrasound should be obtained only if there is an abnormality (mass or enlargement) identified on pelvic exam.

Pain with intercourse requires a careful psychosocial, sexual, and medical history. This patient reports a healthy relationship with one male partner, with good communication, and attempts on their own to decrease pain (lubricants, positional changes). Pelvic examination needs to include visualization of the external genitalia, vaginal introitus, entire vagina, and cervix by using a vaginal speculum, particularly since the patient has reported postcoital bleeding. A cotton swab can be used to test the vestibule for any tenderness. A digital vaginal examination can detect vaginismus, pelvic floor muscle spasms, and/or uterosacral masses/tenderness as well as introital and vaginal caliber. A bimanual examination evaluates for uterine and adnexal size, mobility, and tenderness. Screening for STIs with a cervical swab should be included, both based on patient's age (less than 25 years) and report of postcoital bleeding.

Given her past surgical history and complaints of painful penetrative sex and vaginal bleeding, this patient most likely has introital stenosis. This is easily diagnosed on pelvic examination in the office. Depending on the degree of stenosis, the patient may benefit from vaginal dilation, pelvic floor physical therapy, and/or an introitoplasty to improve her symptoms and accommodate penetrative sexual intimacy.

## 7.2.4 Case 4

A 20-year-old patient has a sigmoid neovagina created during her primary cloacal reconstruction as an infant. She reports success with penetrative sexual intercourse. She does, however, report ongoing vaginal discharge, which requires her to wear a panty liner daily. She has been treated empirically numerous times for both yeast with fluconazole and bacterial vaginosis with metronidazole without improvement in her symptoms. Her urine STI screen is negative.

**What is the next best step in her management?**

    **A.** Vaginal dilation
    **B.** Suppressive antibiotics
    **C.** Examination of her vagina

*Answer:* C

### 7.2.4.1  Learning points

Some patients with more complex cloacal malformations require a bowel neovagina during their primary reconstruction. Sigmoid is the most common type of bowel graft utilized because of its caliber and proximity to the perineum. Additionally, a sigmoid neovagina created in early childhood does not require immediate postoperative dilation. Reported complications of sigmoid vaginoplasty include postoperative ileus, anastomotic leak or obstruction, intra-abdominal adhesions, mucosal prolapse, excessive mucosal discharge, polyps, malignancy, diversion colitis, and development of inflammatory bowel disease.

A potential benefit of a bowel graft is the natural secretions, which can be an effective lubricant. However, these secretions, when excessive, can lead to a copious, malodorous discharge. One-third of patients with bowel neovaginas report a bothersome vaginal discharge and about one in five report malodor.

Patients with bowel neovaginas who report discharge remote from surgery require a complete pelvic examination with inspection of their entire neovagina. Endoscopic evaluation may be particularly helpful. Causes of neovaginal discharge remote from surgery include mucosal trauma, fistula, infection, carcinoma, polyps, and inflammatory colitis. Any suspicious lesions should be biopsied.

If after careful evaluation the discharge is deemed physiologic, vaginal irrigation may help minimize the symptoms. This patient does not need vaginal dilation because she has no problem with penetrative sexual activity. Suppressive antibiotics will not impact the physiologic mucous secretions. Patients with bowel neovaginas require ongoing preventive reproductive care including contraception, screening for STIs, and HPV vaccination. Cytology screening is not recommended if the cervix is absent.

## 7.2.5  Case 5

A 25-year-old woman with a previously repaired imperforate anus with rectoperineal fistula reports she would like to become pregnant. She has normal bowel movements without soiling and normal menstrual cycles. She wants to know if it is safe for her to become pregnant and what she should anticipate.

**Counseling should include which of the following?**

    **A.** Labor and vaginal delivery is contraindicated
    **B.** There are no reports of healthy pregnancy outcomes in women with ARM
    **C.** Preconceptual counseling is paramount

*Answer:* C

### 7.2.5.1  Learning points

- Though limited, there are reports of women with even more complex anorectal malformations with successful pregnancies resulting in live births. There are no reported maternal mortalities; the most common maternal morbidities reported are increased urinary tract infections and worsening chronic kidney disease. These reported pregnancies have been conceived spontaneously as well as with advanced reproductive technologies. All modes of delivery, including spontaneous and operative vaginal delivery and cesarean section, have been reported in this patient population.
- Preconceptual counseling is particularly important in patients with ARM. Like all women, ideally their health should be optimized and their pregnancy planned. Patients with imperforate anus may have additional VACTERL abnormalities. Müllerian anomalies can

impact fertility, risk of preterm labor, and fetal malpresentation. Cardiac anomalies require careful management with cardiology, particularly at the time of delivery, and require fetal echocardiography. Renal function may worsen and if impaired at baseline may increase the risk of preeclampsia. Spinal abnormalities may limit the utility of regional anesthesia.

- Currently no evidence-based guidelines regarding mode of delivery (vaginal vs. cesarean delivery) in women with ARM exist. Recommendations, therefore, are individualized with careful discussion of the inherent risks and benefits of both modes of delivery and shared medical decision-making between obstetrician and patient. Patients with a bowel neo-vagina and/or repaired cloacal malformations are generally encouraged to deliver by cesarean section. Patients with a native vagina and adequate perineal body after repair of IA may consider vaginal delivery. If the patient already has poor anal continence, she may be more willing to risk potential obstetrical anal sphincter injury and attempt a vaginal delivery. Prior to delivery, all previous abdominal and pelvic surgery (including Mitrofanoff appendicovesicostomy and Malone appendicostomy) should be reviewed to determine the best type and location of abdominal and uterine incisions. Pre- and intraoperative collaboration with colorectal surgeons and urologists is beneficial.

# References

1. Minneci PC, Kabre RS, Mak GZ et al. Screening practices and associated anomalies in infants with anorectal malformations: Results from the Midwest Pediatric Surgery Consortium. *J Pediatr Surg*. 2018;53(6):1163–7.
2. Totonelli G, Morini F, Catania VD et al. Anorectal malformations associated spinal cord anomalies. *Pediatr Surg Int*. 2016;32(8):729–35.
3. Halleran DR, Thompson B, Fuchs M et al. Urethral length in female infants and its relevance in the repair of cloaca. *J Pediatr Surg*. 2018; 54(2):303–6.
4. Pena A, Levitt M. Surgical management of cloacal malformations. *Semin Neonatol*. 2003;8(3):249–57.
5. Wood RJ, Reck-Burneo CA, Dajusta D et al. Cloaca reconstruction: A new algorithm which considers the role of urethral length in determining surgical planning. *J Pediatr Surg*. 2017;43(2018):582.
6. Grimsby GM, Menon V, Schlomer BJ et al. Long-term outcomes of bladder neck reconstruction without augmentation cystoplasty in children. *J Urol*. 2016;195(1):155–61.
7. Szymanski KM, Rink RC, Whittam B et al. Long-term outcomes of the Kropp and Salle urethral lengthening bladder neck reconstruction procedures. *J Pediatr Urol*. 2016;12(6):403 e401–403 e407.
8. Caldwell BT, Wilcox DT. Long-term urological outcomes in cloacal anomalies. *Semin Pediatr Surg*. 2016;25(2):108–11.
9. Islam MN, Hasina K, Reza MS, Hasanuzzaman SM, Akter T, Talukder SA. Urinary tract anomalies in patients with anorectal malformation. *Mymensingh Med J*. 2015;24(2):352–5.
10. Sanchez S, Ricca R, Joyner B, Waldhausen JH. Vesicoureteral reflux and febrile urinary tract infections in anorectal malformations: A retrospective review. *J Pediatr Surg*. 2014;49(1):91–4.
11. Giuliani S, Midrio P, De Filippo RE et al. Anorectal malformation and associated end-stage renal disease: Management from newborn to adult life. *J Pediatr Surg*. 2013;48(3):635–41.
12. VanderBrink BA, Reddy PP. Early urologic considerations in patients with persistent cloaca. *Semin Pediatr Surg*. 2016;25(2):82–9.
13. Raveenthiran V, Sam CJ. Epididymo-orchitis complicating anorectal malformations: Collective review of 41 cases. *J Urol*. 2011;186(4):1467–72.
14. VanderBrink BA, Sivan B, Levitt MA, Pena A, Sheldon CA, Alam S. Epididymitis in patients with anorectal malformations: A cause for urologic concern. *Int Braz J Urol*. 2014;40(5):676–82.

# Further reading

1. Breech L. Gynecologic concerns in patients with anorectal malformations. *Semin Pediatr Surg*. 2010;19:139–45.
2. Oelschlager AM, Kirby A, Breech L. Evaluation and management of vaginoplasty complications. *Cur Opin Obstet Gynecol*. 2017;29:316–21.

3. Dietrich JE, Miller D, Quint EH. Obstructive reproductive tract anomalies. *J Pediatr Adolesc Gynecol.* 2014;27:396–402.
4. Dietrich JE, Miller D, Quint EH. Non-obstructive Müllerian anomalies. *J Pediatr Adolesc Gynecol.* 2014;27:386–95.
5. Gebhart JB, Schmitt JJ. Surgical management of the constricted or obliterated vagina. *Obstet Gynecol.* 2016;128:284–91.
6. American College of Obstetricians and Gynecologists, Practice Guideline, No. 651: Menstruation in girls and adolescents: Using the menstrual cycle as a vital sign. *Obstet Gynecol.* 2015;126:143–6.

# 8 A patient with an anorectal malformation who has been previously repaired and who is "not doing well"

Victoria Lane and Jeffrey Avansino

## 8.1 Case study 1

A 4-year-old boy is referred to your clinic for ongoing care of his anorectal malformation. He has undergone surgery for what you suspect may have been a rectobulbar fistula, but the operative notes are missing. The parents inform you that he underwent full VACTERL screening as a newborn infant and no other anomalies were identified. The parents have expressed concerns about fecal incontinence, lower urinary tract infections, and suffering with post-void dribbling.

With regard to the case described, on examination in the office the scars on the abdomen would suggest that the original surgery was performed "laparoscopic assisted" and there is evidence of a colostomy scar.

The next steps for this patient would include which of the following:

A. Spine MRI
B. Spine and pelvis MRI

   **C.** Spine and pelvis MRI and exam under anesthesia
   **D.** Exam under anesthesia only
   **E.** Spine MRI and exam under anesthesia

*Answer:* C

During the work-up a ROOF is identified. The anus appears to be in the anatomically correct position. The treatment of this should be which of the following:

   **A.** No intervention
   **B.** PSARP with rectal mobilization and repair of ROOF
   **C.** Endoscopic transurethral repair
   **D.** Laparoscopic repair of the ROOF

*Answer:* B

From this brief history, you are concerned about:

1. Anal mislocation leading to fecal incontinence.
2. The operation was performed laparoscopic assisted and this places him at increased risk of a ROOF and this would be in keeping with the post-void dribbling and lower urinary tract infections.

## 8.1.1 Learning points

The patient with a previously repaired anorectal malformation (ARM) who is "not doing well" is a vague title for this chapter but is representative of the ARM population, which despite best efforts continues to suffer significant morbidity. Despite significant advances in the medical and surgical care of children over recent years and numerous publications in the literature, a significant number of children are continuing to have problems, many of which are a consequence of the underlying congenital malformations that require careful management (esophageal atresia, congenital cardiac defects, renal pathology); however, many of the anorectal, urological, and gynecological issues are iatrogenic and potentially avoidable [1–5].

Children born with an anorectal malformation (ARM) are known to have the potential to fall under the VACTERL association and it is therefore important to evaluate these children thoroughly to exclude any underlying vertebral, cardiac, tracheo-esophageal, renal, and limb abnormalities, in addition to further evaluation for any concerns regarding the previous anorectal malformation. This requires a multidisciplinary collaborative approach.

The aim of this chapter is to provide a strategy for assessing a child who is "not doing well" following surgical intervention for an anorectal malformation, from a colorectal, urological, or gynecological perspective. In order to be able to evaluate a child, the surgeon must first understand the potential postoperative complications and the reason for their occurrence. Unfortunately, with pediatric colorectal surgery, the complications might not be immediately apparent. The surgeon may not remember the complexities of the case when the toddler returns to the clinic unable to potty train after their repair in the newborn period, or the surgeon may be evaluating the patient of a retired colleague, or a child that has moved pediatric surgical centers or has been adopted.

Efforts continue to improve the education of pediatric surgeons around the world, and there have been many publications in the literature with the aim being to share experience, ideas, and lessons learned [6] to minimize the same mistakes being repeated. Peña et al. [2] reported on the reoperations in anorectal malformations. In order of frequency the complications seen in their series included:

- Stricture or atresia of the rectum
- Mislocated anus

- Recurrent fistula (rectourethral or rectovaginal)
- Persistent urogenital sinus in a cloaca
- Rectal prolapse
- Cloaca/vaginal atresia

Similar complications were reported by Levitt et al. [1] with the indications for redo surgery in cloacal malformations, which included:

- Persistent urogenital sinus
- Rectal atresia/acquired atresia
- Acquired vaginal atresia/stricture
- Mislocated anus
- Urethrovaginal fistula
- Rectal prolapse
- Urethral atresia/stricture
- Rectovaginal fistula

All surgeons will encounter complications secondary to infection and patient disease; however, there are a number of complications that most likely have occurred secondary to:

1. *Diagnosis*: Failure to recognize the complexities of the congenital malformation, leading to poor decision-making. For example, failure to recognize a perineal fistula with an associated vaginal atresia.
2. *Investigations*: Failures to perform/or correctly execute radiological investigations to establish the anatomy leading to poor surgical planning and intraoperative complications. For example, no fistula being assumed secondary to a poorly performed contrast study via the mucous fistula failing to demonstrate a rectourethral fistula due to inadequate pressure.
3. *Operative technique*: Inadequate mobilization of structures, failure to preserve blood supply leading to tension, poor healing, strictures, fistulae, and acquired atresia.

Therefore, when evaluating the child who is "not doing well" consider where things have gone wrong in the following areas:

1. Diagnosis
2. Decision-making
3. Investigations
4. Operative technique

The most common complications are:

- Fecal incontinence
- Constipation
- Obstructed menstruation
- Urinary tract infection
- Stricture or acquired atresia of the rectum
- Mislocated anus outside the sphincter complex
- Fistulae—recurrent or acquired
- Remnant of the original fistula (ROOF)
- Persistent urogenital sinus in cloacal malformations
- Rectal prolapse
- Vaginal atresia
- Urethral atresia, stricture, or injury

- Persistent cloaca
- Renal failure

Children with an anorectal malformation are known to have potential problems with fecal and urinary control [7–9]. Specific questions should be asked to ascertain the functional status with regard to their bladder and bowels using standardized questionnaires where possible. The focus of the evaluation should therefore be:

1. VACTERL associated anomalies
2. Identification of postoperative complications
3. Fecal and urinary continence
4. Gynecologic and reproductive status
5. Long-term renal health [5]

All patients should undergo a clinical examination in the outpatient clinic. This will enable the physician to understand the presenting complaints and establish the severity of the previous anorectal malformation, in addition to the mandatory assessment of global development, blood pressure, and renal function tests.

Postoperative evaluation of a child with a previously repaired anorectal malformation in males and females should initially follow the same protocol:

- Renal evaluation
- Spinal evaluation
- Sacral bony evaluation and calculation of sacral ratio
- Cardiac evaluation

### 8.1.1.1 Male

a. Abdominal examination:

The presence of a colostomy scar indicates that the original anorectal malformation may have been a rectourethral fistula (bulbar, prostatic, bladder neck) initially managed with a colostomy. These patients require careful evaluation to exclude a remnant of original fistula (ROOF) on the posterior wall of the urethra. Male patients who have undergone a laparoscopic-assisted anorectoplasty also require careful evaluation as this technique is known to have an increased risk of leaving a ROOF [10–12]. A ROOF can cause significant problems with post-void dribbling, urinary tract infection, and stone formation. In addition to these infective complications, the ROOF also has malignant potential and if identified should be excised [13,14].

b. Renal tract evaluation:

- *Renal tract US*: To identify anatomical renal anomalies, hydronephrosis, and a measure of the post-void bladder residual.
- *Voiding cystourethrogram*: Performed in cases where there is a concern for vesicoureteric reflux or a ROOF.
- *Urodynamic evaluation*: To assess bladder compliance and volume, detrusor activity, and leak pressures. This is particularly important if the child has associated spinal anomalies but may not be indicated in all children.

c. Spinal cord assessment:

- *Spinal MRI*: To assess for spinal cord tethering and occult spinal dysraphism.

d. Sacral evaluation:

- Lumbosacral radiographs (AP and lateral).
  - *AP*: Looking for evidence of a hemi-sacrum/scimitar sacrum can alert the physician to the presence of a presacral mass.

- *Lateral*: To assess the degree of sacral dysplasia and to calculate the sacral ratio. The sacral ratio can be used to help predict the likelihood that the child will/will not be continent [15–17].
e. Colonic evaluation:
   - *Contrast enema*: To assess the colonic anatomy and also information regarding the presacral space.
f. Pelvic MRI:
   - Presacral space evaluation.
   - ROOF identification.
g. Examination under anesthesia/cystourethroscopy:
   - Assessment of the urethra, identification of ureteric and bladder anomalies.
   - Anal mislocation.
   - Anal stricture.
   - Rectal prolapse.

Considering the limited surgical history available to you, you decide to perform a number of investigations as per the "male" algorithm:

- Sacral radiographs (AP and lateral) to assess the sacral ratio, in order to gain some information with regard to the child's potential for future bowel control.
- *Renal US*: To assess the renal tract as there is a known VACTERL association.
- *Contrast enema*: To assess colonic anatomy.
- *Pelvic MRI*: To assess for a remnant of the original fistula inserting into the urethral tract.
- VCUG to assess for a ROOF and exclude vesicoureteric reflux.
- MRI spine to assess for spinal cord anomalies/tethered cord.
- Cystoscopy to assess:
   - Urethra for a ROOF.
   - Bladder neck competency.
   - Bladder for evidence of trabeculation to suggest a high-pressure neurogenic bladder or cystitis cystica indicative of chronic infection, which would prompt urodynamic investigation.

Results:

- Pelvic MRI:
   - There is an abnormal structure arising from the posterior urethra consistent with a remnant of the original fistula (Figure 8.1).
- Contrast enema:
   - Normal. No evidence of colonic dilatation.
- VCUG:
   - A ROOF is demonstrated (Figure 8.2).
- EUA and cystourethroscopy:
   - Anteriorly mislocated anus outside the sphincter complex.
   - ROOF confirmed at the level of the bulbar urethra.

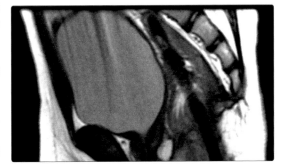

Figure 8.1 Lateral image of the pelvic MRI.

## 8.1.1.2 Female

In the female patient, the algorithm is initially very similar with a detailed history, general assessment, and a more focused history on gynecologic status depending on their age.

Their assessment is similar to that in the male; however there are additional points for consideration:

a. Abdominal examination:
   i. *Scars*: The absence of a colostomy scar would suggest that the original malformation was a perineal or rectovestibular fistula.
   ii. The presence of a vesicostomy/vaginostomy/colostomy would indicate a more complex malformation.
b. Müllerian structures:
   i. Assessment of Müllerian structures is age dependent. In the older child a pelvic US or MRI can be useful to assess for these structures [18–20]; however, every opportunity to assess these structures intraoperatively should be used [21].
c. Examination of the perineum, urethra, vagina, and anus.

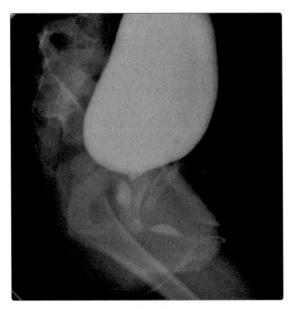

Figure 8.2  VCUG.

Complete anatomical evaluation to assess for (Figure 8.3):

- EUA:
  - Anal mislocation in relation to the sphincter complex
  - Anal stricture
  - Rectal prolapse
  - Perineal body
- Cystovaginoscopy:
  - Urethral and bladder anomalies
  - Remnants of original rectovestibular/vaginal fistula
  - Vaginal septums
  - Assessment of the vaginal introitus
  - Identification of cervix/cervices

## 8.2  Case study 2

This is the case of a 2-year-old girl who has been adopted. The parents present to your outpatient clinic for a full assessment. The parents do not have information about the child's previous medical and surgical history, apart from the fact that their daughter has an anorectal malformation. The parents do not report any particular concerns, the child is thriving and developing normally; however, they do not think the perineal area is normal.

As per the female algorithm, this patient needs a comprehensive VACTERL screen to include spinal assessment, cardiac review and ECHO, and renal assessment.

You are able to examine the child in the outpatient clinic and the findings are demonstrated in the image (Figure 8.4):

- Anal opening
- Urethral opening

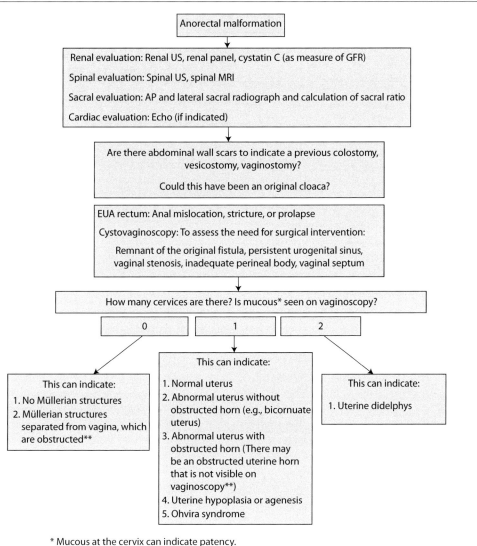

Figure 8.3  Patient algorithm.

- No vaginal opening
- No evidence of a vesicostomy or vaginostomy but the patient did have a colostomy scar

Your initial examination findings are a cause for concern.

The most likely diagnosis is:

A. Cloaca with persistent urogenital sinus
B. Rectovestibularfistulawithvaginalagenesis
C. Urogenital sinus
D. Posterior cloaca

*Answer:* A

### 8.2.1 Learning points

The clinical findings are in keeping with an original cloaca malformation. Originally there would have been a single perineal opening and the original surgeons have simply "created an anus" by performing a pull-through procedure but not addressed the underlying malformation (no correction of the urogenital complex).

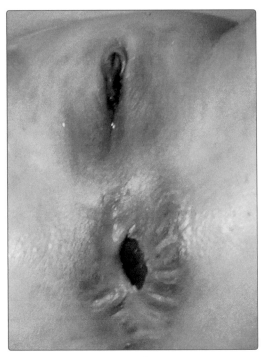

**Figure 8.4** Female perineum.

The patient undergoes cystoscopy and an exam under anesthesia. The anus is properly placed but there was no evidence of a vagina arising from the common channel. The next best step in therapy would be:

A. Redo PSARP
B. Redo PSARP with urogenital mobilization
C. Redo PSARP with creation of neovagina
D. Re-evaluate during adolescence with MRI

*Answer:* D

This child may have vaginal atresia. This would account for the lack of a vaginostomy scar on the abdomen and the reason for the child not developing hydrocolpos, because the vagina is not entering into the common channel and therefore not able to fill with urine.

This child is currently safe; however they need further evaluation of their Müllerian structures. There may be an atretic vagina with functional uterine tissue predisposing her to developing obstructed menses in the future. The timing of any vaginal replacement surgery can be discussed with the family [22].

## 8.3  Case study 3

A 4-year-old male presents to your clinic having previously been operated on for a rectoprostatic urethral fistula. The patient currently has fecal incontinence. The patient is noted to have circumferential prolapse that produces mucous and occasional blood in the underwear. An EUA demonstrates the anal opening to be just outside of the muscle complex. An MRI of the spine demonstrates the conus to be at L4 and there is a fatty filum. The sacral ratio on contrast enema is 0.48. The next best step in management is:

A. Watchful waiting and repair prolapse only if fecal incontinence improves
B. Redo the PSARP
C. Excise the prolapse only

*Answer:* C

### 8.3.1 Learning points

- The morbidity associated with a redo PSARP can be avoided in such a case in a patient with poor potential for bowel control. Patients who have good potential for bowel control would benefit from relocating the anus into the center of the anal muscle complex. If potential for bowel control is unclear, the best option is to redo the PSARP.

You have decided to repair the prolapse only. In order to do this the best approach is:

A. Excise one side, wait for 2–3 months, and excise the other side
B. Do a single circumferential excision
C. Do an anal cerclage (e.g., Thiersch wire)

*Answer:* A

### 8.3.2 Learning points

- Excising one side at a time can be done in an outpatient fashion. Since there is no circumferential anastomosis, dilations can be avoided. This is particularly helpful in older children who tend to be more resistant.
- Anal cerclage has been reported in the management of rectal prolapse in non-ARM patients but does not have a role in this patient population.

## 8.4 Case study 4

A 6-month-old male is in the OR to have their colostomy closed. During the exam under anesthesia, you note that the patient has a skin level stricture and can only accommodate an 8 Hagar dilator. After talking with the family, your next step would be to:

A. Abort the procedure and reschedule a redo PSARP.
B. Abort the procedure and reschedule a Heinicki-Miculicz stricturoplasty.
C. Do a stricturoplasty now and close the colostomy later.
D. Do a stricturoplasty now and close the colostomy under the same anesthetic.
E. Abort the procedure and resume dilations.

*Answer:* C

### 8.4.1 Learning points

- Patients with superficial skin strictures can have an HM stricturoplasty. These can usually be done in the outpatient center. It is the authors' preference to do this during the current anesthetic and close the colostomy after this area has healed, although one could close the colostomy under the same anesthetic as the stricturoplasty.
- A redo PSARP is indicated for a stricture that extends beyond the skin level. A superficial stricturoplasty in this setting is typically not successful.
- Presumably dilations were being done prior to surgery. These are likely not to be successful over the long term and will likely cause undue stress and discomfort to the child.

## 8.5  Case study 5

A 14-year-old female presents with a 1-month history of worsening abdominal pain. She had begun menstruation 3 months prior. Pain is typically worse around the time of menstruation. The patient has a history of a rectovestibular fistula and the rest of her VACTERL work-up is negative. The next best exam to get that day in clinic is:

**A.** An ultrasound of the pelvis
**B.** An MRI of the pelvis
**C.** A radiograph of the abdomen
**D.** A contrast enema
**E.** An exam under anesthesia

*Answer:* A

### 8.5.1  Learning points

- Adolescent women with ARM are at high risk of Müllerian abnormalities that can result in obstruction to menstrual flow. Patients with history of ARM should be seen in the adolescent period to evaluate for Müllerian anomalies.
- The best immediate exam in this setting is a US to determine if the patient has an obstructed uterine horn. An MRI is also reasonable but may be difficult to obtain on the same day and the exam is costlier. Ultimately an MRI will be needed to better define the anatomy. A radiograph and contrast enema are likely to be nondiagnostic. An EUA would be a reasonable next step but could miss an obstructed uterine horn or upper vagina.

The US shows a cystic structure with a normal cervix and uterus above this. Adjacent to the right of these structures are normal Müllerian structures and a normal distal vagina. Digital examination of the patent vaginal vault reveals a large bulge approximately 4 cm from the vaginal introitus. The next step in management is:

**A.** Transperineal vaginal mobilization and vaginoplasty
**B.** Transabdominal sigmoid bowel vaginoplasty
**C.** Hormone suppression
**D.** Transvaginal marsupialization
**E.** Hemihysterectomy

*Answer:* D

### 8.5.2  Learning points

- A transvaginal marsupialization between the patent's right vagina and the obstructed left hemivagina would be the optimal therapy in the previously mentioned scenario.
  - This can be accomplished by incising the common walls between the vagina and then marsupializing them. Needle localization with ultrasound guidance can be used to identify the obstructed vagina. A wire can then be passed followed by a dilator. The wall can be open over the dilator and a section of the common wall removed.
- If there was not a patent introitus, a transperineal vaginal mobilization could be performed, as the vagina was a reasonable distance from the perineum. If the vagina cannot reach, a sigmoid or small bowel vaginoplasty may be performed.
- A hemihysterectomy should be performed if the patient has an obstructed uterine horn without a cervix. Placing a uterus in continuity without a cervix predisposes the patient to ascending infections and nonviable pregnancies.

## 8.6 Case study 6

A 5-year-old male is 5 days out from a redo-PSARP for a misplaced anus. The patient had received a preoperative mechanical bowel preparation with oral antibiotics. The procedure was completed without a protective colostomy. The patient had a liquid bowel movement the evening prior. On rounds you are unable to clearly see the mucosa or the stitches.

The next step is to:

   **A.** Obtain an MRI
   **B.** Obtain a contrast enema
   **C.** Discharge home as he is stooling
   **D.** Perform exam under anesthesia

*Answer:* D

### 8.6.1 Learning points

- At times, it can be difficult to assess a patient's anoplasty. If the anoplasty is not clearly intact in the nondiverted patient then further evaluation is needed. The best next step is an exam under anesthesia. This will allow the surgeon to adequately evaluate the repair. Imaging in this setting is not of use. Sending the patient home would be ill advised, especially in the nondiverted patient.

In the OR, you noticed that the incision is intact but the anoplasty has circumferentially dehisced and retracted 1–2 cm. The next step is to:

   **A.** Redo/reinforce the anastomosis without protective colostomy
   **B.** Redo/reinforce the anastomosis with protective colostomy
   **C.** Protective colostomy only
   **D.** Nothing, you can see the mucosa, it will be fine

*Answer:* B

### 8.6.2 Learning points

- Superficial skin and anastomotic dehiscence are common in patients with ARM. These can be treated with local measures including basic wound care and keeping the area clean. These often heal without incident.
- Poorly perfused tissues with anastomotic tension are a recipe for dehiscence.
  - Dehiscence without retraction can be managed with reinforcement of the anoplasty with debridement of devitalized tissue.
  - Dehiscence with retraction of the rectum requires a diverting colostomy. Reinforcement of the anoplasty is often possible but recurrent dehiscence is high thus a protective colostomy is best.

## References

1. Levitt MA, Bischoff A, Peña A. Pitfalls and challenges of cloaca repair: How to reduce the need for reoperations. *J Pediatr Surg [Internet]*. Elsevier Inc. 2011;46(6):1250–5. Available from: http://linkinghub.elsevier.com/retrieve/pii/S002234681100279X
2. Peña A, Grasshoff S, Levitt M. Reoperations in anorectal malformations. *J Pediatr Surg [Internet]*. 2007;42(2):318–25. Available from: http://linkinghub.elsevier.com/retrieve/pii/S0022346806007627.
3. de Blaauw I, Midrio P, Breech L et al. Treatment of adults with unrecognized or inadequately repaired anorectal malformations: 17 cases of rectovestibular and rectoperineal fistulas. *J Pediatr Adolesc Gynecol*. 2013 Jun;26(3):156–60.

4. Alam S, Lawal TA, Pena A, Sheldon C, Levitt MA. Acquired posterior urethral diverticulum following surgery for anorectal malformations. *J Pediatr Surg.* 2011 Jun;46(6):1231–5.

5. Lane VA, Skerritt C, Wood RJ et al. A standardized approach for the assessment and treatment of internationally adopted children with a previously repaired anorectal malformation (ARM). *J Pediatr Surg.* 2016 Nov;51(11):1864–70.

6. Levitt MA, Pena A. Cloacal malformations: Lessons learned from 490 cases. *Semin Pediatr Surg.* 2010 May;19(2):128–38.

7. Hassett S, Snell S, Hughes-Thomas A, Holmes K. 10-Year outcome of children born with anorectal malformation, treated by posterior sagittal anorectoplasty, assessed according to the Krickenbeck classification. *J Pediatr Surg [Internet].* Elsevier Inc. 2009;44(2):399–403. Available from: http://linkinghub.elsevier.com/retrieve/pii/S0022346808009561

8. Nam SH, Kim DY, Kim SC. Can we expect a favorable outcome after surgical treatment for an anorectal malformation? *J Pediatr Surg.* 2016 Mar;51(3):421–4.

9. Ming A-X, Li L, Diao M et al. Long term outcomes of laparoscopic-assisted anorectoplasty: A comparison study with posterior sagittal anorectoplasty. *J Pediatr Surg.* 2014 Apr;49(4):560–3.

10. Srimurthy KR, Ramesh S, Shankar G, Narenda BM. Technical modifications of laparoscopically assisted anorectal pull-through for anorectal malformations. *J Laparoendosc Adv Surg Tech A.* 2008 Apr;18(2):340–3.

11. Rollins MD, Downey EC, Meyers RL, Scaife ER. Division of the fistula in laparoscopic-assisted repair of anorectal malformations—Are clips or ties necessary? *J Pediatr Surg.* 2009 Jan;44(1):298–301.

12. Bischoff A, Levitt MA, Pena A. Laparoscopy and its use in the repair of anorectal malformations. *J Pediatr Surg.* 2011 Aug;46(8):1609–17.

13. Hidas G, Gibbs D, Alireza A, Khoury AE. Management of rectal stenosis with endoscopic balloon dilatation. *J Pediatr Surg [Internet].* Elsevier Inc. 2013;48(4):e13–6. Available from: http://linkinghub.elsevier.com/retrieve/pii/S0022346813000468

14. Koga H, Okazaki T, Yamataka A et al. Posterior urethral diverticulum after laparoscopic-assisted repair of high-type anorectal malformation in a male patient: Surgical treatment and prevention. *Pediatr Surg Int.* 2005 Jan; 21(1):58–60.

15. Pena A. Anorectal malformations. *Semin Pediatr Surg.* 1995 Feb;4(1):35–47.

16. Levitt MA, Patel M, Rodriguez G, Gaylin DS, Pena A. The tethered spinal cord in patients with anorectal malformations. *J Pediatr Surg.* 1997 Mar;32(3):462–8.

17. Arnoldi R, Macchini F, Gentilino V et al. Anorectal malformations with good prognosis: Variables affecting the functional outcome. *J Pediatr Surg.* 2014 Aug;49(8):1232–6.

18. Junqueira BLP, Allen LM, Spitzer RF, Lucco KL, Babyn PS, Doria AS. Müllerian duct anomalies and mimics in children and adolescents: Correlative intraoperative assessment with clinical imaging. *Radiographics.* 2009; 29(4):1085–103.

19. Robbins JB, Broadwell C, Chow LC, Parry JP, Sadowski EA. Müllerian duct anomalies: Embryological development, classification, and MRI assessment. *J Magn Reson Imaging.* 2015 Jan;41(1):1–12.

20. Chandler TM, Machan LS, Cooperberg PL, Harris AC, Chang SD. Müllerian duct anomalies: From diagnosis to intervention. *Br J Radiol.* 2009 Dec;82(984):1034–42.

21. Breech L. Gynecologic concerns in patients with anorectal malformations. *Semin Pediatr Surg.* 2010 May;19(2): 139–45.

22. Skerritt C, Sánchez AV, Lane VA et al. Menstrual, sexual, and obstetrical outcomes after vaginal replacement for vaginal atresia associated with anorectal malformation. *Eur J Pediatr Surg.* 2016; 27(6):495–502 (EFirst).

# 9 Neonatal diagnosis of Hirschsprung disease

Martin Lacher and Duarte Vaz Pimentel

## 9.1 Case study

The emergency room calls you to see a 2-day-old-boy with bilious vomiting. The patient was born at 37 weeks of gestation. Prenatally trisomy 21 and ventricular septal defect were confirmed. After birth the child was generally well, but now the oxygen saturation is only 90%, so he was put on CPAP. The neonatologist is concerned about the vomiting and a distended abdomen. The patient passed meconium 26 hours after birth after a gentle rectal irrigation. He has bilious nasogastric tube aspirate.

On physical exam his abdomen is distended, nontender to palpation, with no peritonitis. His vital signs are all normal. His leukocyte count, CRP, IL-6, and ABG are normal.

**Looking at the described case, what test is missing for a complete evaluation for suspected Hirschsprung disease (HD)?**

   **A.** Upper GI study
   **B.** Stool cultures
   **C.** Cardiac echo
   **D.** Rectal exam

*Answer:* D

**Learning points**

Infrequent, explosive bowel movements caused by functional colonic obstruction are common in infants with Hirschsprung disease. A rectal examination may demonstrate a tight anal sphincter and explosive discharge of stool and gas (Figure 9.1). This sign significantly increases the likelihood of the child having HD [1].

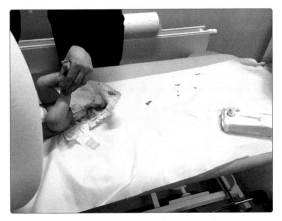

Figure 9.1 Explosive stools on rectal exam.

**After completing your rectal exam, which diagnostic step is next?**

A. Abdominal ultrasound
B. Chest x-ray
C. Abdominal x-ray (AXR)
D. Contrast enema study

*Answer:* C (Figure 9.2)

**Learning points**

Abdominal x-ray: Air fluid levels in the colon are suspicious for HD.

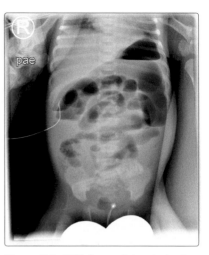

Figure 9.2  AXR shows distended colon, absent gas in the rectum, and an air fluid level in the ascending and descending colon.

**How would you manage this child over the weekend?**

A. Rectal irrigations, resuscitation if needed, no antibiotics
B. Rectal irrigations, broad-spectrum antibiotics, and intravenous fluid
C. No rectal manipulation is allowed; treat with broad-spectrum antibiotics and resuscitation if needed
D. No rectal manipulation is allowed, antibiotics are not needed, perform emergency ileostomy

*Answer:* B

**Learning points**

If the child is stable with rectal irrigations then the case is not considered an emergency.

**Having established a working diagnosis of HD, you start the child on rectal irrigations. How should they be performed?**

A. Warmed isotonic saline solution using a syringe and a large-bore Foley catheter (24Fr) to irrigate 30–50 mL at a time removing stool and air, and repeating this process as often as necessary until the saline comes out clean. No more than 20 mL/kg should remain in the colon. At the end of the irrigation a rectal exam is performed to dilate the sphincter.
B. Warmed ringer lactate using a syringe and a large-bore Foley catheter to irrigate 80–100 mL at a time, and repeating this process until the solution comes out clean. How much solution stays in the colon is not relevant.
C. Warmed isotonic saline solution, irrigate once with a bag connected to a large-bore Foley catheter, hang the bag about 2 ft above the patient until the solution stops flowing. Leave all inside to dissolve hard stool.
D. Warmed isotonic saline solution using a syringe and a large-bore Foley catheter to irrigate 30–40 mL once and leave the solution inside; the patient should be able to pass stool shortly after.

*Answer:* A

**Learning points**

Know how to do rectal irrigations; do NOT delegate rectal irrigations to the nurse right away. Every surgical trainee needs to know how to do them properly. The chance to do rectal irrigations every 8 hours is also the chance to see the patient every 8 hours to make sure he/she is doing well or getting better (Figure 9.3).

## How often should the irrigations be performed?

A. Once a day
B. Twice a day
C. Depending on how distended the abdomen is, perform as often as necessary to decompress the colon
D. None of the above are correct

*Answer:* C

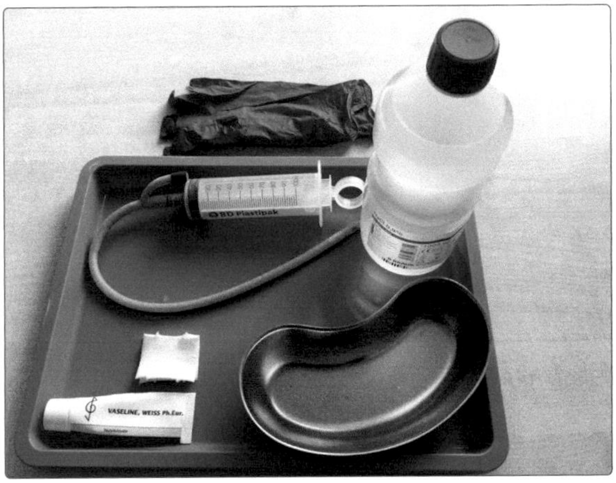

**Figure 9.3** Equipment needed for rectal irrigations.

### Learning points

Irrigations should be performed to empty the colon, whatever it takes.

## How would you achieve the definitive diagnosis in this child?

A. Genetic testing
B. Abdomen x-ray and colonic biopsy only
C. Abdomen ultrasound and colonic biopsy only
D. Contrast enema study and rectal biopsy

*Answer:* D

### Learning points

A rectal biopsy and good histology initially taken from the rectum are the only diagnostic tests that prove HD.

## The following Monday, which diagnostic study in addition to the KUB do you order?

A. Abdominal ultrasound
B. Upper GI
C. Contrast enema with water-soluble media
D. Another AXR

*Answer:* C

### Learning points

Before any rectal biopsy a contrast enema is performed. However, the contrast enema does not show a clear transition zone in a lot of cases. The sensitivity and specificity to see the transition zone on a contrast enema in the neonatal period are 80% and 98%, respectively [2] (Figure 9.4).

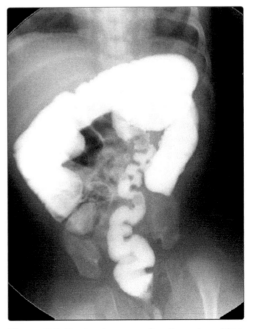

**Figure 9.4** Contrast enema showing a transition zone in the upper sigmoid.

**Learning points**

The surgeon has to recognize whether the contrast enema shows (A) a transition zone distal to the splenic flexure, (B) a transition zone proximal to the splenic flexure, (C) possible total colonic HD, and (D) no obvious transition zone. Every scenario except (D) makes a rectal biopsy mandatory. "Total colonic mapping" needed for long-segment HD cases means sero-muscular or full-thickness colonic biopsies to check whether ganglion cells are present AND that the size of the nerves is less than 40 μm.

**If the transition zone is in the left colon (sigmoid or lower): How long would you continue the treatment of rectal irrigations?**

    **A.** Until the definitive diagnosis is made and if HD is confirmed the surgical treatment is carried out, however long that may be
    **B.** Not more than 4 weeks; the child should start passing stool spontaneously after that
    **C.** Not more than 8 weeks; performing irrigations over this period will condition the colon to not work on its own
    **D.** The patient will surely need irrigations for the rest of his life

*Answer:* A

**Learning points**

Irrigations should be performed to empty the colon, until the time of the pull-through.

**You now want to proceed with obtaining a rectal biopsy. Which is the best method to get a reliable and good histology?**

    **A.** Open rectal biopsy 1 cm above the dentate line
    **B.** Suction rectal biopsy 1–2 cm above the dentate line
    **C.** Laparoscopic biopsy of the upper rectum and histologic mapping of the entire colon
    **D.** Both A and B are correct

*Answer:* D

**Learning points**

The best method to obtain a rectal biopsy is a suction or open technique. The experience of the local pathologist dealing with rectal biopsies or full-thickness open rectal biopsies needs to be considered.

**Scenario 1: After having confirmed the definitive diagnosis of HD by histology, rectal irrigations were performed correctly but the child becomes unwell. The abdomen is distended, tender on palpation; the leukocyte count and CRP are elevated. You order another AXR (Figure 9.5).**

**Learning points**

If a child deteriorates under irrigations, order another AXR to check on colonic dilation and enterocolitis [3,4].

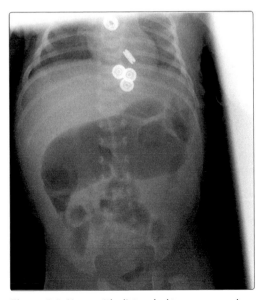

**Figure 9.5** X-ray with distended transverse colon, suspicious for enterocolitis.

Your next step is:

- **A.** Assume this is a transient abdominal problem that can be managed with antibiotics
- **B.** Assume the conservative treatment may have failed and consider an ileostomy or leveling colostomy
- **C.** Assume that CPAP is the problem by filling the small bowel with air and recommend the child be intubated
- **D.** Assume the child has an intravenous catheter-associated sepsis and start antibiotic therapy

*Answer:* B

**Learning points**

Know the limits of managing a patient with HD by irrigations, especially if the transition zone is proximal to the rectosigmoid [4].

**Scenario 2: After having confirmed the definitive diagnosis by histology, rectal irrigations were performed correctly but the child becomes better. You may consider:**

- **A.** Primary (pure transanal) Soave or Swenson pull-through
- **B.** Laparoscopic dissection of the upper rectum and transanal pull-through
- **C.** Continue irrigations for another 8 weeks and schedule the primary (pure transanal) pull-through
- **D.** Primary (pure transanal) pull-through with the technique described by Rehbein
- **E.** A+B+C are correct

*Answer:* E

**Learning points**

Soave or Swenson pull-through with or without laparoscopy are equally fine. If a patient is stable on daily irrigations the pull-through operation may be postponed. The Rehbein pull-through leaves a long segment of aganglionosis and is no longer performed.

**Scenario 3: A contrast enema shows no transition zone, reflux of contrast into a dilated ileum (and retention of contrast on delayed film). Which diagnosis would you consider?**

- **A.** Ultrashort segment HD
- **B.** Long-segment HD
- **C.** Sphincter achalasia
- **D.** Total colonic aganglionosis

*Answer:* D (Figure 9.6)

**Learning points**

The contrast enema is suspicious for total colonic aganglionosis. The management could be ileostomy and biopsies of the entire colon ("total colonic mapping") prior to a later pull-through procedure.

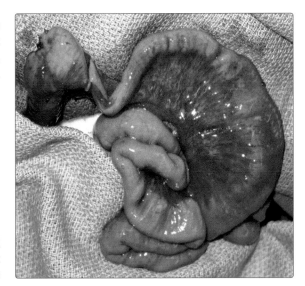

**Figure 9.6** Total colonic aganglionosis with 15 cm of terminal ileum also involved.

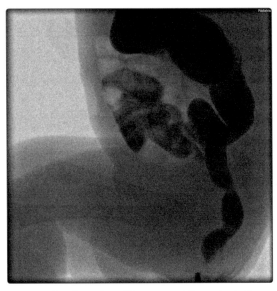

Figure 9.7  Contrast enema showing a transition zone at the splenic flexure or more proximal.

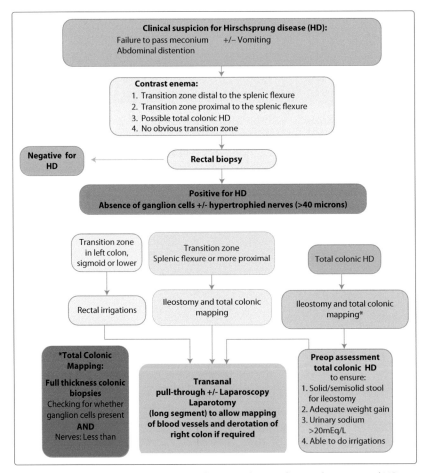

Figure 9.8  Management algorithm for a newborn infant with suspected HD.

**Scenario 4: Contrast enema showing a transition zone at the splenic flexure or more proximal (see Figure 9.7). Which phenotype of HD would you consider?**

   **A.** Ultrashort segment HD
   **B.** Long-segment HD
   **C.** Sphincter Achalasia
   **D.** Total colonic aganglionosis

*Answer:* B

**Learning points**

*Long-segment HD*: The management could be ileostomy and biopsies of the entire colon ("total colonic mapping") prior to a later pull-through procedure (Figure 9.8).

## Suggested references

1. Arshad A, Powell C, Tighe MP. Hirschsprung's disease. *BMJ.* 2012;345:e5521.
2. Putnam LR, John SD, Greenfield SA et al. The utility of the contrast enema in neonates with suspected Hirschsprung disease. *J Pediatr Surg.* 2015;50:963–966.
3. Pastor AC, Osman F, Teitelbaum DH et al. Development of a standardized definition for Hirschsprung's-associated enterocolitis: A Delphi analysis. *J Pediatr Surg.* 2009;44(1):251–256.
4. Gosain A, Frykman PK, Levitt MA et al. Guidelines for the diagnosis and management of Hirschsprung-associated enterocolitis. *Pediatr Surg Int.* 2017;33(5):517–521.

# 10 Hirschsprung disease: Definitive repair with transanal pull-through

Jacob C. Langer, Chris Westgarth-Taylor, Victor Etwire, and Stuart Hosie

## 10.1  Case study 1

A 3-week-old boy presents with bile-stained vomiting and abdominal distention. He was delivered via normal vaginal delivery at 41 weeks. He first passed meconium at 72 hours. He has been exclusively breast-fed and has been having difficulty-passing stool. It is reported that he strains a lot and passes stool every 6 days. On physical examination, the patient is stable, saturating well on room air, but has an obvious distended abdomen that is non-tender and firm. Hernial orifices are clear. Rectal examination confirms a normally sited anus that admits a size 13 Hager. On removal of the Hagar, there is a large release of gas and stool. Abdominal x-ray reveals typical signs of distal bowel obstruction with no air in the rectum.

**What are your next steps in management?**

A. Resuscitation, laparotomy when stable and formation of a defunctioning ostomy
B. Bowel washout with 20 mL/kg of normal saline until decompressed, contrast enema and suction rectal biopsy
C. Irrigations with 10–20 mL aliquots of normal saline until decompressed, contrast enema and suction rectal biopsy
B. Give laxatives to improve passage of stool

*Answer:* C

### 10.1.1  Learning points

The most important thing in managing a patient with Hirschsprung disease after resuscitation is decompression. This is done in the form of irrigations. A volume of 10–20 mL aliquots of normal saline is inserted via a large bore Foley catheter (20F). It is important that the fluid that is instilled must be drained out. The catheter is put past the transition zone and the process is continued until the abdomen is soft, decompressed and the effluent coming out is clear. Rectal stimulations can also be used to assist in the emptying of the rectum. Antibiotics are only indicated if the child has signs of enterocolitis.

Irrigations are initially done 3 times a day. Once the child is decompressed with no signs of enterocolitis, a suction rectal biopsy should be obtained to determine the formal diagnosis.

There is controversy about the need for a contrast enema. Proponents argue that a contrast enema will rule out other causes of neonatal intestinal obstruction such as atresia and meconium obstruction, and opponents of routine contrast enema express concern about the small risk of perforation.

In rare circumstances where it is not possible to decompress with irrigations, an ostomy is indicated. A leveling stoma (a stoma in ganglionated bowel as determined by frozen section) is preferred. In situations in which frozen sections are not available, or in which the pathological transition zone is found to be proximal to the splenic flexure, an ileostomy is indicated. A pitfall in creating a leveling stoma is that the stoma is usually sited in the dilated colon. In this case, the end may have to be tapered. A more proximal colostomy runs the risk of damaging the marginal blood vessels, which may be crucial for the pull-through. In this event an ileostomy is a better option as the colonic blood supply is maintained.

## 10.2  Case study 2

A full term infant presents with possible Hirschsprung disease. A contrast enema suggests a transition zone in the rectosigmoid colon. The plan is to do a transanal pull-through.

**In this child how would you do your leveling biopsies to determine where to do the anastomosis?**

    **A.**  During the transanal resection, you do full thickness biopsies as you go along.
    **B.**  Laparoscopic sero-muscular biopsies prior to the transanal resection.
    **C.**  Laparoscopic full thickness biopsies prior to the transanal resection.
    **D.**  Peri-umbilical incision with full thickness biopsies.
    **E.**  Either C or D are correct.

*Answer:* E

### 10.2.1  Learning points

It is safer to take leveling biopsies prior to the transanal resection, since the pathological transition zone can be different than the radiological transition zone in some cases. Preliminary biopsies can either be done via laparoscopy or an umbilical incision. Full thickness biopsies give the pathologist more tissue (both plexuses) and decrease the chance of a transitional zone pull-through.

## 10.3  Case study 3

A 1-month-old boy weighing 4 kg has a suction rectal biopsy confirming no ganglion cells and hypertrophied nerve trunks (>40 μm). Contrast enema does not show a radiological transition zone, but the child is decompressing well with daily irrigations. A decision is made to do a laparoscopic-assisted transanal Swenson operation. At laparoscopy there appears to be a transition in the mid-ascending colon. This is confirmed on frozen section histology.

**What is your next step?**

   **A.** Continue to laparotomy, resect the aganglionic segment of bowel, reverse the ascending colon down the right side of the abdomen and continue doing a transanal Swenson procedure.

   **B.** Continue to laparotomy, resect the aganglionic segment of bowel, reverse the ascending colon down the right side of the abdomen and continue doing a transanal Duhamel.

   **C.** Abandon procedure and wait for formal histology sections before deciding what to do.

   **D.** Do an ileostomy, do not resect colon and await permanent histology.

*Answer:* D

## 10.3.1  Learning points

Approximately 10% of neonatal contrast enemas will not show a transition zone. When you encounter long segment disease, it is unwise to continue with a definitive procedure. It is difficult to diagnose ganglion cells on frozen section the more proximal one goes, and it is unwise to do an extensive colon resection on the basis of frozen sections. To do a long segment definitive procedure in the neonatal period has the added potential complications of a very vulnerable marginal vessel which may lead to ischemic stenosis at the anastomotic site, and severe excoriation in the nappy area post op.

It is appropriate to bring out a stoma in long segment disease and wait for the ostomy effluent to thicken up so that there is less perineal excoriation after the definitive procedure. Different authors wait variable amounts of time, ranging from 6 months to 3 years.

# 10.4  Case study 4

The suction rectal biopsy result from a 2-month-old baby with possible Hirschsprung disease is reported as the following: No ganglion cells identified, but also no hypertrophied nerve trunks (>40 μm) identified. Calretinin immunohistochemistry is consistent with Hirschsprung disease.

**What are the possibilities and your next investigation?**

   **A.** The child has Hirschsprung disease and a pull-through should be recommended

   **B.** You may have biopsied the anatomical distal zone of aganglionosis; the child needs another biopsy

   **C.** The child may have Hirschsprung disease, but to be sure another biopsy is indicated

   **D.** The child definitely does not have Hirschsprung disease

   **E.** B and C are correct

*Answer:* E

## 10.4.1  Learning points

The diagnosis of Hirschsprung disease requires absence of ganglion cells. In most cases there are also hypertrophied nerve trunks (>40 μm) on the H&E stain. Increased acetylcholine esterase may confirm what the pathologist has identified, but is decreasingly used for diagnosis. Absence of calretinin staining is also supportive of the diagnosis.

There is an anatomical zone of aganglionosis, just proximal to the dentate line that if biopsied may give the false impression of Hirschsprung disease, but there would be no nerve trunk hyperplasia in these specimens either.

On rare occasions patients with very short segment or total colonic Hirschsprung disease may have no hypertrophied nerves identified on histology. Absence of ganglion cells without hypertrophic nerve trunks should usually stimulate a repeat biopsy to confirm the diagnosis. In these situations, it would be appropriate to do a full thickness rectal biopsy to confirm that the biopsy has not been taken too low.

## 10.5  Transanal pull-through

This procedure is suitable for patients with short segment Hirschsprung disease limited to the recto-sigmoid or distal descending colon, and is easier to perform in younger children than older children. We strongly recommend a preliminary biopsy to determine the pathological transition zone prior to beginning the transanal dissection, using either a laparoscopic or umbilical approach, even if the preoperative contrast study suggests a distal transition zone.

### 10.5.1  Preoperative considerations

#### 10.5.1.1  Imaging

Although a contrast enema may be helpful in estimating the level of the pathological transition zone, it is well documented that the sensitivity of determining the transition zone with contrast enema is only about 90% in newborns with Hirschsprung disease, and that the level of the radiological transition zone may not accurately reflect the level of the pathological transition zone in another 10% or so. This is particularly true in those with long-segment disease. This is why we recommend leveling biopsies to be taken prior to beginning the transanal dissection.

The other piece of information from a contrast enema which can be useful is the extent of dilatation of the proximal ganglionic bowel, which may influence the suitability of a coloanal anastomosis. This is particularly true for older children with a delayed diagnosis, who may benefit from a proximal stoma to permit decompression of the dilated colon prior to pull-through surgery.

#### 10.5.1.2  Routine bloodwork

Group and screen blood especially for older children who tend to have more bleeding during procedure.

Histological confirmation of Hirschsprung disease.

#### 10.5.1.3  Bowel preparation and antibiotics

Rectal irrigations should be done to rid the distal bowel of stool prior to the pull-through. This can often be done on the operating table, especially in infants. Mechanical bowel preparation from above is usually difficult and results in abdominal distension, and is usually not necessary.

Prophylactic broad-spectrum antibiotics should be administered at induction of anesthesia. If contamination occurs during the procedure, continued use of antibiotics should be encouraged. The length of time that antibiotics are continued is institution dependent.

### 10.5.2  Intraoperative considerations

#### 10.5.2.1  Positioning

The patient can be positioned in either the prone or the lithotomy position, according to the surgeon's preference. Prone positioning provides better exposure of the anus, but the patient must have a total body prep in order to do the preliminary leveling biopsies in the supine position prior to flipping into prone position. The advantage of the lithotomy position is that the child does not require a total body prep, and it is easier to do the leveling biopsies and any additional colonic mobilization.

### 10.5.2.2 Foley catheter

A catheter can be placed prior to positioning, or after draping in the supine or lithotomy position. A catheter can also be omitted and the bladder intermittently drained manually during the procedure.

### 10.5.2.3 Steps of the procedure

The three common operations performed are the Swenson, Soave, and Duhamel procedures. The transanal approach is only applicable to the former two. There are no strong data to recommend one operation over the others. The choice of procedure must be determined by the operating surgeon's training, experience and expertise in a specific technique. (Figures 10.1 through 10.5 are an example of a transanal Swenson type dissection.)

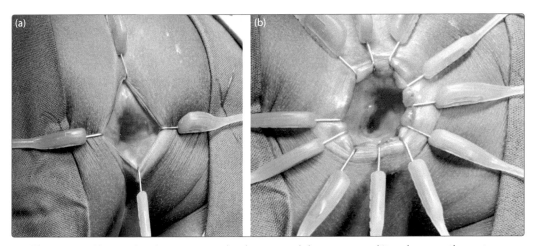

Figure 10.1 Placing the pins to expose the dentate and then to conceal it and expose the rectum.

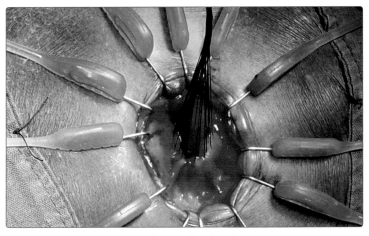

Figure 10.2 Circumferentially placed traction sutures.

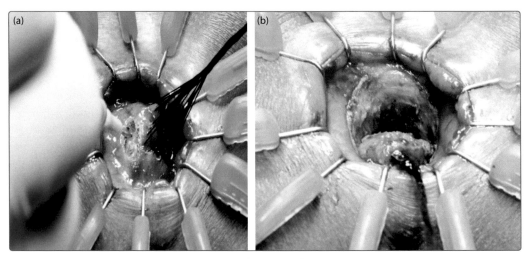

Figure 10.3  Full thickness rectal wall dissection.

*Preliminary biopsy and rectal dissection*: As described above, the transanal dissection should not be started until the pathological transition zone has been identified. This can be done using laparoscopy or through an umbilical incision. The umbilical incision can be made either supra or infra-umbilical, and the muscle can be divided either transversely or in the midline. If an umbilical incision is used, a Hager dilator can be placed transanally and used to push the sigmoid colon up toward the umbilicus. Biopsies ideally should be full-thickness, to provide the pathologist with both submucosal and myenteric plexuses. When using laparoscopy, some surgeons bring the colon out through the umbilical port site when doing the full-thickness biopsy, to prevent intra-abdominal spillage of stool.

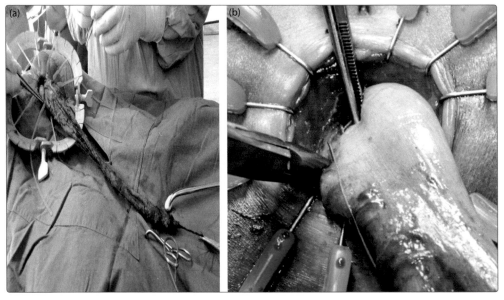

Figure 10.4  After pull-through and placing the outer sutures prior to anastomosis.

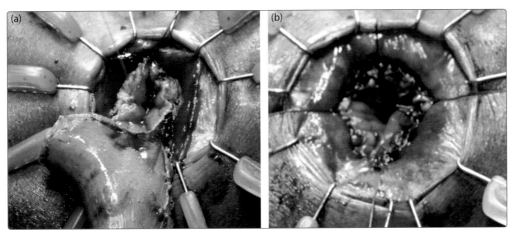

Figure 10.5 Resecting the colon distal to the transition zone and then coloanal anastomosis. Note the retraction pins at the anoderm.

While awaiting frozen section, the mesentery to the distal colon can be divided, either laparoscopically or through the umbilicus. The extent to which this dissection is done depends on surgeon preference and skill.

*Transansal exposure*: The anus is everted, either using a Lonestar retractor or a suture technique. The dentate line must be visualized and protected throughout the operation.

*Incision*: An incision is made above the dentate line. In a neonate this should be approximately 5 mm from the dentate line, and can be up to 10 mm in an older child. For a Swenson procedure the incision is made through the full thickness of the rectal wall. For a Soave procedure the incision is made through the mucosa, and a submucosal dissection is carried out proximally. We believe that this dissection should only be done for 1-2 cm before transitioning through the muscle into the "Swenson" plane on the outside of the rectum, in order to prevent postoperative obstructive problems from the aganglionic cuff. This submucosal dissection theoretically decreases the risk of injury to the vagina or the prostate and urethra that can occur during a Swenson.

*Dissection of the rectum*: The dissection continues on the rectal wall, dividing all of the small vessels as they enter the rectum. When the previously identified biopsy site that documented presence of ganglion cells is reached, the surgeon can divide the colon. Many surgeons go higher than the positive biopsy in order to ensure that the transition zone is not being used for the pull-through. It is also important during the dissection of the rectum to ensure that it does not get twisted. This can be accomplished by placing a right-angle clamp on the distal end of the rectum and maintaining its position throughout the dissection, or by placing sutures on the anterior surface of the bowel as the dissection progresses.

*Mobilization of the colon*: For lower transition zones no mobilization is necessary. However, for a transition zone in the proximal sigmoid or descending colon, the peritoneal attachments of the left colon must be divided, or the splenic flexure mobilized, in order to avoid undue tension. This can be done laparoscopically, through an umbilical incision, or through a laparotomy.

*Anastomosis*: The anastomosis is done using interrupted non-absorbable braided sutures. In cases where there is a size mismatch, it is important to place the 12, 3, 6, and 9 o'clock sutures first and then use a "divide and conquer" technique. It is important to place the sutures into the underlying muscle to anchor the pull-through, and to avoid placing the sutures into the dentate line itself, which will cause pain and interfere with sensation later. The anastomosis should be calibrated with a finger or a Hegar dilator at the end of the procedure.

*Preemptive analgesia*: Either prior to the operation, at the end of the procedure, or both, the child should have some kind of local anesthesia placed. We prefer the use of a caudal block, especially in infants, but local infiltration of the anus and the port sites or umbilicus can also be used.

### 10.5.3  Early postoperative considerations

The Foley catheter should be removed within 48 hours after surgery.

Antibiotics are usually not necessary after surgery if there was no spillage of stool intraoperatively.

As these are transanal operations, bowel function usually returns quite soon. Once this has occurred, feeding can be commenced. It is unusual to need a nasogastric tube in these children.

Aggressive prophylactic perineal care is necessary to prevent excoriation from the frequent stools in the immediate post-operative period.

### 10.5.4  Follow up

Calibration of the anus is done at 2–4 weeks after surgery with a Hegar dilator to ensure patency of the anastomosis. This should be repeated every 1-2 weeks for several months to ensure that a stricture does not develop. Any stricture felt should be treated with daily rectal dilations. Routine dilatation at home by the parents is unnecessary unless the child develops a stricture.

Routine post-operative rectal irrigations have been shown to reduce the incidence of post-operative enterocolitis, especially in long segment disease. This should be considered in such cases.

### 10.5.5  Postoperative complications

Early postoperatively

- Wound infection, anastomotic leak and abscess formation
- Recto-vaginal/urinary tract fistula
- Urinary retention
- Enterocolitis
- Perianal excoriation

Long term

- Soiling
- Obstructive symptoms
- Enterocolitis

## 10.6  Transanal pull-through in a child with a preliminary ostomy

Despite the trend towards primary pull-through, an initial ostomy may be appropriate for patients in whom rectal irrigations are ineffective in ensuring adequate decompression of bowel, patients presenting late with grossly dilated bowel, patients with enterocolitis not resolving on irrigations, patients who present with cecal perforation, and situations in which reliable frozen section diagnosis of the transition zone is unavailable. A leveling colostomy (colostomy in ganglionated bowel proximal to the transition zone) or an ileostomy is recommended in these instances.

For children who have had a colostomy just above the transition zone, the stoma itself is used for the definitive pull-through. In instances where the ostomy is sited significantly proximal to the transition zone (usually an ileostomy), one may consider a pull through just above the transition zone, followed by later closure of the stoma.

## Suggested references

1. Mahajan JK, Rathod KK, Bawa M, Narasimhan KL. Transanal Swenson's operation for recto-sigmoid Hirschsprung's disease. *Afr J Paediatr Surg*. 2011;8:301–5.
2. Bing X, Sun C, Wang Z, Su Y, Sun H, Wang L, Yu X. Transanal pullthrough Soave and Swenson techniques for pediatric patients with Hirschsprung disease. *Medicine (Baltimore)*. 2017 Mar;96(10):e6209.
3. Langer JC, Durrant AC, de la Torre L, Teitelbaum DH, Minkes RK, Caty MG, Wildhaber BE, Ortega SJ, Hirose S, Albanese CT, . One-stage transanal Soave pullthrough for Hirschsprung disease, A multicenter experience with 141 children. *Ann Surg*. 2003 Oct;238(4):569–76.
4. De la Torre-Mondragon L, Ortega-Salgado JA. Transanal endorectal pull-through for Hirschsprung's disease. *J Pediatr Surg*. 1998;33:1283–86.
5. De la Torre L, Ortega A. Transanal versus open endorectal pull-through for Hirschsprung's disease. *J Pediatr Surg*. 2000 Nov;35(11):1630–2.
6. Peyvasteh M, Askarpour S, Ostadian N, Moghimi M, Javaherizadeh N. Diagnostic accuracy of barium enema findings in Hirschsprung's disease. *Arq Bras Cir Dig*. Jul-Sep 2016;29(3):155–8.

Jonathan H. Sutcliffe, Alejandra Vilanova-Sánchez, and Jacob C. Langer

## 11.1 When to suspect TCA

### 11.1.1 Case 1

Your colleague asks for advice about a 1-month-old term baby boy who has presented with distention and failure to thrive. He is otherwise well, and having excluded an anorectal malformation, washouts were initially successful. A rectal biopsy was obtained and the results have caused a fair amount of discussion; although no ganglion cells were seen, the size of the nerve fibers was described as "normal," all less than 40 μm. Since the baby was doing well, the diagnosis of Hirschsprung disease seemed unclear.

Washouts have recently become less effective and the family are increasingly frustrated. The mother herself had Hirschsprung disease ("long segment" according to available records) and so is very aware of this as a potential diagnosis. They have asked your colleague if they think this is Hirschsprung disease or not. What can be done to move things forward and would a contrast study help?

**Which of the following answers is correct?**

A. A diagnosis of Hirschsprung disease requires both aganglionosis and hypertrophied nerve fibers (>40 microns). This can't be Hirschsprung disease.

B. Babies with short segment Hirschsprung disease always present later than long segment or total colonic aganglionosis because less bowel is affected.

C. The mother's diagnosis is highly relevant here, particularly since she had long segment disease, and the baby is male.

D. A contrast enema can differentiate well between short segment disease and total colonic aganglionosis.

E. None of the above.

*Answer:* C

### 11.1.1.1 Learning points

- The diagnosis of HD rests on aganglionosis in an adequate biopsy. The use of calretinin staining is very useful i.e., presence of calretinin rules out Hirschsprung disease. Acetyl-cholinesterase staining may also be used to identify thickened nerve fibers [1,2].
- The presence of normal sized nerve fibers has been recognized in some patients with total colonic aganglionosis (TCA).
- Long segment disease may present later than those with classic segment disease.
- The "recurrence rates" (i.e., risk of HD in a first degree relative) for HD have been described; there is a higher risk if the mother has TCA, particularly if she delivers a boy. The overall risk for a sibling of an affected child is 4%, but this varies with the gender of the proband and the length of affected bowel. The highest recurrence risk is for a male sibling of a female proband with long segment disease (33%), with the lowest being for a female sibling of a male proband with classical HD (1%) [3].
- Contrast enemas are used to a variable extent in different centers. Approximately 8% of infants with HD do not have a radiological transition zone, and transition zones are sometimes seen in children without HD. Although the colon in TCA classically has a "question mark" appearance, this is not present in all cases. Some surgeons feel that having an indication about the site of the transition zone can help with operative planning. The diagnosis of HD must be proven with a rectal biopsy [4].

## 11.2  Approach to a child struggling with washouts

The contrast enema has demonstrated a slightly foreshortened colon shaped like a "question mark" colon suggestive of total colonic aganglionosis. The nurse specialists you work with have been unable to decompress the child with washouts, and the baby has been put on continuous nasogastric feeds to help him grow. Your colleague has asked if you could take over care. You meet with the family to discuss your plan.

You recommend an urgent laparotomy, colonic mapping and formation of a stoma.

In the frozen section the cecum was aganglionic however the terminal ileum was ganglionated. An ileostomy at the level of the ileal biopsy was performed. No colonic resection was performed.

**Which of the following answers is correct?**

A. This procedure must be performed through an upper transverse incision

B. Seromuscular biopsies will confirm that you are proximal to the transition zone

C. A frozen section is as good as definitive pathology to diagnose Hirschsprung disease

D. Sending the appendix is a good way to test for total colonic aganglionosis

E. None of the above

*Answer:* E

## 11.2.1 Learning points

- The incision might be lower midline, upper transverse or Pfannensteil over a bladder catheter. An alternative approach is through an umbilical incision, using Hagar dilators transanally to facilitate retrieval of the sigmoid into the wound and making the stoma in the umbilicus.
- Although seromuscular biopsies can demonstrate ganglion cells in the myenteric plexus, full thickness biopsies are needed to show normal nerve fibers since this can only be done reliably in the submucosal plexus. Even then, tissues from the around the circumference must at some point be made available to the pathologist to ensure that you are completely above the transition zone.
- The appendix can be misleading; aganglionosis of the appendix has been described in the presence of a normally innervated ascending and transverse colon. This might mean that the patient is mislabelled as total colonic aganglionosis [5].
- An ileostomy will be needed. Biopsies should taken from the dilated segment if present, since they are more likely to be above the transition zone. Both an end ileostomy and a loop have been advocated; an end ileostomy will reduce overspill, and a loop can act to vent the downstream segment.
- Irrigations of the distal bowel may be considered; this is to avoid accumulation of stools in the defunctioned colon. Secondly, if parents are used to perform irrigations before the definitive repair it will be easier for them to do them properly to avoid enterocolitis. With 1 or 2 irrigations a week should be enough to maintain the distal colon clean.
- A colectomy should not be done at this time based on a frozen section diagnosis of the transition zone level, since frozen sections may be incorrect.
- Skip areas of ganglion cells may be found in the colon in cases of TCA, and this can be very confusing. Biopsies must be done in multiple parts of the colon and in the small bowel to avoid error.

## 11.3 Once the stoma is done, what is your next step in management?

Stoma placement has meant that your patient has decompressed, and after a few days of high output, has been able to go home on full feeds to grow. Parents are happier but want to catch up to discuss ongoing management. What are your recommendations about the timing of surgery and choice of procedure and why? Would you consider a long-term stoma if this was your child?

**Which of the following answers is correct?**

A. A pull-through should be delayed and is often done around 8–12 months
B. A Duhamel pull-through is best
C. A Swenson pull-through is best
D. He will need a colectomy and terminal ileostomy with no other surgical options
E. None of the above

*Answer:* A

## 11.3.1 Learning points

To discuss
- Timing of surgery; ensure that the child is thriving, has an ileostomy output of <20 mL/kg and with an appropriate stool consistency (apple sauce). Ensure the home environment is as stable as possible. From 8 to 12 months is a good rule of thumb [6].

- All infants with an ileostomy require sodium supplementation. Adequacy of supplementation can be monitored by maintaining a urine sodium > 25 mEq [7].
- A range of procedures have been undertaken often with similar results. The experience of the surgeon and the institution is an important factor. A "straight" Swenson or Duhamel pull-through would be the most common currently. Although different modifications have been tried, the Duhamel pouch should be short. J-Pouches have also been used [8].
- The colon patch procedures (Martin and Kimura) are usually associated with late complications including chronic enterocolitis and poor emptying, and in most cases are not recommended [9].
- Discuss long term outcomes candidly with the family. In addition to the complications of surgery for short segment disease, long segment disease is associated with an increased risk of high output, perianal excoriation, soiling, HD-associated enterocolitis and HD-associated inflammatory bowel disease.
- There are some patients for whom a long-term stoma is best. Many patients with aganglionosis extending well into the small bowel, with resultant short bowel syndrome have persistently loose, high output effluent. Other patients may have significant co-morbidity such that continence would be unlikely e.g., Mowat-Wilson syndrome, associated high anorectal malformation, and a pull-through would not confer any benefit. Acceptable outcomes in children with Down syndrome have however been reported, and careful discussion with families is required [10].

## 11.4  The ileal Duhamel

Your patient is approaching their 12 months of age and you and the family have planned admission. You have recommended an ileal Duhamel. Your colleague wants to come to the operating room to be involved. They are less familiar with the Duhamel procedure and asks exactly what you will do.

### 11.4.1  Preoperative

1. Ensure original pathology specimens from initial rectal biopsy and from leveling procedure are reported and have been reviewed.
2. Ensure experienced pathologist requested for the frozen section. Ask for them to call when the specimen has been received as well as to report.
3. Ensure an experienced assistant is available.
4. Consent.
5. Review images and have up in the operating room.
6. There is usually no need for bowel prep when the patient already has an ileostomy.

### 11.4.2  Intraoperative

1. NGT.
2. Appropriate antibiotics.
3. Write path forms.
4. Place in lithotomy position with legs elevated enough to visualize anus but not so much that the abdomen cannot be accessed. Child should be at bottom of the operating table.
5. Prep and drape with clear drapes for legs to remain visible.
6. Catheter in once draped.

### 11.4.3 Approach and assessment

1. Take down ileostomy first. Excise most distal 1–2 cm and send for frozen section to ensure presence of normal ganglion cells. Use a stapler for to transect the ileum in a mesenteric–antimesenteric orientation. Divide the mesentery as needed to allow sufficient length. Bulldog clips may be used to test perfusion prior to dividing arcades.

2. Often the entire operation can be done through the ileostomy incision. However, an additional incision can be used if the surgeon has difficulty accomplishing the colectomy or developing the retrorectal space through the ileostomy incision alone. Options include:
   - Pfannensteil with transverse skin incision and either transverse muscle-cutting incision (better access) or midline muscle incision up to umbilicus (less pain).
   - Umbilical incision with either transverse muscle-cutting incision or midline incision above umbilicus.
   - Laparoscopy.
   - Midline incision from above umbilicus to above pubis.

3. Colectomy
   Identify and mobilize the colon and aganglionic ileum, which is distal to the ileostomy. It is often easiest to start proximal and work your way to the distal sigmoid, dividing the mesentery and the omentum as you go.

4. Developing the retrorectal space
   - Hold up on the sigmoid colon to create tension. Confirm position of ureters bilaterally.
   - Divide peritoneum along the rectum down to the peritoneal reflection. Here the two leaves of mesentery diverge. Between them is the retrorectal space. This is a filmy, fatty layer.
   - Develop the retrorectal space. This dissection can be done bluntly using blunt dissection with a finger, a kittner/kilner or laparoscopic graspers or suction.
   - When down to sphincters, sweep 3–9 o'clock around anus. If possible, use a finger.
   - Second surgeon to bottom of table.
   - Place Lonestar retractor. For a Duhamel, place the pins at the anocutaneous junction rather than higher up the canal. This will still allow good visualization of the dentate line without prolapsing the dentate over the internal sphincters and distorting the anatomy. Since the incision in the mucosa will be closer to the dentate than for other techniques, this is of importance.

### 11.4.4 Pull-through and anastomosis

- From above, pass a clip with a pledget loaded through retro-rectal space and position in midline to not more than 5 mm above dentate line.
- Make transverse incision in the posterior rectal wall, cutting directly onto the pledget. Extend circumferentially to both sides for a total length of approximately 1 cm. Make sure to stay 5 mm from the dentate line for the length of the incision—there is a tendency to get more distal when extending the incision laterally. This rectal incision should look like a smile rather than a straight line.
- Place the 11:00 and 1:00 stitches (4-0 polyglycolic) through the posterior rectal wall incision (passing from the mucosal surface outwards through the serosa) and leave the needles on.
- Grasp the kittner with a long Babcock clamp and gently withdraw the kittner while passing the Babcock proximally in the retrorectal space.
- When the Babcock is visualized from the abdomen, grasp the antimesentic corner of the ileal staple line and pull it down and slightly through the retrorectal incision. Ensure that the pulled-through ileum is not twisted.

- Excise the antimesenteric corner of the staple line, creating an opening which is approximately the same size as the posterior rectal incision.
- Use the previously placed sutures at 11:00 and 1:00 to take bites from the pulled-through ileum (passing from the serosal surface through to the mucosal surface) and tie them down. This fixes the pull-through in the correct position.
- Complete the anastomosis by placing sutures in the 3:00 and 9:00 positions and initially leaving them untied. The 6:00 position contains a staple line. Sutures are therefore placed on either side at the 5:30 and 6:30 position. Use a "divide and conquer" approach to fill in the gaps.
- Once the anastomosis has been completed, place a 60 mm linear stapler between the 11:00 and 1:00 sutures with one arm in the native rectum and the other in the pulled-through ileum. Linear staplers suitable for laparoscopic use are generally slimmer and easier to use transanally.
- The person at top confirms nothing is in between e.g., ovary, fallopian tubes, vas, ureters. Fire once. Usually one or two more loads will be necessary to get to the top of the native rectum. There is always a small "spur" because the stapler doesn't divide all the way to the end of the instrument, but in total colonic disease this is acceptable. An important concept for a Duhamel procedure is the length of the pouch. For 'classic' segment disease, removal of the native rectum from a point just above the staple line will leave a 5–6 cm pouch, this needs a formal laparotomy. For TCA, the length of the pouch can safely be left 1–2 cm longer. This means that the native rectum can be removed slightly further away from the staple line and in turn this means that the whole abdominal procedure can be performed through the ileostomy incision.
- Test the Duhamel anastomosis with a finger. Place a bowel clamp across the ileum above the anastomosis, fill the pelvis with saline, and gently blow some air into the neo-rectum with a bulb syringe to ensure that there is no leak.

### 11.4.5 Closure

- Close incisions and laparoscopic port sites in the usual fashion.
- Consider protecting with a proximal loop ileostomy if there is a leak, if there is concern about blood supply or tension, or if there is any other concern about healing of the anastomosis.

### 11.4.6 Postoperative

- Nasogastric tube until regains bowel function
- Analgesia
- Foley catheter for 24–48 hours
- Antibiotics per institutional protocol for clean-contaminated gastrointestinal procedure
- Liberal use of buttock paste to protect perineal skin; can also use loperamide if stools are very frequent

### 11.4.7 Follow up

- See again at approximately 2 weeks postop. Perform digital rectal examination to ensure that the Duhamel staple lines haven't become fused. The rectal exam will solve this problem.
- There is no need for dilatation by parents at home.
- Return to clinic every 2–4 weeks for a few visits, then spread out as long as child is well.
- Some older children develop difficulty-passing stools, with retention and obstructive symptoms. Use of intrasphincteric botulinum toxin may be helpful until they figure it out.

## 11.5 What to do if there is an unexpected on table finding

### 11.5.1 Case 2

You have started a pure transanal pull-through in a 5 month old baby using a Swenson technique. You have dissected up into the peritoneal cavity and all biopsies so far have come back as aganglionic. You have called the family from theater and explained you need to take biopsies from the rest of the colon. Total colonic aganglionosis is identified on frozen section. What are you now going to do and why?

#### 11.5.1.1 Learning points

Beginning the pelvic dissection for a pull-through without knowing how long the affected segment is carries a risk that you will face this situation. Although a contrast enema can provide useful information, it is insufficiently sensitive to exclude TCA. Some centers would therefore never commence a pull-through without first obtaining a leveling biopsy to avoid the situation described here (e.g., transumbilical biopsy at the level of the potential radiological Transition Zone). While not every center would undertake this approach, there are a number of problems to be considered should one find oneself in this position:

- A patient with TCA will have a pull-through earlier than they would otherwise.
- There is clear potential to worsen parental anxiety.
- There are important technical considerations. Once a resection of the rectum has been performed, the anal canal has been dissected in a way that means that a Duhamel is no longer an option. A Swenson, however, can be a good option.
- If you end up performing a colectomy in such a situation it would be done based on a frozen section and this is not recommended.

For all these reasons a leveling biopsy is recommended before starting the dissection in any type of HD, even in those which are likely to be short segment.

Careful discussion with the family on table is mandatory. Once the Swenson has been performed, a covering ileostomy should be performed as the output onto the perineum is likely to be high. Careful attention to technique is required to reduce the risk of stoma prolapse over the next few months before it is closed. The marginal artery must be preserved when closing the stoma.

## References

1. Kapur RP, Reed RC, Finn LS, Patterson K, Johanson J, Rutledge JC. Calretinin immunohistochemistry versus acetylcholinesterase histochemistry in the evaluation of suction rectal biopsies for Hirschsprung Disease. *Pediatr Dev Pathol.* 2009;12:6–15.
2. Kapur RP. Submucosal nerve diameter of greater than 40 μm is not a valid diagnostic index of transition zone pull-through. *J Pediatr Surg.* 2016;51:1585–91.
3. Moore SW, Zaahl M. Clinical and genetic correlations of familial Hirschsprung's disease. *J Pediatr Surg.* 2015;50:285–8.
4. Muller CO, Mignot C, Belarbi N, Berrebi D, Bonnard A. Does the radiographic transition zone correlate with the level of aganglionosis on the specimen in Hirschsprung's disease? *Pediatr Surg Int.* 2012;28:597–601.
5. Lane VA, Levitt MA, Baker P, Minneci P, Deans K. The appendix and aganglionosis. A note of caution—how the histology can mislead the surgeon in total colonic hirschsprung disease. *Eur J Pediatr Surg Reports.* 2015;03:003–6.
6. Sanchez AV, Ivanov M, Halleran DR et al. Total colonic Hirschsprung's disease: The hypermotility and skin rash protocol. *Eur J Pediatr Surg.* 2019. doi:10.1055/s-0039-1694744.
7. O'Neil M, Teitelbaum DH, Harris MB. Total body sodium depletion and poor weight gain in children and young adults with an ileostomy: A case series. *Nutr Clin Pract.* 2014;29:397–401.

8. Marquez TT, Acton RD, Hess DJ, Duval S, Saltzman DA. Comprehensive review of procedures for total colonic aganglionosis. *J Pediatr Surg*. 2009;44:257–65; discussion 265.
9. Escobar MA, Grosfeld JL, West KW et al. Long-term outcomes in total colonic aganglionosis: A 32-year experience. *J Pediatr Surg*. 2005;40:955–61.
10. Catto-Smith AG, Trajanovska M, Taylor RG. Long-term continence in patients with Hirschsprung's disease and down syndrome e. *J Gastroenterol Hepatol*. 2006;21:748–53.

# 12 Total colonic Hirschsprung: Pre- and postoperative care

Alejandra Vilanova-Sánchez, Carlos A. Reck-Burneo, and Brenda Ruth

## 12.1 Ileostomy, growth, and high output: What do pediatric surgeons need to know about high output ostomy management?

### 12.1.1 Case 1

A 5-month-old patient with a diagnosis of total colonic Hirschsprung disease (TCHD) and an ileostomy in place presents to your outpatient clinic. He is having high liquid ileostomy output, 50 mg/kg/day. His mother reports that he is eating formula normally but he is not gaining weight well. There is no history of abdominal distension or pain or any other signs of enterocolitis. He is on the 10th percentile for weight.

**What would you do?**

- A. Check urine sodium
- B. Consult with the GI team
- C. Start on pectin
- D. Check the ostomy for stricture
- E. All the above

*Answer:* E

### 12.1.1.1  Learning points

1. *Urine sodium, glucose, growth, and ileostomy*: Sodium is the most abundant electrolyte in the extracellular space. It is acquired through dietary intake, and most of it gets absorbed actively in the ileum and passively in the jejunum. Sodium co-transports glucose and electrolytes and is thus fundamental for absorption of those nutrients in the small intestine. When a diverting ileostomy is present sodium losses can be significant, and the oral sodium intake needs to be increased to prevent weight loss and failure to thrive.

   The easiest way to establish if enough sodium is being absorbed is by checking the urinary output of sodium. This value is pretty constant and mostly dependent on the amount of sodium in the plasma. Even though studies are ongoing as to the normal excretion in infants, it is generally accepted that supplementation should be added when sodium levels fall below 40 meq/L. When starting sodium supplements, it should be started with 1 g/day and increased as needed until the urinary levels have normalized.

2. *Ostomy stricture and liquid stools*: An ostomy stricture can cause a high liquid stool output. Different mechanisms of action have been proposed. The most common one is an obstruction and thus "filtration" of only liquid with retention of solid particles. This leads to small bowel distention and a compensatory increase in peristalsis and thus decreased absorption of fluid. An ostomy stricture can be easily diagnosed with digital examination or checking with Hagar dilator and should be excluded as the first step in every physical examination of an ostomy patient presenting with high output.

3. *Pectin and difference with insoluble fiber, and loperamide*: Two elements influence stool consistency and thickness. One is the dietary elements such as the amount of fiber and glucose in the diet and another one is the motility of the intestine. Both have a direct relationship to the amount of water absorbed from the dietary bolus and can be influenced by a myriad of factors such as the microbiome, bile acids, the pH of food, diet, and irritants among others. Osmotic agents such as glucose will absorb water and thus not allow stool to thicken fast enough when not enough time is given to be exposed to the intestinal mucosa such as in ileostomies or short segments of colon. Fiber works by absorbing water and retaining it in the intestinal lumen within its fibers. It is a bulk-forming agent as it expands with water and increases the bulk of stool so that it can more easily be pushed further by peristalsis. Fiber can be dosed as "age plus 5–10 g" or 0.5 g/kg of body weight. Pectin is a soluble fiber that works by two mechanisms. It will soften stool by retaining water, and it will bind bile acids further increasing stool bulk and decreasing peristalsis. It is also considered a pre-biotic as it will re-balance a healthy intestinal microbiome. The dose of pectin studied in children that is effective is at 4 g/kg of oral intake. Another commonly used medication to decrease stool output is loperamide. Loperamide is a transit slowing medication that acts by decreasing intestinal motility. It is an opioid that does not cross the blood−brain barrier and thus only slows the gut. Its use in children under 2 years of age is off-label, and patients who are receiving loperamide should be followed carefully. The dose is 0.08–0.24 mg/kg and should not exceed 3 mg/day in children under 3 years of age. Contraindications to its use are obstruction such as in the case of a stoma stricture, enterocolitis or bloody stools. Care should also be taken not to exceed the maximum dose as central nervous system symptoms such as drowsiness may ensue.

## 12.1.2  Case 2

A 6-month-old patient with ileostomy in place and previous colonic mapping confirming TCHD presents to your clinic to schedule the ileoanal pull-through. He is on 50th percentile for weight and height. He is eating well with no abdominal pain or distension. His mother reports that his ostomy output is very stable around 35 mL/kg/day but is very loose. When you check the ostomy bag the output is completely liquid.

**When do you schedule the patient for their pull-through?**

    A. The patient is ready to perform the pull-through as the ostomy output is normal for an ileostomy.

    B. The patient is ready when he is continent for urine. This will be around 1 and 1.5 years old.

    C. The pull-through should not be done until the ostomy output has applesauce consistency, otherwise the perineal rash in the postoperiod will be untreatable.

    D. Start on pectin or imodium to thicken the stools.

    E. C and D.

*Answer:* E

### 12.1.2.1 Learning points

If a patient has liquid output throughout the ileostomy the pull-through should be delayed until the output gets a thick consistency. If a PT is done in a patient with liquid stools the perineal rash will be very difficult to treat. Because of perianal pain the patients do not want to pass stool and performing irrigations will be very painful. This increases the likelihood of stool retention, enterocolitis and the need to reopen the ileostomy. On the other hand, the pull-through does not have to be delayed until the age of toilet training (around 2 years of age). It does not have any impact on the future fecal continence, enterocolitis or perineal rash in these patients.

## 12.2 TCHD: Hypermotility and diaper dermatitis management before and after the definitive pull-through

### 12.2.1 Case 3

A 10-month-old patient with TCHD who had an ileoanal pull through 1 month ago is having 7–9 liquid stools a day. There is no abdominal distension and no enterocolitis symptoms. His weight has been stable for the last month.

**The perineal skin is very excoriated (Figure 12.1). How do you proceed?**

    A. The patient needs a permanent ileostomy

    B. He is too young to have had a pull-through. He will need an ileostomy and wait 1 year and close the ostomy.

    C. He will need a combination of perineal skin care, irrigations, water-soluble fiber, and loperamide.

    D. If he does not improve we need to contact the GI team.

    E. C and D.

*Answer:* E

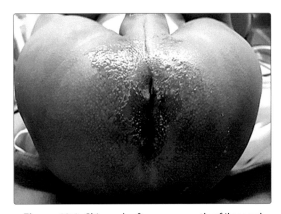

**Figure 12.1** Skin rash after one month of ileoanal pull-through with no treatment for hypermotility.

### 12.2.1.1 Learning points

Frequent liquid stools from hypermotility caused maceration of the skin, inflammation due to the enzymes, and irritants in the stool. This situation is very common in the postoperative period after an ileoanal pull-through. This is not only due to the lack of colon but also what is relevant is that most of the patients with TCHD have been with ileostomy since the neonatal period and the skin is not prepared for acidity and moisture in the perianal region. There are a few important parts of the treatment for these complex patients to minimize skin damage. First, families must be prepared for what to expect after the pull-through. The first months will be very challenging with regard to skin care. Also, it is very important to teach families on how to perform irrigations because in the postoperative period they may need to do them even without the symptoms of enterocolitis, to treat any distension.

Many barrier creams have been commercialized to treat hypermotility skin rash. Moisture barriers including liquid skin sealants (cyanoacrylate based) and other products such as ostomy bags with adhesives creams are good to prevent and treat the rash. The recommendation is to start treating and moisturizing the skin from day 0 after the pull-through. For example, start applying the cyanoacrylate-based cream right after finishing the pull-through to make a barrier between the skin and stools from the very first day. In every institution it is important to have a standardized protocol that addresses cleansing, and consistent use of barrier products for preventing and treating incontinent-associated dermatitis.

As mentioned previously, irrigations are part of the skin care treatment. Besides its use for preventing enterocolitis they help reduce the number of bowel movement and therefore improve skin status as they empty the most distal part of the bowel. Irrigations starting from day 7–10 after the pull-through can be very useful.

Another important step is a constipating diet. Avoiding sugar, juices, raw fruits, raw vegetables helps to decrease the bowel movement and therefore the skin rash.

Sometimes all these measures are not enough to reduce the bowel movements and improve perineal skin and water-soluble fiber (pectin) or imodium to bulk the stools should be added to decrease the number of bowel movements. Pectin twice a day at least 3 weeks after surgery is a helpful adjunct. If the skin does not improve, loperamide could be added alone or in combination with pectin (see protocol).

If after all these steps the hypermotility is not manageable and the patient passes stools a number of times, then a GI team with experience should be consulted for short bowel syndrome (Table 12.1).

### 12.2.2 Case 4

The same patient as discussed previously. You start on pectin, irrigations, loperamide and a cyanocrylate-based barrier cream. After 1 month, the perineum looks much better (Figure 12.2). His mother reports that he is doing well but sometimes he gets distended and she thinks he holds onto the stools. Once she passes a rectal catheter a large amount of stools comes out and the distension improves.

**What do you think is happening?**

A. The loperamide needs to be decreased.
B. This is a side effect of the water-soluble fiber.
C. He will need an examination under anesthesia to check if the anastomosis is not strictured. If the anastomosis is okay he will need a Botox injection in the internal anal sphincter.

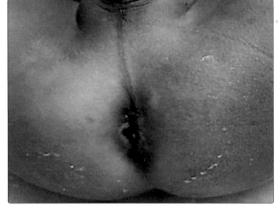

**Figure 12.2** Same patient as in Figure 12.1 after using loperamide, pectin and skin care for hypermotility.

  **D.** He needs more loperamide.
  **E.** A and B.

*Answer:* C

### 12.2.2.1  Learning points

The role of Botulinum toxin in TCHD is vital. Enterocolitis is more common in TCHD than in shorter segment HD. The cause of HAEC is unknown, although several hypotheses have been proposed based on experimental evidence. These include dysbiosis of the intestinal microbiome, impaired mucosal barrier function, altered innate immune responses, and bacterial translocation which are more compromised in children with TCHD and particularly those with Down syndrome (Gosain PSI 2017) (Barrena). Our protocol is to inject 100 UI of Botulinum toxin into the internal anal sphincter after surgery in every patient having a ileoanal pull-through in order to decrease the rate of HAEC. We repeat the injections as needed. Injecting the internal anal sphincter does not cause constant stools leaking because the external anal sphincter is still competent and does not worsen the skin status.

## 12.3  Protocol for TCHD

*Table 12.1* Bowel management protocol for hypermotility in patients with TCHD

1. ***Prepare Ileostomy prior to the definitive PT (if liquid or high output >30 mL/kg) or liquid stool causing skin problems around the stoma:***
    i. Pectin or methylcellulose 1–2 months before pull-through or ileostomy closure to thicken the ileostomy output
    ii. If ileostomy output is >30 mL/kg/day start on loperamide 0.5 mg/kg with maximum dose of 0.8 mg/kg/day
    iii. If the ileostomy output does not have an adequate consistency the ileostomy closure or pull-through should be delayed
2. ***Medical management after definitive pull-through without leaving a protective ileostomy/or ileostomy closure after definitive pull-through:***
    i. On postoperative day 0; application on the buttocks and perineal area of cyanoacrylate-based barrier liquid. Repeat application every 2–3 days as needed until the hypermotility is controlled.
    ii. Proton pump inhibitors to reduce acidity of stool.
    iii. Start on irrigation after 2 weeks of surgery and continue for the first 6 months.
    iv. Encourage constipating diet. Avoid laxative food, mainly non-absorbable sugar-based food and oily food.
    v. Water-soluble fiber. Pectin or methyl-cellulose from 2 weeks to 1 month after surgery.
    vi. Loperamide started if there are more than 5 liquid stools a day.
    vii. If night accidents: 100 mL saline enema before bedtime and/or increase loperamide dose before going to bed.
    viii. Examination under anesthesia and 100 UI of Botulinum toxin injection after 1 month of pull-through.
    ix. Monitoring growth curve and urine Na+.
3. ***Medical treatment if all the above do not resolve hypermotility:***
    i. Involve GI specialist
    ii. Cholestyramine (maximum 8 gr divided daily)
    iii. Diphenoxylate/atropine
    iv. Hyoscyamine—0.125 mg tab/6 hours
    v. Clonidine

# 13 The post pull-through Hirschsprung patient who is not doing well with obstructive or incontinence symptoms

Jacob C. Langer and Marc A. Levitt

Most children thrive after operative management of Hirschsprung disease (HD). However, there is a small subset of patients who do not do well after their pull-through procedure.

These children can be categorized into three groups: (1) those who are soiling, and (2) those who suffer from obstructive symptoms, including severe constipation or distention and (3) those who present with recurrent episodes of enterocolitis. There is often overlap among these groups, and an individual child may have more than one of these symptoms. It is important for the surgeon to follow these children closely, at least until they are through the toilet training process, in order to identify and provide timely treatment for these problems. Most of these issues can be systematically treated with a combination of bowel management, dietary changes, and laxatives, and, potentially, a redo operation, with the goal of having a child who reliably empties their colon, and is clean. The purpose of this chapter is to describe our algorithm for the work-up and management of such post Hirschsprung disease pull-through patients.

## 13.1 Case study 1

An 18-month-old child had a transanal Soave pull-through at age 3 months. The operation went well, and initially he was stooling well and thriving. For the past 9 months, however, he has had intermittent distension and is requiring daily irrigations in order to pass stool.

### 13.1.1 Obstructive symptoms

Obstructive symptoms may take the form of abdominal distension, bloating, vomiting, or ongoing severe constipation. There are five major reasons for these symptoms following a pull-through: mechanical obstruction, abnormal innervation of the pulled-through bowel, disordered motility in the residual colon or small bowel, internal sphincter achalasia, or functional megacolon caused by stool-holding behavior. The clinician will have much greater success in managing these difficult patients if an organized approach is taken (Figure 13.1).

*Mechanical obstruction*: The most common cause of mechanical obstruction after a pull-through operation is a stricture (Figure 13.2). This problem is more common after a Swenson or Soave operation. Patients undergoing a Duhamel procedure may have a retained "spur" consisting of the anterior aganglionic bowel, which may fill with stool and obstruct the pulled-through bowel (Figures 13.3 and 13.4). In other cases, there may be obstruction secondary to

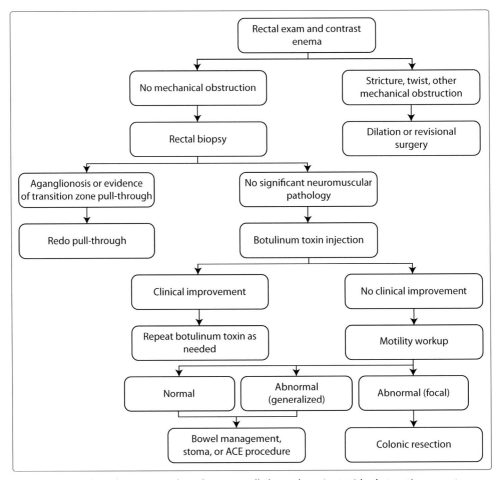

**Figure 13.1** Algorithm; approach to the post pull-through patient with obstructive symptoms.

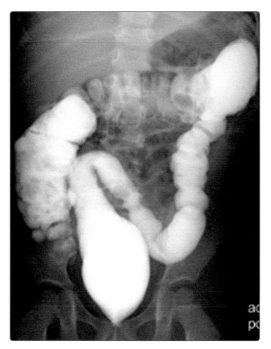

Figure 13.2 Stricture of a pull-through.

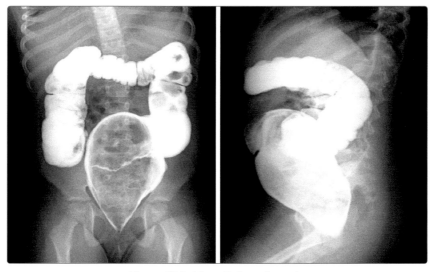

Figure 13.3 Mega Duhamel pouch.

a twist in the pulled-through bowel (Figure 13.5), or narrowing due to a long muscular cuff in children who have had a Soave operation (Figure 13.6).

Obstruction can be discovered with digital rectal examination and a contrast enema. Initial management of an anastomotic stricture involves repeated dilatation using a finger, dilator, or balloon. For recalcitrant strictures, antegrade dilatation using Tucker dilators, intralesional steroid, or topical mitomycin C can be tried. In some cases, redo of the pull-through is necessary. Duhamel spurs can be resected from above or managed by extending the staple

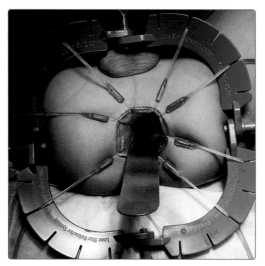

Figure 13.4 Duhamel spur.

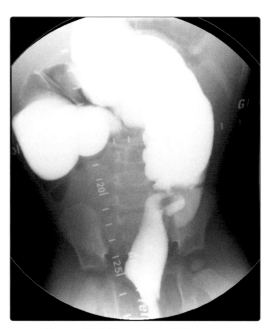

Figure 13.5 Twist of a pull-through.

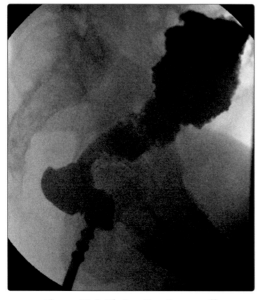

Figure 13.6 Obstructing Soave cuff.

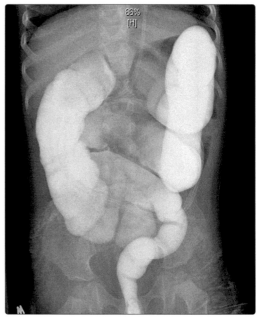

Figure 13.7 Transitional zone pull-through.

line from below. Twisted pull-throughs and narrow muscular cuffs usually require a repeat pull-through. A muscular cuff can occasionally be divided laparoscopically, but in many cases it needs to be removed transanally.

Abnormal innervation of the pulled-through bowel may be due to an error in histological analysis, a transition zone pull-through (Figure 13.7), or loss of ganglion cells, and can be diagnosed by performing a biopsy above the colo-anal anastomosis looking for the presence

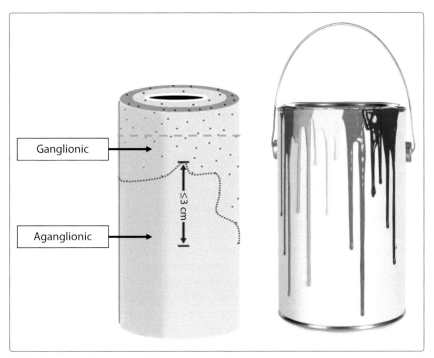

**Figure 13.8** Paint can illustration of the asymmetry of ganglionated bowel.

and number of ganglion cells. Measurement of nerve trunk diameter is a useful marker for a transition zone pull-through in patients under one year of age but its meaning is unclear for older patients. The specimen from the original operation should be reviewed and further sections should be taken circumferentially at the resection margin since the transition zone can be asymmetrical (Figure 13.8). In most cases, the best treatment for persistent or acquired aganglionosis is a repeat pull-through.

This complication is potentially avoided with experienced pathology guidance during the initial pull-through. During frozen section analysis, the pathologist must confirm normal ganglion cells and normal nerve trunks (less than 40 μm for patients under one year of age) at the site of the planned anastomosis. The specimen must be full thickness because if submucosa is not analyzed, hypertrophic nerves might be missed. The common practice of sending only the muscularis layer, often done during a laparoscopic biopsy, is helpful to guide the surgery but a full thickness piece must be analyzed before sewing in the pull-through.

## 13.1.2 Motility disorder

Children with HD often have abnormal motility throughout the intestinal tract, including gastroesophageal reflux and delayed gastric emptying. A major gap in our understanding of HD is why some ganglionated bowel does not function normally. These abnormalities may be focal, usually involving the left colon, or they may be generalized. Techniques for diagnosing motility disorders include radiological shape study, radionuclide colon transit study, and colonic manometry. Diffuse dysmotility is best treated with bowel management, which may include antegrade enemas through a cecostomy tube or Malone appendicocecostomy (MACE). In some children prokinetic agents may also be helpful.

### 13.1.3  Internal sphincter achalasia

This term refers to obstructive symptoms caused by the lack of a normal recto-anal inhibitory reflex which is found in all children with HD. Most children eventually "grow out" of this problem, usually by the age of 5 years. The diagnosis can be confirmed by demonstrating a clinical response to intrasphinteric botulinum toxin. The traditional operative approach for internal sphincter achalasia had been internal sphincterotomy or myectomy, but since this problem may resolve on its own, and there is concern about sphincter-cutting operations leading to incontinence, chemical sphincterotomy with intrasphincteric botulinum toxin makes more sense. In many cases, repeated injection of botulinum toxin, or applications of nitroglycerine paste or topical nifedipine, are necessary while waiting for resolution of the problem.

### 13.1.4  Functional megacolon

Functional megacolon is the result of stool-holding behavior, which is very common in normal children. This behavior may be more common in children with HD because of their predisposition to constipation, and is a problem best treated with a bowel management regimen consisting of laxatives and behavior modification strategies. In severe cases, the child may require antegrade enemas, or even a stoma. In many cases, the cecostomy or stoma can be reversed when the child reaches adolescence.

## 13.2  Case study 2

A 5-year-old child had a transanal Swenson pull-through as a neonate. She is passing stool on a daily basis, but is experiencing "accidents" at least once per day. She has had no distension or enterocolitis episodes. She does not know when she is about to have an accident, and her parents are worried about her starting school.

### 13.2.1  Soiling

There are three broad causes for soiling after a pull-through: abnormal sphincter function, abnormal sensation, or "pseudo-incontinence." Abnormal sphincter function may be due to sphincter injury during the pull-through or to a previous myectomy or sphincterotomy, and can usually be identified using visual inspection, anorectal manometry, or endorectal ultrasound (Figure 13.9). There are two forms of abnormal sensation. The first is lack of sensation of a full rectum, which can also be identified using anorectal manometry, and the other is an inability to detect the difference between gas and stool. This problem is usually due to loss of the transitional epithelium because the anastomosis was performed below the dentate line (Figure 13.10). This distinction is usually evident on physical examination. Both sphincter weakness and abnormal sensation are iatrogenic and preventable problems which are not currently amenable to a surgical solution. Most of these children are best managed using a bowel routine which may include a constipating diet, stimulant laxatives, and rectal or antegrade enemas. Biofeedback training has been advocated, especially for those children with sphincter weakness. In some cases, the child is best served by a stoma.

If both the sphincter and sensation mechanisms are intact, the most likely cause of soiling after a pull-through is pseudo-incontinence. This may be caused by severe obstipation with a massively distended rectum and overflow of liquid stool (Figure 13.11). Other patients leak small amounts of stool through the day, creating "skid marks" in the underwear. Some children can suffer from hyperperistalsis of the pulled-through bowel (Figure 13.12), which results in the inability of the anal sphincter to achieve control despite normal sphincter function. The

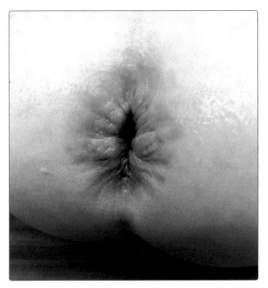

Figure 13.9 Photograph of an anus that is patulous, representing overstretched sphincters.

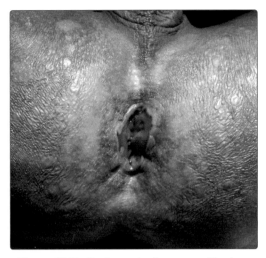

Figure 13.10 Photograph of an anus with a loss of the dentate line resulting from a pull-through started too low.

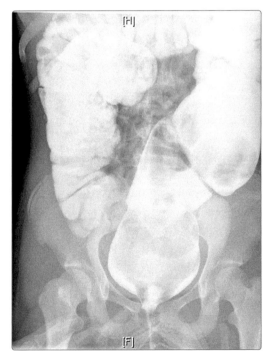

Figure 13.11 Example of a dilated colon.

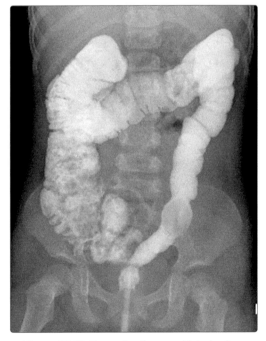

Figure 13.12 Example of a non-dilated colon.

difference between the obstipation and hyperperistalsis forms of pseudo-incontinence can be inferred on contrast enema, and confirmed using colonic motility studies.

Successful management of soiling in a child with HD depends on a clear understanding of the reasons for the soiling. Evaluation requires a careful history and physical examination (often best done under general anesthesia), and investigations such as abdominal films, contrast enema, anorectal manometry, and in some cases, colonic motility studies. Children with severe constipation will benefit from laxative therapy. However, if the sphincter and/or sensation are inadequate, passive laxatives such as lactulose or PEG 3300 will make the problem worse. The child instead should be treated with stimulant laxatives such as senna or bisacodyl; with added fiber for bulking of the stool. If these are inadequate in achieving rectal emptying the child may require a mechanical program using retrograde or antegrade enemas. On the other hand, children with stool-holding behavior who have normal sphincter function and sensation will often experience exacerbation of the behavioral problem after retrograde enemas or any other kind of anal manipulation. Children without constipation who have hyperperistalsis of the pulled-through bowel or abnormal sphincter function or sensation will benefit from a constipating diet and medications such as loperamide.

## 13.3   Case study 3

A 1–year-old child had a Duhamel pull-through at age 1 month. The operation went well, and he has been stooling well and thriving. At 4 months of age he developed a viral respiratory illness, which was followed by an episode of abdominal distension, fever, and diarrhea. He was admitted to the hospital with a provisional diagnosis of enterocolitis and was treated with irrigations and antibiotics; over 4 days he went back to his normal bowel pattern. He has had two additional episodes of enterocolitis over the past 8 months, which have both resolved with irrigations and antibiotics in hospital.

### 13.3.1   Enterocolitis

Although the exact cause of enterocolitis is unknown, certain factors, such as fecal stasis, can precipitate and aggravate the problem. It can occur after any of the HD operations (Figure 13.13). The stasis can result in proliferation and mucosal invasion by intraluminal flora resulting in a local and systemic inflammatory response and bacterial translocation. The clinical criteria for enterocolitis include fever, abdominal distention, and diarrhea; however, this broad definition makes it difficult to determine its actual incidence. Individual reports in the published data quote an incidence of up to half of patients. The presence of chronic enterocolitis can lead to failure to thrive. Enterocolitis may be present both before and after operative correction, and can range in severity from mild to life threatening. It is more common in younger children, longer segment disease, and trisomy 21. A reliable guide to defining enterocolitis is shown in Figure 13.14.

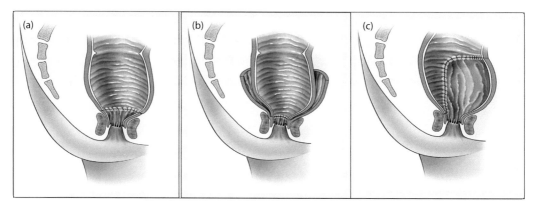

Figure 13.13 Schematic drawings of the Swenson (a), Soave (b), and Duhamel (c) procedures.

| History | |
|---|---|
| Diarrhea with explosive stool | 2 |
| Diarrhea with foul-smelling stool | 2 |
| Diarrhea with bloody stool | 1 |
| History of enterocolitis | 1 |
| Physical examination | |
| Explosive discharge of gas and stool on rectal examination | 2 |
| Distended abdomen | 2 |
| Decreased peripheral perfusion | 1 |
| Lethargy | 1 |
| Fever | 1 |
| Radiologic examination | |
| Multiple air fluid levels | 1 |
| Dilated loops of bowel | 1 |
| Sawtooth appearance with irregular mucosal lining | 1 |
| Cutoff sign in rectosigmoid with absence of distal air | 1 |
| Pneumatosis | 1 |
| Laboratory | |
| Leukocytosis | 1 |
| Shift to left | 1 |
| Total | 20 |
| | HAEC ≥ 10 |

Figure 13.14 Langer score for enterocolitis.

The etiology of Hirschsprung associated enterocolitis (HAEC) is unknown, and is probably multi-factorial. Stasis caused by functional obstruction permits bacterial overgrowth with secondary infection. Infectious agents such as *Clostridium difficile* or rotavirus have been postulated as being causative, but there are few data to support a specific pathogen. There is some evidence implicating alterations in intestinal mucin production and the mucosal production of immunoglobulins, which presumably result in the loss of intestinal barrier function and allows bacterial invasion.

The treatment of HAEC involves nasogastric drainage, intravenous fluids, broad-spectrum antibiotics, and decompression of the rectum and colon using rectal stimulation or irrigations. The risk of HAEC may be decreased by using preventive measures such as routine irrigations or chronic administration of metronidazole or probiotic agents, particularly in those who are thought to be at higher risk for this problem based on clinical or histological grounds. Since enterocolitis is the most common cause of death in children with HD and can occur postoperatively even in children who did not have it preoperatively, it is very important that the surgeon educates the family about the risk of this complication and urges early intervention if the child develops concerning symptoms. Although rarely necessary, one should be prepared to open a proximal diverting colostomy or ileostomy in patients with persistent, severe enterocolitis not manageable with irrigations.

## 13.3.2 Long-term outcomes

Despite the relatively common occurrence of postoperative soiling, obstructive symptoms, and enterocolitis, most resolve after the first five years of life. Studies of teenagers and adults with HD suggest that sexual function, social satisfaction, and quality of life all appear to be relatively normal in the vast majority of patients once they reach their late teens. Exceptions include children with long-segment disease, who have a higher risk of enterocolitis, incontinence, and dehydration than children with shorter segment disease, children with trisomy 21 who have a greater risk of enterocolitis and incontinence, and children with other co-morbidities such as those with congenital central hypoventilation syndrome, congenital heart disease, and syndromes that are associated with developmental delay or other forms of disability.

## 13.4  Conclusions

The optimal long-term outcome for patients after surgery for Hirschsprung disease is to be fecally continent and to have normal bowel movements without abdominal distention or enterocolitis. Usually, this outcome is achieved; however, there is a small subset of patients who have difficulty after their primary operation. These patients should be evaluated with a systematic approach to determine the etiology of their problems, which informs the appropriate therapeutic approach. Most children eventually overcome these problems with appropriate treatment, and long-term outcomes are usually excellent.

## Further reading

1. Langer JC, Rollins MD, Levitt M, Gosain A, Torre L, Kapur RP, Cowles RA, Horton J, Rothstein DH, Goldstein AM; American Pediatric Surgical Association Hirschsprung Disease Interest Group. Guidelines for the management of postoperative obstructive symptoms in children with Hirschsprung disease. *Pediatr Surg Int.* 2017 May;33(5):523–6.
2. De La Torre L, Langer JC. Transanal endorectal pull-through for Hirschsprung disease: technique, controversies, pearls, pitfalls, and an organized approach to the management of postoperative obstructive symptoms. *Semin Pediatr Surg.* 2010 May;19(2):96–106.
3. Langer JC. Persistent obstructive symptoms after surgery for Hirschsprung's disease: Development of a diagnostic and therapeutic algorithm. *J Pediatr Surg.* 2004 Oct;39(10):1458–62.
4. Gosain A, Frykman PK, Cowles RA, Horton J, Levitt M, Rothstein DH, Langer JC, Goldstein AM; American Pediatric Surgical Association Hirschsprung Disease Interest Group. Guidelines for the diagnosis and management of Hirschsprung-associated enterocolitis. *Pediatr Surg Int.* 2017 May;33(5):517–21.
5. Levitt MA, Dickie B, Peña A. The Hirschsprungs patient who is soiling after what was considered a "successful" pull-through. *Semin Pediatr Surg.* 2012 Nov;21(4):344–53.
6. Levitt MA, Dickie B, Peña A. Evaluation and treatment of the patient with Hirschsprung disease who is not doing well after a pull-through procedure. *Semin Pediatr Surg.* 2010 May;19(2):146–53.
7. Wester T, Granström AL. Botulinum toxin is efficient to treat obstructive symptoms in children with Hirschsprung disease. *Pediatr Surg Int.* 2015 Mar;31(3):255–9.
8. Han-Geurts IJ, Hendrix VC, de Blaauw I, Wijnen MH, van Heurn EL. Outcome after anal intrasphincteric Botox injection in children with surgically treated Hirschsprung disease. *J Pediatr Gastroenterol Nutr.* 2014 Nov;59(5):604–7.

# 14 Long-term outcomes of anorectal malformations and Hirschsprung disease

Tomas Wester, Mikko Pakarinen, and Risto Rintala

## 14.1  Case 1: Hirschsprung disease

A 3-year-old boy with non-syndromic, rectosigmoid Hirschsprung disease was operated on at 4 weeks of age with total transanal endorectal pull-through. He has had several episodes of mild Hirschsprung-associated enterocolitis (HAEC), with foul-smelling, explosive diarrhea. He has responded well to rectal irrigations and oral metronidazol. Recently, he had one of these episodes. The parents describe that he needs irrigations almost every day, also between the enterocolitis episodes, to pass stools.

## 14.2  Case 2: Hirschsprung disease

A 14-year-old boy with rectosigmoid Hirschsprung disease underwent transanal pull-through at approximately 3 months of age. He has had significant problems with frequent loose stools and soiling. He has been continent as long as he has used loperamide and a bulking agent. He has now stopped using the drugs, because it is difficult to remember. He now presents with incontinence, particularly when he is playing soccer and also at school.

## 14.2.1  Learning points

### Short-term outcomes

Early postoperative complications are important because, for instance, anastomotic leaks and severe strictures may have a negative impact on long-term functional outcomes. It has been shown that 11%–14% of the patients experience at least one early complication [1]. Some patients with anastomotic leaks, severe strictures, twisted pull-through, residual aganglionosis, and transition zone pull-through need a redo pull-through. Redo pull-through probably has a negative impact on the functional outcome, although data are conflicting [2–4].

HAEC is a serious complication of HSCR, which is associated with worse functional outcome and lower bowel function score than healthy controls [5]. The etiology of HAEC is complex. Postoperative HAEC has been reported to occur in 6%–45% of HSCR patients [6]. Clinically, HAEC is characterized by abdominal distension and explosive, foul-smelling diarrhea. HAEC usually occurs within the first few years after pull-through. Treatment consists of fluid and electrolyte resuscitation, bowel irrigation, and antibiotics. Attempts have been made to prevent HAEC. There is no strong evidence that prophylactic antibiotics prevent recurrent HAEC. There are conflicting data with respect to probiotics. It has been shown that botulinum toxin injections in the anal sphincter reduce the number of readmissions related to HAEC [6].

It is generally considered that stooling pattern changes and the number of daily bowel movements decreases with increasing age [1]. Recent studies have shown that a significant proportion of patients have fecal incontinence, and/or constipation during childhood. Neuvonen et al. showed that children aged 4–12 years had significantly lower bowel function score compared to healthy controls. The patients had worse rectal sensation, more abnormal defecation frequency, more fecal accidents, more problems withholding defecation, more soiling, and were more socially restricted than healthy controls [5].

### Outcomes beyond childhood

It has been shown that bowel function score was significantly better after transanal pull-through in patients over 18 years of age compared to younger patients. In adult patients, rectal sensation, fecal accidents, problems to withhold defecation, and fecal soiling did not differ compared to healthy subjects. The only significant finding was that stool frequency was higher in HSCR patients [5].

Fecal incontinence is a very distressing symptom with severe psychosocial consequences. Fecal incontinence in patients with HSCR can be caused by sphincter injuries due to the stretching of the sphincters during transanal dissection, abnormal anal sensation due to injuries to the anal canal, or it may be incontinence secondary to constipation. The reported incidence of fecal incontinence in adolescent and adults vary from 8% to 71%, which probably reflects how bowel function was assessed [6]. Patients with an intact anal canal and fecal incontinence after pull-through should receive medical management as the first-line treatment. In patients with a dilated colon and constipation, oral laxatives and a short course of enemas are often sufficient. In patients without colonic dilatation and a tendency to loose stools (hypermotility), a constipating diet, loperamide, and bulking agents may improve symptoms. The management of patients with abnormal sphincter function, and/or damaged anal canal is more complex and consists of bowel management programs, antegrade continence enemas, and occasionally a stoma.

Long-term studies have shown that 1%–50% of patients with HSCR have constipation [6]. Neuvonen et al. evaluated bowel function in patients at a median age of 15 years having undergone transanal endorectal pull-through and showed that 9% of the patients reported constipation [5]. Most of the patients respond to oral laxatives, but occasionally need enemas.

It has usually been found that constipation improves with time in patients with HSCR. It is important to exclude anatomical and innervation abnormalities. Constipation after surgical repair of HSCR may be caused by a stricture, residual aganglionosis, transition zone pull-through, colonic motility disorders, or stool-holding behavior. Mechanical complications can often be detected with digital examination in combination with contrast enema. Strictures can usually be managed with repeat anal dilatations. Rectal biopsies will show the presence of residual aganglionosis or a remaining transition zone. If symptomatic, these conditions need redo pull-through.

Hartman et al. showed in a review article that patients with HSCR report slightly more quality of life problems than comparison groups. Compared with children, adolescents reported worse quality of life but better disease-specific functioning. It was concluded that the relationship between disease-specific functioning and quality of life remains unclear [7]. Data on the quality of life in adults are slightly conflicting. Jarvi et al. [8] could not show that symptom-specific quality of life was affected compared to controls, while Granström et al. [9] showed that HSCR had a significant impact on symptom-specific quality of life, but not on generic quality of life.

## 14.3  Case 3: Anorectal malformation in males

A 12-year-old boy with a history of a repaired rectourethral bulbar fistula presents for a routine yearly checkup. The child underwent an uneventful open posterior sagittal anorectoplasty (PSARP) with a covering sigmoidostomy during the first 6 months of life. No associated structural anomalies of the heart, genitourinary tract, or limbs were detected. Screening MRI of the spinal cord at the age of 2 years revealed a low-lying conus medullaris ending at the level of the L-3 end plate associated with a thoracolumbar syrinx and a filum terminal lipoma as well as mild sacral dysplasia with three sacral segments remaining. Bilateral grade II vesico-urethral reflux had resolved spontaneously by second year of life. He has been continent for urine from early on with good bladder emptying without urinary tract infections and the parents have noted erections. He completed toilet training for stools at the age of 4 years. Despite development of voluntary bowel movements and effective treatment of constipation with laxatives and enemas, an appendicostomy for antegrade colonic enema (ACE) washouts was performed due to frequent soiling and uncertain fecal control at the age of 5 years before starting school. Currently, he stays clean with ACE washouts performed every day or every other day, although he is able to recognize the urge to defecate and sometimes empties the bowel spontaneously between washouts. The boy goes to normal school and thrives as a defender in a local football team. He feels that 1 hour with each ACE washout takes too much of his busy life and is wondering whether he could further reduce the frequency or stop ACE washouts entirely. With approaching puberty, the boy's mother raises concerns about the possibilities to father children and general expectations of sexual functions and social life.

### 14.3.1  Learning points

Rectourethral fistula represents some 40% of all anorectal malformations in males, while the fecal continence outcomes remain less optimistic than for lower types of anorectal malformations [10,11]. Although 75% of the patients with rectourethral fistula develop voluntary bowel movements following PSARP, rectal sensation, ability to withhold defecation, fecal soiling, and fecal accidents are all clearly inferior when compared to age-matched normal population controls. These functional impairments in fecal control affect 33, 54, 70 and 54% of the patients, although they are reported infrequently, less than once a week, by most [12]. Of all patients with rectourethral fistula some 30% achieve total spontaneous fecal continence, one-quarter benefit from formal bowel management such as ACE washouts and occasional patients end up with end-ostomy [10,12]. The outlook is much better among those patients who develop voluntary bowel movements. Only 5%–15% of them report frequent impairments in rectal sensation, inability to withhold defecation, fecal soiling, or fecal accidents occurring more often than once a week. Patients with operated rectourethral fistula complete toilet training for stools much later than normal controls normally at a median age of 5 years. Overall, social continence as defined by soiling or fecal accidents less than once a week and no requirement for protective aids is achieved in three quarters of the patients [12].

The development of voluntary bowel movements and fecal control is affected by the level of the rectourethral connection and patient age [10–13]. Of patients with bulbar, prostatic, or vesical rectourethral fistula, 82%–92%, 73%–76%, and 25%–28% develop voluntary bowel movements, while respective proportion of patients free from soiling or fecal accidents is 42, 29, and 0% [10,12,13]. Spontaneous fecal control appear to improve with increasing age in patients with rectourethral fistula after PSARP, which allows the discontinuation of ACE washouts in a significant proportion of patients after gaining more secure fecal control. The overall frequency of soiling and fecal accidents decreased from 99% among patients less than 12 years old to 59% and 37% among patients older than 12 years (range 13–29 years) [12]. Frequent soiling and fecal accidents, occurring more often than once a week, were reported by 33% of the younger patients compared to 13% and 8% in the older patient group. Nearly all younger patients required laxatives or bowel management, whereas only 30% of the patients older than 12 years required such therapeutic measures, enabling total spontaneous fecal continence and voluntary bowel movements in 42% [12]. When assessed separately, 44% of the younger patients had constipation as opposed to 13% of the older patients, suggesting that significant improvement in constipation also occurs with increasing age [10].

Associated anomalies of the spinal cord and sacral dysplasia were observed in 28% and 25% of 40 patients with rectourethral fistula when screening MRI of the spinal cord was uniformly performed [14]. Prevalence of filum terminal lipoma, low-lying conus medullaris inferior to the L-2 end plate, and thoracolumbar syrinx was 23, 10, and 5%, respectively. Sacral dysplasia was mild to moderate since all patients had 3–4 sacral segments remaining. Interestingly, the presence of any spinal cord anomalies was unrelated to bowel functional outcomes or lower urinary tract symptoms assessed during childhood or adolescence [14]. These findings favor expectant conservative approach to spinal cord anomalies in the absence of abnormal neurological findings in the lower limbs. The overall frequency of urinary incontinence was 23%, mostly urge incontinence, while 26% had a history of urinary tract infections. Overall, 61% reported urge and 39% straining, while 74% of patients reported any lower urinary tract symptoms.

Sexual function seems well preserved in most patients with rectourethral fistula following PSARP. In a recent study including 20 rectourethral fistula patients after PSAR with a median age of 22 years, 90% reported normal erections and ejaculations [15]. Frequency of stable relationships and sexual activity were comparable to age-matched normal controls, and the majority reported normal orgasm during intercourse. However, the median age of coital debut was significantly higher among the patients at 18 years as opposed to 16 years among controls. Ejaculations were absent in two patients and one had azoospermia despite normal ejaculations, comprising 15% of patients with rectourethral fistula, which should be taken into account especially if infertility is suspected.

Social issues are not uncommon in patients with rectourethral fistula even in the PSARP era, although they report gastrointestinal quality of life comparable to matched controls [12,15]. The overall prevalence of social problems is around 35%, which is not affected by patient age [12]. These may be severe enough to limit social life and occasionally even cause psychological disturbances, underlining the importance of continuing multidisciplinary support aiding to cope with all aspects of the illness. In this respect, early and efficient management of fecal incontinence to avoid consequences of social discrimination cannot be overemphasized.

# 14.4  Case 4: Anorectal malformation in females

A female newborn presented with a missing anus right after birth, the clinical diagnosis was rectovestibular fistula. A decision to proceed with fecal diversion was made and the child underwent a divided sigmoid colostomy. Screening for associated malformations did not reveal any other defects. The patient thrived well and was discharged home at the age of 7 days. At 3 months of age she underwent distal colostogram that confirmed the diagnosis. A definitive repair was performed by anterior sagittal anorectoplasty. The postoperative phase was uneventful. The anal dilatation regime was continued until Hegar probe size 14 was reached and the diverting sigmoid colostomy was taken down.

The baby had frequent bowel movements, 3–6 per day, for several months after the closure of the stoma. She thrived and gained weight and height within normal limits. At the age of 1 year the bowel frequency started to decrease as she progressed to more and more solid foods. She maintained acceptable bowel movements every 2–3 days. At the age of 2 years bowel movement became more infrequent and significant soiling, both day and nighttime, occurred. A diagnosis of fecaloma formation was made and subsequently confirmed by barium enema. At clinical examination, the anus appeared normal without stenosis or stricture. The child underwent bowel washouts with docusate enemas and oral stimulant laxative treatment (sodium picosulfate) was initiated. Oral medication alleviated symptoms of constipation but attempts to stop or taper laxative treatment were unsuccessful. Following successful management of constipation the child was toilet trained for bowel movements and urine. She remained completely continent for urine. The girl had occasional slight soiling episodes, however, there was no need for protective nappies. The soiling was managed by change of underwear. The soiling was not associated with any social issues. The patient started her primary school at normal age. The minor soiling episodes that occurred 2–3 times per week did not cause any social embarrassment or activity restrictions. The girl was actively engaged in hobbies such as ballet dancing and soccer. Oral laxatives were continued as attempts to taper or stop the medication resulted in exacerbation of symptoms of constipation. At the age of 12 years the patient started have menstruations, the physical and sexual maturation were within normal range. Since the initiation of puberty, the need for laxatives decreased remarkably and they were completely stopped at the age of 13 years. The patient had 4–6 bowel movements per week and no soiling. At last follow-up at the age of 17 years the bowel function was normal without any soiling or symptoms of constipation. She has a boyfriend and has had sexual intercourse without problems.

## 14.4.1  Learning points

The functional outcomes in female patients with vestibular fistula are better than those with more severe malformations such as rectourethral fistula in males or cloacal malformations in females [10]. On the other hand, patients with perineal fistulas or anteriorly placed anus have clearly better bowel function in the long term [16]. Approximately 75% of children and 95% of adolescents or adults with vestibular fistula are socially continent (soiling episodes less than once a week), respectively [17]. Constipation requiring treatment is a common complication in these patients affecting more than half of the patients during childhood. Constipation tends to decline with age [10]. Urinary continence is usually preserved following surgery for rectovestibular fistula if major sacral defects are lacking. As adolescents or adults, patients with vestibular fistula have sexual functions that are largely comparable to healthy controls. The proportion of patients having stable relationships and with experience of sexual intercourse and normal orgasms is similar to controls. Only the coital debut is somewhat delayed [15]. The overall quality of life of patients with vestibular fistula is comparable to their healthy peers, although a negative effect on sexual life has been observed [15]. The fertility prospects of patients with vestibular fistula should be good but delivery by cesarean section is recommended by most authors.

## 14.5 Case 5: Anorectal malformation in female with a cloaca

A female newborn presented with distended abdomen, no anus, and only one opening in the perineum. A clinical examination disclosed the diagnosis of persistent cloaca. Abdominal ultrasound showed moderate hydrometrocolpos with duplicated Müllerian structures that extended to the level of umbilicus, bilateral hydronephrosis, and dilated ureters. A cardiac echography was also performed and revealed a hemodynamically significant ventricular septal defect. On day 1 after birth the patient underwent cloacoscopy. The opening of the common channel was just posterior to the slightly enlarged clitoris. The length of the common channel was estimated to be about 3 cm and the length of the urethra was 1.5 cm. The patient had two vaginas and both were significantly dilated. The rectocloacal fistula drained to the septum between both vaginas. As vaginal reconstruction using native vaginas appeared to be feasible, the patient underwent divided colostomy formation to the proximal sigmoid colon. Urinary drainage was secured by suprapubic catheter cystostomy. The hydrometrocolpos rapidly decompressed by urinary diversion, also the dilatation of upper urinary tract decreased significantly. The patient stabilized with cardiac medication and was discharged home at the age of 3 weeks. She underwent cardiac catheterization at the age of 2 months and repair of the symptomatic ventricular septal defect under cardiopulmonary bypass at the age of 3 months. She recovered from cardiac surgery uneventfully. At the age of 6 months, a distal colostogram was performed and confirmed the findings of previous cloacoscopy in the newborn period. At the age of 8 months the patient underwent repair of the cloacal anomaly by PSARVUP, additional transabdominal mobilization was not necessary. The cloacal confluence was left *in situ* as urethra, the vaginal halves were mobilized from the urethra and bladder neck and tapered significantly posteriorly. The vaginal septum was partially resected. The rectocloacal fistula was easily mobilized and pulled to the anal site that was identified with a muscle stimulator. The repaired vagina reached without undue tension to the perineum just posteriorly to the common channel that was left untouched as a urethra. The repair was finalized by forming a wide perineal body between the neoanus and vaginal introitus. The perineal wounds healed well. The neoanus was gradually dilated to accept Hegar probe size 14 and after this the diverting colostomy was taken down. After stoma closure the bowel function was variable. The patient had several bowel movements per day and also staining of the nappies between bowel movements. Urinary flow appeared unobstructed with good stream. Follow-up urinary tract echographies showed somewhat dilated upper tracts but good bladder emptying. Because of recurrent pyuria the patient was kept on antibiotic prophylaxis with trimethoprim. At the age of 2 years the bowel function became irregular and soiling between bowel movements increased. A barium enema showed fecal impaction and the patient was prescribed oral laxatives that regularized the bowel movements. However, daily soiling of the nappies continued but with lesser degree. At the age of 3.5 years the patient became dry for urine and voided voluntarily. She still used nappies for fecal soiling. Because of daily soiling the patient underwent a Malone appendicostomy operation for antegrade bowel washouts at the age of 6 years. After the surgery the patient remained clean with washouts 3–4 times a week. The patient underwent an urodynamic examination before the Malone operation. It showed acceptable detrusor function but relatively high urine residuals. Because the patient was dry and asymptomatic, no treatment was offered.

The patient started to have menstruations at the age of 13. They became regular within a year, the patient did not have any gynecological symptoms. At follow-up echography, however, a pelvic cyst formation was detected. This was interpreted as a paraovarian cyst and followed up by yearly echography. The urinary continence was perfect and there were no urinary tract infections despite relatively high urinary residuals (50–100 mL). The patient continued to use bowel washouts through Malone appendicostomy but on an irregular basis. She could stay clean with voluntary bowel movements at least 1–2 weeks but opted to keep her appendicostomy as a safeguard. At the age of 17 years the patient underwent laparoscopic resection of the paraovarian cyst that was found to be growing at follow-up echographies; the histology disclosed a simple cyst. At gynecological examination the vaginal introitus was somewhat scarred but accepted a Hegar probe size 27. There was a shallow proximal septum between the vaginal halves but this was considered not to interfere with normal sexual life. Despite relative narrowing of the vaginal introitus the patient was capable of painless sexual intercourse.

### 14.5.1  Learning points

In the literature there is scarcity of reports on long-term follow-up of cloacal malformations. Most reports present only small number of cases or the outcomes are displayed as a part of general population of anorectal malformations.

A recent systematic review on the functional outcomes in cloaca patients pooled the data on anorectal function for a total of 263 patients [18]. In the collective series voluntary bowel movements were reported in 57% of the patients, ranging between 41% and 60%. Total continence was reported in only one study of this systematic review. Pena et al. found 17% of the patients to be totally continent at last follow-up [19]. Some degree of fecal soiling was reported in 71% of the patients (range in the studies 14%–83%) in this systematic review. Frank fecal incontinence was found in 33% of the patients (range in the studies 14%–41%). In 17% of the patients (range in the studies 5%–22%) the quality of bowel control was so poor that the patients chose a permanent colostomy.

Constipation was reported to be a common problem in patients with cloaca. Overall, more than half of the patients suffered from constipation requiring medical management or enema program. The incidence of constipation ranged between 30% and 88% [18].

Bowel management for fecal incontinence or recalcitrant constipation, either by retrograde bowel washouts or by antegrade washouts appendicostomy, was used on average by 38% (range 14%–65%) of the patients in this systematic review [18].

The reported bowel function outcomes in adolescents and adults are somewhat different than in the series that have pooled functional data from all age groups. Davies et al. [20] had 15 cloaca patients with a mean follow-up of 26 years. Of these patients 27% were spontaneously continent, 33% had an appendicostomy or used retrograde washouts, 13% used medication to augment continence, and 27% had a permanent stoma. Couchman et al. [21] identified 19 cloaca patients with a mean follow-up of 22 years. Fecal continence was reported by 58%, the remaining 42% had an ileostomy or colostomy, or ACE conduit. In the authors' personal series 27 patients are adolescent or adults [22]. The mean age of the patients is 23 years (range 13–40 years). Of these 27 patients 52% had developed spontaneous continence and do not require any medications or protective aids, 22% had an appendicostomy for bowel emptying, and 11% had opted for a permanent stoma formation.

Patients with cloaca commonly have urinary tract dysfunction. Urological as well as spinal and spinal cord anomalies are very common. Moreover, the extensive surgery required to repair a cloacal malformation may deteriorate the bladder function [23]. In a systematic review [18] concerning cloaca patients of all ages, urinary tract function was reported in 332 patients, pooled from nine studies. Spontaneous voiding was achieved on average by 46% (range 22%–54%) of the assessed patients. Intermittent catheterization to empty the bladder was reported by 42% of the patients (range 12%–100%) and 22% had undergone urinary diversion (range 18%–27%). Urinary incontinence was reported in 23% (range 9%–41%) of the patients.

The bowel functional outcomes in adolescent and adult patients appeared better than those in the series including patients of all ages, but this is not the case in terms of urinary tract function. Davies et al. [20] found that only 20% of the adult or adolescent cloaca patients were fully continent for urine. Couchman et al. [21] reported urinary tract function in 19 adolescent or adult patients with cloaca. Of the 19 patients 47% were able to void spontaneously, the remaining 10 required catheterization via the urethra or a continent Mitrofanoff vesicostomy. In the authors' own series of 27 adolescent or adult patients 63% voided spontaneously and were continent for urine [22], 11% had undergone bladder augmentation and bladder neck closure, 11% stayed dry by intermittent catheterizations, and 15% had slight daily wetting that required the use of protective pads.

Renal function has been reported to be impaired in a significant proportion of patients with cloaca [24]. Chronic renal failure measured by decreased glomerular filtration rate has been found in 25%–75% of adolescent or adult patients with cloaca [22]. On the other hand, in the authors' series of 27 adolescent or adult patients with cloaca only 11% had renal impairment. Not unexpectedly renal failure has been more common in patients with significant urological abnormalities. It is evident that regular monitoring of renal function including echographic imaging is warranted in all patients with cloaca, also during adult life.

All patients with cloacal anomalies have abnormal genital tract. Approximately, 40% of patients have duplicated Müllerian system with two vaginas and uteri. Approximately, 20%–25% of patients have absent or vestigial uterus, these patients are affected by amenorrhea. Most of these patients have also vaginal agenesis or very small blind ending vaginas.

In the literature the reports on long-term gynecological outcomes in patients with a cloaca are even scarcer than those concerning anorectal or urinary tract function. In a systematic review [18] gynecological function was reported by 71 patients who were pooled from three reports. Normal menstruations were found in only 35% of the patients. Obstructed menstruations were a common finding affecting 38% (24/63) of the patients. The causes of obstruction have been variable. Some patients had a stenosis in the persistent urogenital sinus; these patients had not undergone any genital tract reconstruction [25]. Another group of patients who had undergone genital reconstruction but still developed partial or complete obstruction of the menstrual flow are usually related to [26] asymmetric duplicated Müllerian systems. Couchman et al. [21] found obstructed menstruation in 26% of their 19 adolescent or adult patients with a cloaca. In the authors' own series of 27 adolescent or adult patients 60% had normal menstruations, 16% had amenorrhea due to Müllerian agenesis or other causes, and 11% had had obstructed menstruations.

The obstructed genital organs usually require surgical management that sometimes needs to be performed emergently. The usual presentation is a cystic abdominal mass. Typical procedures for patients with obstructed double systems include resection of the obstructed hemiuteri and adnexa, and eradication of the abdominal collections of blood or endometriosis [25,26]. In addition to obstructions in menstrual flow, cloaca patients have commonly other cystic problems in the internal genital organs. Of the authors' 27 adult or adolescent cloaca patients 20% required surgical interventions for large cystic collections that involved uteri and adnexal tubes. Histologically these collections were benign paraovarian cysts [22].

The vaginoplasty that was performed at the time of the primary repair of the cloaca requires revision in a significant percentage of patients to allow normal sexual activity. Couchman et al. [21] reported that 56% of the patients who underwent vaginal reconstruction in infancy required a secondary or even tertiary surgery. The authors questioned the rationale of total urogenital reconstruction during infancy and suggested that genital reconstruction could be delayed until there is full clarity of the anatomy of Müllerian structures. However, most pediatric surgeons and urologists who have experience in reconstructions of cloacas strongly advise full reconstruction in infancy [19,27,28]. It is logical to reconstruct the vagina at the same time as the rectum and urinary tract. The findings in the report of Warne et al. [25] support this as the patients with early vaginal repair had a stricture rate of 15% which compared favorably with the patients having postpubertal vaginoplasty and a stricture rate of 42%. Of the authors' 27 adolescent and adult patients secondary vaginal procedures were required in 50% of the 22 patients who had elected the definitive vaginal repair [22]. Of the secondary vaginal repairs eight were simple introitus plasties, two required a redo-colovaginoplasty due to severely strictured distal vagina following ileo-vaginoplasty, and one redo total urogenital mobilization to create an adequate vaginal introitus.

The rate of sexual activity in patients with cloaca has been reported only in three studies. Of Hendren's 154 patients [27] 24 were adults and 71% of these had had sexual intercourse. Warne et al. [25] found that 57% of their 21 patients (age range 17–34 years) had been sexually active. Adequate vagina for sexual intercourse as assessed by a gynecologist was found in 86% of the patients. In the study of Couchman et al. [21] 42% of 19 patients (age range 13–35 years) were reported to be sexually active, of whom 1 had experienced difficulties in penetration. Of the author's 27 patients (age range 13–30) 52% reported sexual activity [22]. Two of these had occasionally problems with penetration requiring lubrication.

In the literature there are only few reports concerning fertility and pregnancies in patients with a cloaca. Of Hendren's [27] 24 adult patients 6 had gone successfully through pregnancies. Five of these delivered by cesarean section and one vaginally. In the report of Couchman et al. [21] three of the eight patients with sexual activity were attempting to conceive with assisted conception methods and one patient had a complex preterm delivery. Of the authors' 14 sexually active patients 3 had delivered healthy babies by cesarean section [22]. Cesarean section as the method of delivery is recommended by most experts as vaginal delivery, even if possible, may damage the repaired vagina and interfere with urinary and fecal continence. The quality of life of cloaca patients has been studied in particular only by Versteegh et al. [29]. The QoL of children and adolescents with cloaca was comparable with that of female patients with rectoperineal and rectovestibular fistula using a standardized and validated scoring instrument for QoL evaluation (PedsQL 4.0 inventory). The reported QoL scoring did not differ significantly from the reference values obtained from a healthy population with similar age distribution. On the other hand, parents of patients with cloaca reported more problems on several psychosocial domains compared with the healthy children and adolescents. There are no studies on quality of life of adult patients with cloaca.

## 14.6  Conclusions

Despite significant developments in the understanding of the pathological anatomy and physiology of ARM and HD the results of surgical therapy remain far from perfect. The functional defects and psychosocial difficulties that occur commonly in children with ARM and HD continue in adulthood in a significant proportion of patients. An essential part of the management of anorectal malformations and Hirschsprung disease should be multidisciplinary long-term follow-up that, in addition to medical issues, provides support to the patients and their families at each stage of development. The team required includes pediatric surgeons, urologists and nephrologists, adolescent gynecologists, specialized nursing staff, and psychological and psychosocial support specialists. A critical stage is transition to adult services that is required to be smooth with close collaboration with adult medical and support staff who need to be aware of the multiple problems that these patients may encounter as adolescents and adults.

## References

1. Kim AC, Langer JC, Pastor AC et al. Endorectal pull-through for Hirschsprung's disease—A multicenter, long-term comparison of results: Transanal vs transabdominal approach. *J Pediatr Surg*. 2010;45:1213–20.
2. Friedmacher F, Puri P. Residual aganglionosis after pull-through operation for Hirschsprung's disease: A systematic review and meta-analysis. *Pediatr Surg Int*. 2011;27:1053–7.
3. Dingemans AJM, van der Steeg HJJ, Rassouli-Kirchmeier R et al. Redo pull-through surgery in Hirschsprung's disease: Short-term clinical outcome. *J Pediatr Surg*. 2017;52:1446–50.

4. Ralls MW, Freeman JJ, Rabah R et al. Redo pull-through for Hirschsprung disease: A single surgical group's experience. *J Pediatr Surg*. 2014;49:1394–9.

5. Neuvonen MI, Kyrklund K, Rintala RJ et al. Bowel function and quality of life after transanal endorectal pull-through for Hirschsprung's disease: Controlled outcomes up to adulthood. *Ann Surg*. 2017;265:622–9.

6. Wester T, Granström AL. Hirschsprung disease—Bowel function beyond childhood. *Semin Pediatr Surg*. 2017;26:322–7.

7. Hartman EE, Oort FJ, Aronson DC et al. Quality of life and disease-specific functioning of patients with anorectal malformations and Hirschsprung's disease: A review. *Arch Dis Child*. 2011;96:398–406.

8. Järvi K, Laitakari EM, Koivusalo A et al. Bowel function and gastrointestinal quality of life among adults operated for Hirschsprung's disease during childhood: A population-based study. *Ann Surg*. 2010;252:977–81.

9. Granström AL, Danielson J, Husberg B et al. Adult outcomes after surgery for Hirschsprung's disease: Evaluation of bowel function and quality of life. *J Pediatr Surg*. 2015;50:1865–9.

10. Kyrklund K, Pakarinen MP, Rintala RJ. Long-term bowel function, quality of life and sexual function in patients with anorectal malformations treated during the PSARP era. *Semin Pediatr Surg*. 2017;26:336–42.

11. Rintala RJ, Pakarinen MP. Outcome of anorectal malformations and Hirschsprung's disease beyond childhood. *Semin Pediatr Surg*. 2010;19:160–7.

12. Kyrklund K, Pakarinen MP, Koivusalo A, Rintala RJ. Long-term bowel functional outcomes in rectourethral fistula treated with PSARP: Controlled results after 4–29 years of follow-up: A single-institution, cross-sectional study. *J Pediatr Surg*. 2014;49:1635–42.

13. Levitt MA, Pena A. Outcomes from the correction of anorectal malformations. *Curr Opin Pediatr*. 2005:17:394-401.

14. Kyrklund K, Pakarinen MP, Taskinen S, Kivisaari R, Rintala RJ. Spinal cord anomalies in patients with anorectal malformations without severe sacral abnormalities or meningomyelocele: Outcomes after expectant, conservative management. *J Neurosurg Spine*. 2016;25:782–9.

15. Kyrklund K, Taskinen S, Rintala RJ, Pakarinen MP. Sexual function, fertility and quality of life after modern treatment of anorectal malformations. *J Urol*. 2016;196:1741–6.

16. Pakarinen MP, Rintala RJ. Management and outcome of low anorectal malformations. *Pediatr Surg Int*. 2010 Nov;26(11):1057–63.

17. Kyrklung K, Pakarinen MP, Koivusalo A, Rintala RJ. Bowel functional outcomes in females with perineal or vestibular fistula treated with anterior sagittal anorectoplasty: Controlled results into adulthood. *Dis Colon Rectum*. 2015; 58:97–103.

18. Versteegh HP, van Rooij IA, Levitt MA, Sloots CE, Wijnen RM, de Blaauw I. Long-term follow-up of functional outcome in patients with a cloacal malformation: A systematic review. *J Pediatr Surg*. 2013 Nov;48(11):2343–2350.

19. Peña A, Levitt MA, Hong A, Midulla P. Surgical management of cloacal malformations: A review of 339 patients. *J Pediatr Surg*. 2004 Mar;39(3):470–9.

20. Davies MC, Liao LM, Wilcox DT, Woodhouse CR, Creighton SM. Anorectal malformations: What happens in adulthood? *BJU Int*. 2010 Aug;106(3):398–404.

21. Couchman A, Creighton SM, Wood D. Adolescent and adult outcomes in women following childhood vaginal reconstruction for cloacal anomaly. *J Urol*. 2015 May;193(5 Suppl):1819–22.

22. Rintala RJ. Congenital cloaca: Long-term follow-up results with emphasis on outcomes beyond childhood. *Semin Pediatr Surg*. 2016 Apr;25(2):112–6.

23. Warne SA, Godley ML, Wilcox DT. Surgical reconstruction of cloacal malformation can alter bladder function: A comparative study with anorectal anomalies. *J Urol*. 2004 Dec;172(6 Pt 1):2377–81.

24. Warne SA, Wilcox DT, Ledermann SE, Ransley PG. Renal outcome in patients with cloaca. *J Urol*. 2002 Jun;167(6):2548–51.

25. Warne SA, Wilcox DT, Creighton S, Ransley PG. Long-term gynecological outcome of patients with persistent cloaca. *J Urol*. 2003 Oct;170(4 Pt 2):1493–96.

26. Levitt MA, Stein DM, Peña A. Gynecologic concerns in the treatment of teenagers with cloaca. *J Pediatr Surg*. 1998 Feb;33(2):188–93.

27. Hendren WH. Cloaca, the most severe degree of imperforate anus: Experience with 195 cases. *Ann Surg*. 1998 Sep;228(3):331–46.

28. Levitt MA, Peña A. Cloacal malformations: Lessons learned from 490 cases. *Semin Pediatr Surg*. 2010 May;19(2):128–38.

29. Versteegh HP, van den Hondel D, IJsselstijn H, Wijnen RM, Sloots CE, de Blaauw I. Cloacal malformation patients report similar quality of life as female patients with less complex anorectal malformations. *J Pediatr Surg*. 2016; 51(3):435–9.

# 15 Antegrade access as an adjunct to bowel management: Appendicostomy and neoappendicostomy

Rebecca M. Rentea, Devin R. Halleran, and Alejandra Vilanova-Sánchez

## 15.1 Case study 1

A 9-year-old patient with a 7-year history of severe functional constipation with soiling presents for evaluation. He participated in a bowel management program after several years of minimal success on multiple laxative-based regimens. Physical examination revealed an abdomen that was softly distended and a normal-sized and well-positioned anus. His work-up included a contrast enema, which showed that the child had a moderately dilated rectosigmoid colon. Because he failed medical management he underwent motility evaluation which included anal manometry (AMAN), colonic manometry (CMAN), and a rectal biopsy. All of these studies were completely normal. The child was placed on rectal enemas with a regimen of 400 mL of Saline and 20 mL of glycerin, because laxatives had been ineffective. These improved his emptying dramatically and resolved his soiling, but the enemas were traumatic and he became anally defensive. The patient is continent of urine and has no underlying urinary dysfunction or renal disease.

**What is your next step in management?**

- **A.** Perform colonoscopy to evaluate for a structural lesion as the cause of the child's symptoms
- **B.** Offer Malone appendicostomy
- **C.** Attempt a laxative trial

*Answer:* B

### 15.1.1  Learning points

- The Malone appendicostomy, or MACE procedure, was first described in 1990 as a technique to create a catheterizable channel through which a patient or caregiver can deliver an antegrade colonic enema flush to reliably empty the colon in children with severe constipation or fecal incontinence [1].
- Antegrade enema access allows for flushes to be performed in patients who are uncomfortable with the rectal route and allows for children to become more independent in their care. For a patient to be successful with antegrade enemas, they are ideally clean first with retrograde enemas, but this is not always possible.
- In patients with functional constipation, Hirschsprung disease should be ruled out with a rectal biopsy that shows the presence of ganglia with normal nerves. An AMAN (if over age 1) can also rule out Hirschsprung disease. The absence of a history of failure to thrive or episodes of enterocolitis make this diagnosis very unlikely. Additionally, a contrast enema, anal manometry, and colonic manometry can be very useful in the work-up of patients with functional constipation prior to any surgical intervention.
- The normal colonic manometry predicts success with antegrade flushes. Sometimes if colonic manometry shows a dysmotile segment (usually the sigmoid), a resection may be needed, but even for these cases starting with antegrade flushes only is recommended as daily flushes can improve the motility and often allow the patient to use laxatives in the future at a lower dose. If a colon resection is ultimately needed, a shorter segment of colon may need to be removed after a period of successful flushes.

## 15.2  Case study 2

A 6-year-old male with a history of an anorectal malformation (rectobladder neck fistula), tethered cord, sacral ratio 0.3 (meaning a very underdeveloped sacrum) presents with severe constipation and soiling. The child had a posterior sagittal anorectoplasty (PSARP) during the first year of life. An examination under anesthesia (EUA) demonstrated that the anus was adequately sized and centered within the sphincter complex. There was no stricture or prolapse. The child participated in bowel management program and is currently managed on a successful rectal enema regimen.

**What is your next step in management?**

- **A.** Offer Malone appendicostomy
- **B.** I do not have enough information
- **C.** Offer a laxative trial

*Answer:* B

### 15.2.1  Learning points

- Prior to performing an appendicostomy, a complete understanding of the patient's urinary status and the potential need for future urologic reconstruction is required. If there is no underlying urologic dysfunction or foreseeable need for urologic reconstruction, then an appendicostomy can be performed.

- If the urologic status is not clear, then it is preferable to wait until the child is older and the need for urologic reconstruction is elucidated for several reasons:
  - To determine need for bladder neck tightening and/or appendicovesicostomy (Mitofanoff).
  - To determine need for bladder augmentation which could be performed at the time of colon resection if one is needed.
  - Ability to perform a split appendicostomy to utilize the appendix for both the appendicovesicostomy and appendicostomy. If the appendix can only be used for one channel then the Mitofanoff is preferable. The colon access could then be created with a neoappendicostomy.
  - A laxative trial would not be affective as this patient would not be predicted to have bowel control given the type of malformation and the quality of the spine and sacrum (ARM continence index) (Figure 15.1).

## 15.3 Case study 3

A 5-year-old male with a history of a previously repaired rectobulbar fistula presents for evaluation of severe constipation and fecal incontinence over the last year. On examination, the child is noted to have an adequately sized anus located within the sphincter complex. There is no stricture or prolapse. The sacrum and spine are normal. The child is currently managed successfully with rectal enemas, although his parents state the child is becoming less cooperative with enemas and they would like to discuss an antegrade option. He had several urinary tract infections in infancy but has not had any in nearly 3 years. He remains diapered and has several wet diapers daily along with nightly bedwetting. He is followed regularly by a pediatric urologist who recommends continued surveillance for now.

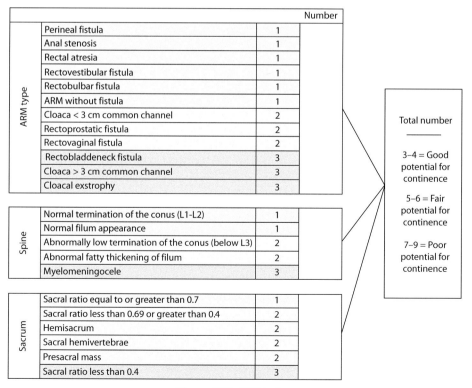

| ARM type | | Number |
|---|---|---|
| Perineal fistula | 1 | |
| Anal stenosis | 1 | |
| Rectal atresia | 1 | |
| Rectovestibular fistula | 1 | |
| Rectobulbar fistula | 1 | |
| ARM without fistula | 1 | |
| Cloaca < 3 cm common channel | 2 | |
| Rectoprostatic fistula | 2 | |
| Rectovaginal fistula | 2 | |
| Rectobladdeneck fistula | 3 | |
| Cloaca > 3 cm common channel | 3 | |
| Cloacal exstrophy | 3 | |

| Spine | | |
|---|---|---|
| Normal termination of the conus (L1-L2) | 1 | |
| Normal filum appearance | 1 | |
| Abnormally low termination of the conus (below L3) | 2 | |
| Abnormal fatty thickening of filum | 2 | |
| Myelomeningocele | 3 | |

| Sacrum | | |
|---|---|---|
| Sacral ratio equal to or greater than 0.7 | 1 | |
| Sacral ratio less than 0.69 or greater than 0.4 | 2 | |
| Hemisacrum | 2 | |
| Sacral hemivertebrae | 2 | |
| Presacral mass | 2 | |
| Sacral ratio less than 0.4 | 3 | |

Total number
____

3–4 = Good potential for continence

5–6 = Fair potential for continence

7–9 = Poor potential for continence

Figure 15.1 ARM index.

**What would you recommend?**

- A. Offer appendicostomy
- B. Offer appendicostomy, appendicovesicostomy
- C. Offer laparoscopic cecostomy
- D. Recommend continued rectal enemas

*Answer:* D

### 15.3.1 Learning points

- The urologic status is unknown in this child at this point, and thus it is not clear whether he will require any future urinary reconstruction.
- A cecostomy in this patient offers the child an antegrade enema route, while preserving the valuable appendix for future urinary reconstruction if needed.
  - If an appendicovesicostomy is needed in the future, the cecostomy can be taken down simultaneously and an appendicostomy can be created using the split appendix technique.
  - If an appendicovesicostomy is not needed, the cecostomy can be taken down and an appendicostomy can be created using the in situ technique if the parents desire.
- Appendicostomy should not be performed until the urologic status is fully known, with the appendicovesicostomy preferentially using the appendix.

## 15.4 Case study 4

A 12-year-old child with a history of myelomeningocele presents for evaluation. The child is currently on high dose laxatives and fiber and has several accidents throughout the day. He is incontinent of urine, has frequent urinary tract infections, and was recently diagnosed with chronic kidney disease (CKD) stage 2. Urologic evaluation including ultrasound and urodynamics demonstrates that he is a good candidate for a Mitrofanoff without the need for augmentation or bladder neck tightening.

**What is your next step in management?**

- A. Offer appendicostomy
- B. Offer appendicostomy along with the appendicovesicostomy using the split appendix technique

*Answer:* B

### 15.4.1 Learning points

- There are several benefits to collaboration between pediatric colorectal and urologic surgeons in these complex patients with concomitant bowel and bladder dysfunction. If bowel and bladder reconstruction is needed, this can be performed simultaneously using the split appendix technique (Figure 15.2).
- The appendicovesciostomy can be brought to the skin through the umbilicus as the bladder is a midline structure, and the appendicostomy brought through the right lower quadrant as the cecum is located laterally, thus orienting the structures in a more anatomically natural configuration.

**Intraoperatively, you find that the appendix measures only 3 cm. What do you do?**

- A. Perform appendicostomy only.
- B. Perform appendicovesicostomy only.

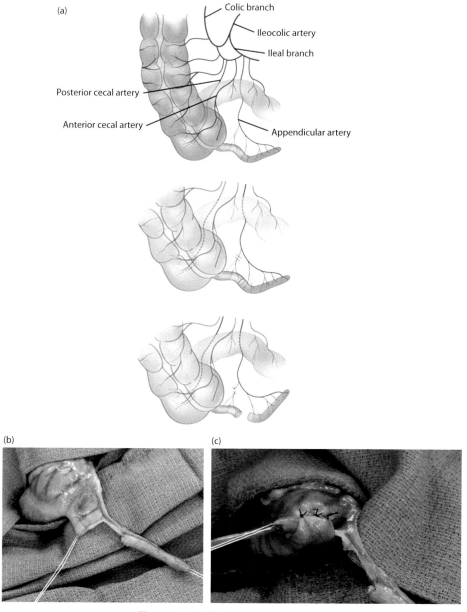

(a)

Colic branch

Ileocolic artery

Ileal branch

Posterior cecal artery

Anterior cecal artery

Appendicular artery

(b)

(c)

Figure 15.2  Split appendix technique.

C. Perform appendicostomy and ileovesicostomy.
D. Perform appendicostomy and colovesicostomy.
E. Perform neoappendicostomy and appendicovesicostomy.

*Answer:* E

## 15.4.2  Learning points

- In cases where the appendix is of inadequate length to be used for both the appendicostomy and appendicovesicostomy, it is preferable to use the appendix for the

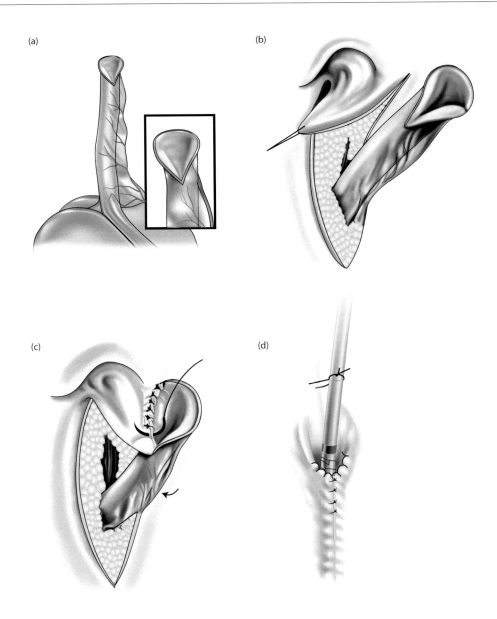

(a)

(b)

(c)

(d)

**Figure 15.3** V-shaped incision in the skin and the appendix.

appendicovesicostomy. The appendix is the most durable structure for the Mitrofanoff. In these patients, it is possible to perform a neoappendicostomy using a cecal flap to recreate the appendix (Figure 15.3).

## 15.5 Technical aspects for the Malone appendicostomy

### 15.5.1 Patient selection

*ARM*: Patients with fecal incontinence due to true fecal incontinence with poor potential for bowel control (high malformation, SR ratio <0.6 or tethered cord) or chronic constipation (pseudo-incontinence).

*Hirschsprung disease (HD)*: Patients with loss of the dentate line and/or impaired sphincters with true incontinence.

*Functional constipation:* Patients with severe chronic constipation who do not tolerate rectal route in whom colonic manometry has revealed normal colonic motility.

*Spinal patients:* Patients with true fecal continence due to spinal causes (e.g., spina bifida or traumatic spinal injury).

## 15.5.2  Preoperative considerations

### 15.5.2.1  Urologic evaluation

Prior to performing an appendicostomy, a complete understanding of the patient's urinary status and the potential need for future urologic reconstruction is required (especially in patients with ARM and spinal problems). The collaboration between both services facilitates (1) sharing of the appendix in cases where an appendicovesicostomy is needed using the split appendix technique, (2) minimization of abdominal procedures, (3) minimization of general anesthetic events, and (4) overlay of the postoperative recovery [2].

A.  If there is no urologic dysfunction present or no reconstruction is anticipated, a Malone appendicostomy can be performed.

   In cases where urologic dysfunction is present and reconstruction is needed:

B.  A split appendix technique can be performed if the appendix is long enough to be used for both appendicovesicostomy and appendicostomy (Figure 15.2).

C.  If the appendix is not of adequate length or is not of adequate quality to utilize for both channels, it is preferable to use the appendix as an appendicovesicostomy and create a neoappendicostomy. The neoappendicostomy may also be performed in cases where there is no needed urologic reconstruction needed and a previous appendectomy was performed (for example if an appendicectomy was performed during a Ladd's procedure).

### 15.5.2.2  Bowel preparation and antibiotics

A mechanical bowel preparation is needed if the patient is planned to receive a neoappendicostomy or if it is unknown whether the patient has an appendix and therefore a neoappendicostomy may be performed.

A mechanical bowel preparation is not routinely performed in patients who present for a planned appendicostomy, assuming that the patient is on a successful flush regimen that keeps the colon empty of stool.

Preoperatively, the patient receives one dose of broad-spectrum antibiotics.

## 15.5.3  Intraoperative considerations

Key steps for laparoscopic Malone appendicostomy are as follows:

1.  Open the umbilical skin in a V fashion (Figure 15.3).
2.  Use this access for pneumoperitoneum access.
    Insert a 4 mm trocar in the left lower quadrant. Mobilize the cecum and right colon from their retroperitoneal attachments. If more dissection is needed, a third 4 mm trocar in the supraumbilical access is helpful. Trocars can be often placed in locations of previous scars.
3.  Once the cecum reaches the umbilicus easily, then vertically incise the infraumbilical fascia approximately 3–4 cm, cauterizing into the trocar.
4.  Bring the cecum and appendix through the umbilical incision.
5.  Open the tip of the appendix in a V fashion. Insert a 10 Fr. feeding tube.

(a)                    (b)

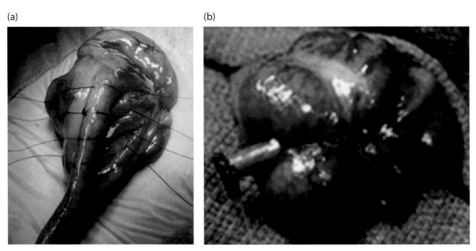

Figure 15.4 Plication of the cecum.

6. Plicate the cecum (with the tube in place) around the appendix opening a window in the appendix mesentery if needed, using non-absorbable suture to create a valve mechanism (Figure 15.4).
7. Transect the distal appendix if it is too long.
8. Close the fascia with 2-0 long-term absorbable suture.
9. Perform a V to V anastomosis of the appendix to the umbilical skin with 5/0 absorbable suture.
10. Place a 10 Fr. feeding tube into appendix lumen, securing it to skin.

*Note*: If there is a previous history of multiple laparotomies and laparoscopy is not feasible, a previous incision can be used to access the abdomen. In such a case a circle anastomosis is a good technique as no umbilical fascial incision is required, just passage of the appendix through the umbilical ring.

Key steps for neoappendicostomy are as follows:

1. Mobilize the right colon and cecum from their retroperitoneal attachments.
2. Incise a U-shaped flap of cecum over a single vessel.
3. Tubularize the flap over a 10 Fr. feeding tube (Figure 15.4).
4. Close the cecal defect in two layers with 4/0 absorbable sutures.
5. Vertically incise the infraumbilical fascia approximately 2 cm or a right lower quadrant if a Mitrofanoff is being placed in the umbilicus.
6. Plicate the cecum around the neoappendix using non-absorbable sutures to create a valve mechanism, ensuring plication stitches do not allow the neoappendix to lie against the closed colostomy.
7. Close the fascia with long-term absorbable suture.
8. Perform anastomosis of the appendix to the skin.
9. Placement of a 10 Fr. feeding tube into neoappendix lumen, securing to skin.

The umbilicus is the common location for the appendicostomy to anastomosed to the skin, as it provides an optimal cosmetic result (Figure 15.5). In patients in whom a simultaneous appendicovesicostomy is performed, the Mitrofanoff is commonly brought to the umbilicus as the bladder is a midline structure, and the Malone is brought to the skin in the right lower quadrant.

### 15.5.4 Postoperative considerations

#### 15.5.4.1 For appendicostomy

Postoperatively, patients receive additional two doses of broad-spectrum antibiotics, and are started on a clear liquid diet once the effects of general anesthesia have worn off. On post-operative day #1, the patient is advanced to a regular diet and flushes are started at the same volume and concentration as was used preoperatively. An abdominal film is taken before discharge to check the colon is empty.

#### 15.5.4.2 For neoappendicostomy

Postoperatively, patients receive additional two doses of broad-spectrum antibiotics. The patient is kept NPO for 1–3 days. Once the patient is on a regular diet we divide the enema volume in 2, giving one half the total enema volume every 12 hours. This is done so as to not overstretch the suture lines. After 1 month we start the patient on once daily full volume enema flushes.

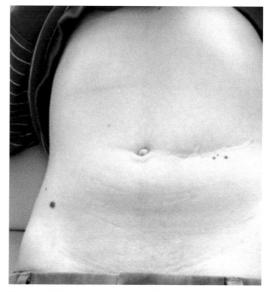

Figure 15.5 Cosmetic result of the appendicostomy.

### 15.5.5 Follow up

Our practice is to remove the 10 Fr. feeding tube at 1 month, and at that time place an ACE stopper which remains for a period of 6 months. The ACE stopper (Figure 15.6) maintains patency of the tract and prevents stenosis. After that point, the channel needs regular intubation in order to remain patent and to minimize the risk of stenosis.

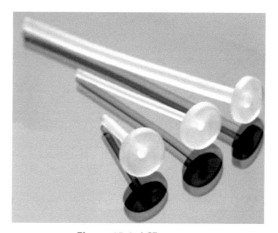

Figure 15.6 ACE stopper.

### 15.5.6 Common complications

Before the procedure, the patient should be informed on the complication profile associated with the MACE procedure and the management of those complications.

1. *Stenosis*: Malone orifice stenosis is a complication associated with up to 20% of MACE procedures and is the result of the natural healing process at the skin level [3–5]. This is commonly the result of failure to regularly intubate the stoma. A superficial revision can be performed in order to widen the orifice.
2. *Leakage*: Leakage is a result of disruption of the valve-like mechanism. When present, this complication can be managed with re-plication of the cecum around the base of the appendix to recreate the valve.

# References

1. Malone PS, Ransley PG, Kiely EM. Preliminary report: The antegrade continence enema. *Lancet*. 1990:336(8725):1217–8.
2. Halleran DR, Wood RJ, Vilanova-Sanchez A et al. Simultaneous robotic assisted laparoscopy for bladder and bowel reconstruction. *J Laparoendosc Adv Surg Tech A*. 2018: Dec;28(12):1513–6.
3. Rangel, SJ and de Blaauw I. Advances in pediatric colorectal surgical techniques. *Semin Pediatr Surg*. 2010;19(2): 86–95.
4. Rangel SJ, Lawal TA, Bischoff A et al. The appendix as a conduit for antegrade continence enemas in patients with anorectal malformations: Lessons learned from 163 cases treated over 18 years. *J Pediatr Surg*. 2011;46(6):1236–42.
5. VanderBrink BA, Cain MP, Kaefer M et al. Outcomes following Malone Antegrade Continence Enema and their surgical revisions. *J Pediatr Surg*. 2013;48(10):2134–9.

# 16 Severe functional constipation: Surgery and gastroenterologic collaboration

Peter L. Lu, Desalegn Yacob, and Carlo Di Lorenzo

## 16.1  Introduction

The majority of children with functional constipation respond to conventional treatment with laxatives and behavioral modification. However, children with severe functional constipation refractory to conventional treatment often require specialized care from gastroenterologists and surgeons working in collaboration. Anorectal and colonic manometry testing can provide the medical team a better understanding of the physiological mechanisms contributing to a child's defecation problem and can be used to guide subsequent medical or surgical treatment. Anorectal manometry measures the neuromuscular function of the anus and rectum using a catheter placed through the anal canal into the rectum, and can be used to evaluate for the presence of Hirschsprung's disease, internal anal sphincter achalasia, and pelvic floor dyssynergia. Colonic manometry measures the neuromuscular function of the colon using a catheter placed in the lumen of the colon, and can be used to evaluate for the presence of colonic motor dysfunction, including colonic inertia and segmental colonic dysmotility.

## 16.2  Case study 1

A 12-year-old female with severe constipation presents for evaluation. Her constipation began around the time of starting school and has persisted for the past 7 years despite years of oral laxative treatment. She spends hours each day straining to pass even small amounts of soft stool. She often reports the feeling of incomplete evacuation after bowel movements. Physical examination shows an abdomen that is mildly full in the suprapubic area but is otherwise soft, non-distended, and non-tender. Her anus is normally positioned and digital rectal exam is remarkable for soft, formed stool in the rectum. Her prior evaluation includes a contrast enema demonstrating dilation of her rectosigmoid colon, which prompted her gastroenterologist to refer her to the colorectal surgery team. She has since had an anorectal manometry test that showed a normal anal resting pressure and normal squeeze mechanism. She had a normal recto-anal inhibitory reflex (RAIR) and her rectal sensory thresholds were slightly increased. However, she had significant increases in anal sphincter pressure with several attempts to push and failed a balloon expulsion test.

**What is your next step in management?**

> **A.** Resection of the dilated sigmoid colon
> **B.** Malone appendicostomy for antegrade continence enemas
> **C.** Pelvic floor biofeedback therapy
> **D.** Anal sphincter botulinum toxin injection

*Answer:* C

## 16.2.1 Learning points

- **Anorectal manometry** testing evaluates the neuromuscular function of the anus and rectum following trans-anal placement of a specialized catheter. A recent consensus document describes in detail the performance and interpretation of this test in children [1]. For the older, cooperative child, anorectal manometry testing generally begins with measurement of the resting anal pressure and the length of the anal canal. This is followed by evaluation of the child's squeeze and bear down (or push) mechanisms, measurement of rectal sensation, and evaluation for the presence or absence of a RAIR during gradual rectal balloon inflation. The RAIR is present when internal anal sphincter relaxation is observed during rectal balloon inflation. The absence of a normal RAIR raises suspicion for Hirschsprung's disease or internal anal sphincter achalasia. Children with an absent RAIR should undergo rectal biopsy, which differentiates subjects with Hirschsprung's disease from those with internal anal sphincter achalasia. Rectal biopsy of a child with internal anal sphincter achalasia should show morphologically normal ganglion cells. For the younger or uncooperative child, anorectal manometry testing can be performed under sedation. Sedation limits the test to measurement of resting anal pressure and evaluation of the RAIR, and certain anesthetic medications like propofol can decrease the accuracy of measured resting anal pressure [2].
- **Pelvic floor dyssynergia** or dyssynergic defecation occurs when there is incomplete relaxation or paradoxical contraction of the pelvic floor and external anal sphincter during defecation [3]. Children with pelvic floor dyssynergia can describe prolonged straining with limited passage of stool and report the feeling of incomplete evacuation. In children with pelvic floor dyssynergia, anorectal manometry shows an increase in anal pressure during attempts to bear down or push (Figure 16.1). Children with this condition may also be unable to pass a rectal balloon during the balloon expulsion test [1,4].
- **Pelvic floor biofeedback therapy** aims to restore a normal pattern of defecation using verbal and visual feedback. In children with pelvic floor dyssynergia, this involves training the child to increase abdominal pressure while relaxing the pelvic floor and the external anal sphincter during efforts to defecate. Visual feedback is generated either by using an anorectal manometry catheter or surface electromyography leads placed externally. Pelvic floor biofeedback therapy is generally recommended for adults with pelvic floor dyssynergia and has been demonstrated to be superior to laxative treatment [5,6]. Although there is

less evidence for the benefit of pelvic floor biofeedback therapy in children with constipation, a recent randomized-controlled trial demonstrated that the addition of biofeedback therapy to conventional treatment led to significant clinical improvement and decreased laxative use [7–10]. In the child with pelvic floor dyssynergia and persistent constipation despite conventional treatment, pelvic floor biofeedback therapy should be considered prior to surgical treatment.

## 16.3  Case study 2

A 16-year-old female with severe constipation and anxiety disorder presents for evaluation. For the past several years, she has had hard bowel movements 1–2 times per week. She also complains of daily abdominal pain that improves with defecation but at times persists even when constipation is better controlled. She can spend hours in the bathroom with a persistent urge to defecate, often in the mornings

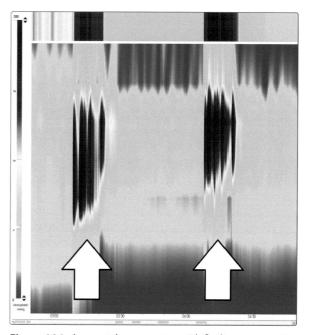

**Figure 16.1**  Anorectal manometry with findings suggestive of pelvic floor dyssynergia. This study was performed using a solid state, high-resolution manometry catheter and pressure is depicted using color. The horizontal band of higher pressure in the middle of the figure reflects the pressure of the anal canal. With both attempts to bear down or push (identified by the two white arrows), the pressure of the anal canal increases significantly.

before school. Attempts to use stimulant laxatives have been limited by abdominal cramping and pain. Physical examination shows an abdomen that is soft, non-distended, and non-tender. Her anus is normally positioned and digital rectal exam is remarkable for soft, formed stool in the rectum. Her prior evaluation includes a normal contrast enema. Her anorectal manometry showed decreased rectal sensory thresholds, suggesting increased rectal sensitivity, but was otherwise normal.

**What is your next step in management?**

    **A.**  Malone appendicostomy for antegrade continence enemas
    **B.**  Anal sphincter botulinum toxin injection
    **C.**  Colonic manometry
    **D.**  Refer back to GI given concern for irritable bowel syndrome with constipation

*Answer:* D

## 16.3.1  Learning points

- **Irritable bowel syndrome (IBS)** is a functional gastrointestinal disorder that involves abdominal pain associated with defecation, a change in stool frequency, or a change in stool form or appearance. It is the most common pediatric functional abdominal pain disorder, with an estimated worldwide prevalence of approximately 8.8% [11]. The diagnosis of IBS is made using the Rome criteria, which categorizes children with IBS into subtypes based on a child's predominant stool pattern [12]. In this case, our patient meets Rome criteria for the diagnosis of IBS with constipation. A feature that distinguishes her presentation from that of functional constipation is that her pain persists even when her constipation improves. Anxiety and depression are associated with the diagnosis of IBS and likely contribute to its pathophysiology [11,13,14]. Our patient's anorectal manometry suggesting rectal hypersensitivity is evidence of visceral hyperalgesia, a common finding in children with IBS. Visceral hyperalgesia can lead to a persistent urge to defecate and abdominal pain in response to use of stimulant laxatives [15,16].

- Traditional pharmacological treatment for children with constipation has included osmotic laxatives, stimulant laxatives, and lubricants [17]. However, newer pharmacological treatments used in adults with constipation and IBS with constipation show promise for children with similar conditions, particularly when abdominal pain limits stimulant laxative use. **Lubiprostone** is a prostaglandin E1 derivative that promotes intestinal fluid secretion, softening stool and promoting intestinal motility through luminal distention [18]. Several randomized-controlled studies have demonstrated the efficacy and safety of lubiprostone in adults with constipation [19–21]. An open-label study of lubiprostone in children with functional constipation found it to be well tolerated and effective in improving bowel movement frequency, but improvements in abdominal pain were not significant [22]. **Linaclotide** is a peptide agonist of the intestinal guanylate cyclase-C receptor, which also promotes intestinal fluid secretion. Linaclotide not only softens stool and accelerates intestinal transit, but can also decrease visceral sensitivity in animal models [18,23]. Several randomized-controlled studies in adults have demonstrated improvements in constipation symptoms and abdominal pain [23–25]. Although research is ongoing, no studies have been published yet on the use of linaclotide for children with constipation-predominant IBS, and its use is contraindicated in children younger than 6 years of age because of the risk of severe dehydration.

## 16.4 Case study 3

A 10-year-old male with severe constipation and fecal incontinence presents for evaluation. He has infrequent stools that are large, hard, and difficult to pass and has daily stool leakage in his underwear. His symptoms persisted despite increasing laxative use, and a few months prior he began using daily rectal enemas with good evacuation. However, he is becoming increasingly oppositional to rectal enema administration. Physical examination shows an abdomen that is full but soft, non-distended, and non-tender. His anus is normally positioned and digital rectal exam is remarkable for hard stool in the rectum. Prior evaluation includes a contrast enema demonstrating rectosigmoid dilation and a redundant sigmoid colon. His anorectal manometry was normal, with normal resting anal sphincter pressure, normal squeeze and bear down mechanisms, and an intact RAIR. His colonic manometry showed a series of high-amplitude propagating contractions (HAPCs) progressing from the ascending colon through the sigmoid colon in response to a stimulant laxative. The HAPCs were associated with the urge to defecate and passage of a large amount of stool.

**What is your next step in management?**

A. Resection of the dilated sigmoid colon
B. Malone appendicostomy for antegrade continence enemas
C. Pelvic floor biofeedback therapy
D. Sacral nerve stimulation

*Answer:* B

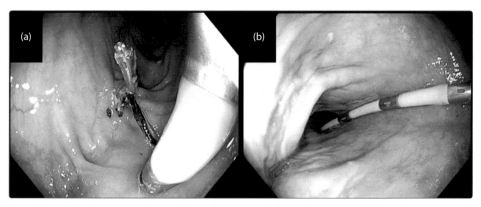

Figure 16.2 Colonic manometry catheter placement during colonoscopy. (a) Once the manometry catheter has been appropriately positioned in the lumen of the colon, the tip of the catheter can be secured to the colonic mucosa using an endoscopic clip and a loop of suture tied to the catheter. (b) During withdrawal of the endoscope, the manometry catheter can be seen positioned within the lumen of the colon. This particular catheter has 36 sensors, each spaced 3 cm apart.

## 16.4.1  Learning points

- **Colonic manometry** testing evaluates the neuromuscular function of the colon using a specialized catheter placed in the lumen of the colon. A recent consensus document describes in detail the performance and interpretation of this test in children [1]. Catheter placement is performed under anesthesia during colonoscopy or with fluoroscopic guidance. In some cases, an endoscopic clip is used to secure the catheter to the colonic mucosa to prevent migration during the study (Figure 16.2). Once the child has recovered from anesthesia, the test generally begins with recording of colonic motor activity during the fasting period. This is followed by ingestion of a meal and assessment for a gastrocolonic response, which is characterized by a postprandial increase in motor activity and tone. HAPCs are contractions that are generally >60 mm Hg in pressure and propagate in an organized, antegrade manner. They can be seen in all phases of the colonic manometry, including as part of the gastrocolic response. Provocative testing is often performed in cases when HAPCs are absent or limited following a meal, most commonly by assessing manometric and clinical response to intraluminal administration of stimulant laxatives like bisacodyl (Figure 16.3).
- For the child with severe functional constipation refractory to conventional treatment, colonic manometry testing is used to diagnose an underlying **colonic motility disorder** and guide subsequent treatment. An absence of HAPCs throughout the colon is consistent with **colonic inertia**. Premature termination of HAPCs before reaching the distal sigmoid colon suggests **segmental colonic dysmotility** (Figure 16.4), and the length of affected colon can be estimated by correlating manometric patterns with an abdominal radiograph taken after catheter placement [1]. A normal colonic manometry, as in our case, is associated with an improved response to antegrade continence enema treatment [26–29]. Clinical observations during colonic manometry testing can be informative as well. Children with constipation who report being unable to sense the urge to defecate often react to these strong propagating contractions through non-verbal communication like grimacing, posturing, or volitional stool retention. In these circumstances, it can be helpful for the children to recognize that the sensation felt during HAPCs should serve as a signal that it is time to have a bowel movement [30].

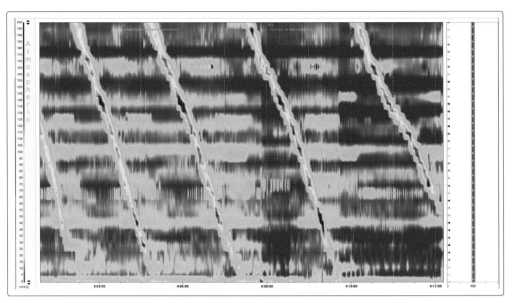

Figure 16.3  Colonic manometry showing several series of high-amplitude propagating contractions. This study was performed using a solid state, high-resolution manometry catheter and pressure is depicted using color. After administration of bisacodyl, the colon generates several series of contractions that begin at the most proximal sensor (the top of the figure) and propagate in an antegrade manner to the distal sensors (the bottom of the figure).

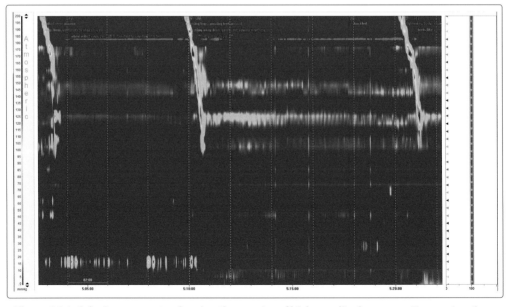

Figure 16.4  Colonic manometry showing three series of high-amplitude propagating contractions in a child with segmental colonic dysmotility. Unlike the response shown in Figure 16.3, this child had contractions that begin at the most proximal sensor but terminate prematurely. By correlating these findings with an abdominal radiograph taken immediately prior to bisacodyl administration, we estimated that the distal 40 cm of colon did not generate propagating contractions.

## 16.5  Case study 4

A 14-year-old male with severe constipation and fecal incontinence presents for evaluation. Four years prior, an anorectal manometry was normal and colonic manometry showed a limited segment of sigmoid dysmotility. He underwent Malone appendicostomy creation and started to use antegrade continence enemas with a satisfactory initial clinical response. However, over the past two years, his response to this treatment has been waning despite several adjustments of his enema components. He sits on the toilet for up to 3 hours after enema administration with only limited stool output. He is having stool leakage several times a day. A recent contrast enema with contrast administered through his appendicostomy shows mild dilation of the ascending colon and unchanged appearance of a redundant sigmoid colon compared to a previous study before creation of the appendicostomy. Physical examination shows an abdomen that is full in the lower abdomen but soft, non-distended, and non-tender. His anus is normally positioned and digital rectal exam is remarkable for hard stool in the rectum.

**What is your next step in management?**

- **A.** Resection of the dilated ascending colon
- **B.** Resection of sigmoid colon based on prior colonic manometry
- **C.** Anal sphincter botulinum toxin injection
- **D.** Repeat colonic manometry

*Answer:* D

### 16.5.1  Learning points

- Although our patient has had a colonic manometry test in the past, it is important to recognize that colonic motility can change over time, particularly if there has been a prolonged period of time with incomplete emptying and colonic stool retention. In a child with a prior colonic manometry demonstrating segmental colonic dysmotility several years prior, it would be appropriate to repeat a colonic manometry to re-evaluate the extent of colonic dysmotility. Estimation of the length of the dysmotile colon by correlating manometry results with an abdominal radiograph after catheter placement can be helpful if colonic resection is needed [31].

## References

1. Rodriguez L, Sood M, Di Lorenzo C, Saps M. An ANMS-NASPGHAN consensus document on anorectal and colonic manometry in children. *Neurogastroenterol Motil: Off J Eur Gastrointest Motil Soc.* 2017;29(1).
2. Tran K, Kuo B, Zibaitis A, Bhattacharya S, Cote C, Belkind-Gerson J. Effect of propofol on anal sphincter pressure during anorectal manometry. *JPGN J Pediatr Gastroenterol Nutr.* 2014;58(4):495–7.
3. Bharucha AE, Dorn SD, Lembo A, Pressman A. American Gastroenterological Association medical position statement on constipation. *Gastroenterology.* 2013;144(1):211–7.
4. Belkind-Gerson J, Surjanhata B, Kuo B, Goldstein AM. Bear-down maneuver is a useful adjunct in the evaluation of children with chronic constipation. *JPGN J Pediatr Gastroenterol Nutr.* 2013;57(6):775–9.
5. Rao SS, Benninga MA, Bharucha AE, Chiarioni G, Di Lorenzo C, Whitehead WE. ANMS-ESNM position paper and consensus guidelines on biofeedback therapy for anorectal disorders. *Neurogastroenterol Motil: Off J Eur Gastrointest Motil Soc.* 2015;27(5):594–609.
6. Chiarioni G, Whitehead WE, Pezza V, Morelli A, Bassotti G. Biofeedback is superior to laxatives for normal transit constipation due to pelvic floor dyssynergia. *Gastroenterology.* 2006;130(3):657–64.
7. van Engelenburg-van Lonkhuyzen ML, Bols EM, Benninga MA, Verwijs WA, de Bie RA. Effectiveness of pelvic physiotherapy in children with functional constipation compared with standard medical care. *Gastroenterology.* 2017;152(1):82–91.

8. Loening-Baucke V. Biofeedback treatment for chronic constipation and encopresis in childhood: Long-term outcome. *Pediatrics*. 1995;96(11):105–10.

9. van der Plas RN, Benninga MA, Buller HA et al. Biofeedback training in treatment of childhood constipation: A randomised controlled study. *Lancet*. 1996;348(9030):776–80.

10. Jarzebicka D, Sieczkowska J, Dadalski M, Kierkus J, Ryzko J, Oracz G. Evaluation of the effectiveness of biofeedback therapy for functional constipation in children. *The Turkish J Gastroenterol: The Off J Turkish Soc Gastroenterol*. 2016;27(5):433–8.

11. Korterink JJ, Diederen K, Benninga MA, Tabbers MM. Epidemiology of pediatric functional abdominal pain disorders: A meta-analysis. *PLOS ONE*. 2015;10(5):e0126982.

12. Hyams JS, Di Lorenzo C, Saps M, Shulman RJ, Staiano A, van Tilburg M. Functional disorders: Children and adolescents. *Gastroenterology*. 2016;S0016–5085(16)00181–5.

13. Shelby GD, Shirkey KC, Sherman AL et al. Functional abdominal pain in childhood and long-term vulnerability to anxiety disorders. *Pediatrics*. 2013;132(3):475–82.

14. Drossman DA, Hasler WL. Rome IV-Functional GI disorders: Disorders of gut-brain interaction. *Gastroenterology*. 2016;150(6):1257–61.

15. Chitkara DK, Bredenoord AJ, Cremonini F et al. The role of pelvic floor dysfunction and slow colonic transit in adolescents with refractory constipation. *The Am J Gastroenterol*. 2004;99(8):1579–84.

16. Simren M, Tornblom H, Palsson OS et al. Visceral hypersensitivity is associated with GI symptom severity in functional GI disorders: Consistent findings from five different patient cohorts. *Gut*. 2018;67(2):255–62.

17. Tabbers MM, DiLorenzo C, Berger MY et al. Evaluation and treatment of functional constipation in infants and children: Evidence-based recommendations from ESPGHAN and NASPGHAN. *J Pediat Gastroenterol Nutr*. 2014;58(2):258–74.

18. Koppen IJ, Di Lorenzo C, Saps M et al. Childhood constipation: Finally something is moving! *Expert Rev Gastroenterol Hepatol*. 2016;10(1):141–55.

19. Johanson JF, Ueno R. Lubiprostone, a locally acting chloride channel activator, in adult patients with chronic constipation: A double-blind, placebo-controlled, dose-ranging study to evaluate efficacy and safety. *Aliment Pharmacol Ther*. 2007;25(11):1351–61.

20. Johanson JF, Morton D, Geenen J, Ueno R. Multicenter, 4-week, double-blind, randomized, placebo-controlled trial of lubiprostone, a locally-acting type-2 chloride channel activator, in patients with chronic constipation. *Am J Gastroenterol*. 2008;103(1):170–7.

21. Barish CF, Drossman D, Johanson JF, Ueno R. Efficacy and safety of lubiprostone in patients with chronic constipation. *Dig Dis Sci*. 2010;55(4):1090–7.

22. Hyman PE, Di Lorenzo C, Prestridge LL, Youssef NN, Ueno R. Lubiprostone for the treatment of functional constipation in children. *J Pediatr Gastroenterol Nutr*. 2014;58(3):283–91.

23. Schoenfeld P, Lacy BE, Chey WD et al. Low-dose linaclotide (72 mug) for chronic idiopathic constipation: A 12-week, randomized, double-blind, placebo-controlled trial. *Am J Gastroenterol*. 2018;113(1):105–14.

24. Lembo AJ, Kurtz CB, Macdougall JE et al. Efficacy of linaclotide for patients with chronic constipation. *Gastroenterology*. 2010;138(3):886–95 e1.

25. Lembo AJ, Schneier HA, Shiff SJ et al. Two randomized trials of linaclotide for chronic constipation. *The N Engl J Med*. 2011;365(6):527–36.

26. van den Berg MM, Hogan M, Caniano DA, Di Lorenzo C, Benninga MA, Mousa HM. Colonic manometry as predictor of cecostomy success in children with defecation disorders. *J Pediatr Surg*. 2006;41(4):730–6; discussion -6.

27. Mugie SM, Machado RS, Mousa HM et al. Ten-year experience using antegrade enemas in children. *J Pediatr*. 2012;161(4):700–4.

28. Rodriguez L, Nurko S, Flores A. Factors associated with successful decrease and discontinuation of antegrade continence enemas (ACE) in children with defecation disorders: A study evaluating the effect of ACE on colon motility. *Neurogastroenterol Motil: Off J Eur Gastrointest Motil Soc*. 2013;25(2):140–e81.

29. Gomez-Suarez RA, Gomez-Mendez M, Petty JK, Fortunato JE. Associated factors for antegrade continence enemas for refractory constipation and fecal incontinence. *Journal J Pediatr Gastroenterol Nutr*. 2016;63(4):e63–8.

30. Firestone Baum C, John A, Srinivasan K et al. Colon manometry proves that perception of the urge to defecate is present in children with functional constipation who deny sensation. *J Pediatr Gastroenterol Nutr*. 2013;56(1):19–22.

31. Wood RJ, Yacob D, Levitt MA. Surgical options for the management of severe functional constipation in children. *Curr Opin Pediatr*. 2016;28(3):370–9.

# 17 | Colonic resection in children with colonic dysmotility

Karen A. Diefenbach, Desalegn Yacob,
Rita D. Shelby, and Richard J. Wood

## 17.1  Case study 1

A 13-year-old male presents with a 7-year history of intractable constipation and encopresis and has had an extensive evaluation. His workup consisted of a contrast enema, a rectal biopsy, and colonic and anorectal manometries. His colonic manometry (CMAN) was normal with high-amplitude propagating contractions (HAPC) and his anorectal manometry (AMAN) was also unremarkable with normal resting pressure, push test, and intact recto-anal inhibitory reflex (RAIR). The rectal biopsy was also normal with ganglion cells present while the contrast enema demonstrated moderately dilated rectosigmoid colon. He has previously participated in a bowel management program, first with an oral laxative regimen with minimal success followed by a regimen of saline and glycerin enemas. The rectal enema regimen was minimally successful due to noncompliance and parents reported that they were traumatic making this option not feasible. He now presents for consideration for possible operative management of his condition. He is continent of urine and has no underlying urinary dysfunction or renal disease. Physical examination revealed an abdomen that was mildly distended but soft, and a normal perianal exam.

**What are the next steps in management?**

- A. Proceed to the OR for colonic resection
- B. Continue the current medical management
- C. Offer an alternate combination of laxatives or flushes
- D. Recommend Malone appendicostomy for antegrade continence enema (ACE)

*Answer:* D

### 17.1.1 Learning points

- Patients with chronic functional constipation with no or limited distal colonic dysmotility may be managed with daily administration of ACE through a Malone appendicostomy or cecostomy. This option allows the patient to reliably and easily administer therapeutic antegrade flushes without the discomfort of rectal enemas. It also has the advantage of evacuating the entire colon in one sitting.
- Colonic resection for functional constipation remains controversial. However, indications for resection include poor response to medical management with antegrade flushes and a discrete colonic segment with dysmotility or a significantly dilated rectosigmoid colon that interferes with effectiveness of an antegrade flush. It can also be considered in older children and young adults with chronic constipation who have done well with ACE but fail transition to oral laxative and do not wish to be dependent on antegrade flushes.
- Patients who have total colonic dysmotility and fail medical management with flushes may benefit from a diverting ileostomy to give the colon an opportunity to recover before a total colonic resection is done.

### 17.1.2 Preoperative considerations

#### 17.1.2.1 Imaging

All children should have baseline posteroanterior (PA) and lateral sacral imaging to rule out sacral malformations. Contrast enema is required in these patients prior to determining treatment plan. Contrast enema allows for anatomic evaluation of the colon.

#### 17.1.2.2 Testing

Majority of these patients present with manometry already completed. However, if not already done, anorectal and colonic manometry should be performed. These manometric studies are helpful in identifying defecation problems caused by motility disorders. Colonic manometry can assess the contractile activity of the colon in a fasting state, postprandially, and after the administration of a stimulant medication. Furthermore, it can assist in determining if the dysmotility is pan-colonic or localized to a specific segment. Anorectal manometry when performed without sedation can assess the internal and external sphincter function, sensation, and pelvic floor dysfunction. A clinician ultimately has to interpret the manometric study results in the context of the patient's clinical presentation and form a therapeutic plan.

#### 17.1.2.3 Bowel preparation and preoperative antibiotics

Mechanical bowel preparation is not usually required if the patient has been on a successful bowel regimen. If a Neo-Malone, performed in patients without an appendix, is planned a bowel prep is indicated. If the patient is noncompliant with bowel regimen or present with impaction, they may be made to undergo a bowel prep.

- Preoperatively, the patient typically receives one dose of broad-spectrum antibiotics.

### 17.1.3 Intraoperative considerations

1. The laparoscopic approach is well accepted for this procedure.
2. The patient is positioned in a supine position.
3. A V-incision is placed at the inferior margin of the umbilicus and the umbilical skin flap is raised. A 5 mm port is placed through this incision.

4. Additional laparoscopic ports are placed to allow access to the appendix and the right lower quadrant.
5. The appendix and cecum are mobilized to reach the umbilicus without tension.
6. The blood supply to the appendix is inspected and windows in the mesoappendix performed to allow preservation of the blood supply to the base of the appendix.
7. Plication of the cecum around the base of the appendix is performed using 3-0 silk sutures with the catheter in the appendix to maintain the lumen.
8. The appendix is brought out through the umbilical port site and the distal portion of the appendix is resected to be flush with the base of the umbilicus.
9. The wall of the appendix is split at the location that lines up with the tip of the umbilical skin flap. The appendix is sewn into the base of the umbilicus with interrupted 4-0 Vicryl sutures.
10. The catheter is placed within the appendicostomy and secured to the abdominal wall with a nonabsorbable stitch. We use a 10 FR, Counsel tip Foley for this with the balloon inflated with 3 mL of water to prevent dislodgement.

### 17.1.4 Postoperative considerations

#### 17.1.4.1 Diet

Patients are often started on a clear liquid diet once the effects of general anesthetics have worn off. On postoperative day 1, the patient is advanced to a regular diet. Once the patient is on regular diet, antegrade flushes are started. If patient has previously been on an enema program, the enema will determine flush volume and additives. If patient has never been on a flush, the typical flush used is a mixture of 400 mL of saline and 20 mL of glycerin.

The patient and parent(s) undergo teaching about catheter care and flush administration. Discharge of the patient takes place once the patient is on a regular diet and tolerating flushes.

### 17.1.5 Follow-up

#### 17.1.5.1 Long-term follow-up

Long-term follow-up is necessary to monitor for success and the first follow-up visit is scheduled at 1 month post discharge for changing the catheter and the placement of an ACE stopper in the appendicostomy. The patient is followed for at least 6 months before an oral laxative trial is attempted.

## 17.2 Case study 2

A 10-year-old female with a history of severe intractable functional constipation and soiling presents for evaluation. She has previously participated in a bowel management program involving multiple laxatives of various doses with minimal success. After failure with retrograde enemas, she had a Malone appendicostomy placed. Unfortunately this approach has also failed to address her inability to successfully evacuate her colon. She now presents for consideration for further management. A contrast enema has already demonstrated a redundant and dilated sigmoid colon. A full thickness rectal biopsy shows normal ganglion cells and no hypertrophic nerves. She was eventually sent for an evaluation with a colonic manometry and was found to have dysmotility in a significant portion of the left colon including the sigmoid. The proximal colon down to the splenic flexure was normal manometrically and also had normal appearance on the contrast enema. An anorectal manometry study done awake was unremarkable and of no concern.

**What is your next step in management?**

    **A.** Offer an alternate bowel regimen
    **B.** Offer an extended left colon resection
    **C.** Offer an ileostomy

*Answer:* B

### 17.2.1 Learning points

- Motility studies are a key part of the workup of a patient with severe intractable constipation and are critical in determining where to resect.
- Once the patient fails medical management and antegrade continence enema, the next step is resection of problematic bowel. The appendicostomy should be retained and used especially in the early post-resection period. It is possible that the patient will be able to quickly wean off the antegrade flushes and do well with oral laxatives. It is also possible that the antegrade continence flushes will be needed for a longer period of time. The flush required may change after the anatomy is altered by resection.
- Ileostomy is a viable option. However, in a patient with segmental dysmotility, it may not be the preferred option as it does not address the problem. Furthermore most patients would prefer to not have a stoma permanently or for a prolonged period of time if it can be avoided. Resection allows the possibility for normal bowel function and a quality of life that meets the patient's expectation.

## 17.3 Case study 3

A 5-year-old female with a history of severe functional constipation with soiling presents for evaluation. She was recently diagnosed with failure to thrive secondary to severe intractable functional constipation. She has unfortunately failed medical management and has continued to decline after Malone appendicostomy. She now presents for further workup and intervention to address her ongoing defecation difficulties that is impacting her life severely. A contrast enema was mostly unremarkable with a mildly dilated sigmoid colon and a full-thickness rectal biopsy was normal. She underwent manometric evaluation with both colonic and anorectal studies. The colonic study demonstrated the absence of motility in the entire colon despite the administration of high-dose stimulants of bisacodyl and glycerin directly into the colon through the central lumen of the catheter. Anorectal manometry was normal.

**What is your next step in management?**

    **A.** Offer an alternate bowel regimen
    **B.** Offer a subtotal colectomy
    **C.** Offer an ileostomy

*Answer:* C

### 17.3.1 Learning points

- Ideally an ileostomy is a temporary solution. It allows the colon to decompress and potentially improve the colonic motility and avoid an extended resection.
- These patients require a close follow-up with repeat manometry in 1–2 years. If motility is improved on follow-up then stoma can be reversed and attempts at medical management of bowel function can be reattempted.

- Patients with intractable constipation that leads to failure to thrive are in the extremes. If a comprehensive evaluation rules out other etiologies for their nutritional problems and constipation is deemed to be reason, the most efficient way to improve their health status is diversion with an ileostomy.

## 17.4  Case study 4

A 5-year-old female with a history of severe intractable functional constipation presents for evaluation. She has developed fecal incontinence over the past 6 months and is currently been managed with rectal enemas. She has however recently begun to become less cooperative with the rectal enemas and parents are seeking an alternate management plan. A contrast enema demonstrated a moderately dilated rectosigmoid. As part of the work up a rectal biopsy was done and it was abnormal with absent ganglia but normal nerves. Furthermore, motility studies demonstrate some dysmotility in the distal areas of the colon.

**What is your next step in management?**

A. Offer an alternate bowel regimen
B. Offer a Malone appendicostomy or cecostomy
C. Offer an ileostomy
D. Treat this as you would treat Hirschsprung disease (HD)

*Answer:* D

### 17.4.1  Learning points

The presentation of normal nerves and no ganglion is concerning for HD or for a biopsy taken too low and could therefore represent the physiological zone of hypoganglionosis just above the anal canal. A repeat rectal biopsy should be performed to confirm Hirschsprung disease either present or absent. Proceeding to bowel surgery such as segmental resection or ileostomy without accurate diagnosis would be inappropriate management for this patient. Once Hirschsprung is effectively ruled in or out treatment could follow appropriately.

## 17.5  Case study 5

A 5-year-old female presents with a history of severe functional constipation now complicated by the failure to thrive. She also has developed fecal incontinence over the last 6 months. She is currently managed on rectal enemas with some success. She has started to become less cooperative. She now presents for consideration for further management. A contrast enema demonstrated a moderately dilated rectosigmoid. After consideration for possible surgical management, a rectal biopsy was completed. This was abnormal and demonstrated abnormal nerves, but normal ganglia. Furthermore, motility studies demonstrate dysmotility of some areas of the colon.

**What is your next step in management?**

A. Offer an alternate bowel regimen
B. Offer a Malone appendicostomy or cecostomy
C. Offer an ileostomy
D. Treat this as you would treat Hirschsprung disease (HD)

*Answer:* C

### 17.5.1 Learning points

The presentation of abnormal nerves and normal ganglion is consistent with chronic constipation without an organic etiology such as HD. The presence of failure to thrive in a patient with intractable constipation that is not responsive to medical management is an indication for colonic diversion with an ileostomy. The post-ileostomy follow-up should include repeat colonic manometry study in a year or longer based on the provider clinical assessment. If the repeat manometry study shows normalization of colonic motility, the stoma may be taken down along with the creation of a Malone appendicostomy, a Neo-Malone, or a cecostomy in order to initiate antegrade flushes as a part of a bowel management program.

## Further reading

1. Di Lorenzo C, Youssef NN. Diagnosis and management of intestinal motility disorders. *Semin Pediatr Surg.* 2010;19:50–8.
2. Eradi B, Hamrick M, Bischoff A et al. The role of a colon resection in combination with a Malone appendicostomy as part of a bowel management program for the treatment of fecal incontinence. *J Pediatric Surg.* 2013;48(11):2296–300.
3. Gassior A, Reck C, Vilanova-Sanchez A et al. Surgical management of functional constipation: An intermediate report of a new approach using laparoscopic sigmoid resection combined with Malone appendicostomy. *J Pediatr Surg.* 2018;53(6):1160–2.
4. Villarreal J, Sood M, Zangen T et al. Colonic diversion for intractable constipation in children: Colonic manometry helps guide clinical decisions. *J Pediatr Gastroenterol Nutr.* 2001;33(5):588–91.
5. Wood RJ, Yacob D, Levitt MA. Surgical options for the management of severe functional constipation in children. *Curr Opin Pediatr.* 2016;28:370–79.

# 18 Importance of collaboration in pelvic reconstruction: How to avoid complications and extra interventions

Molly E. Fuchs, Kate McCracken, and Daniel G. DaJusta

## 18.1 Case study 1

A 1-day-old female is born at 37 weeks gestation by spontaneous vaginal delivery. Her mother received no prenatal imaging. Examination reveals a single perineal orifice and absent anus. Her abdomen is distended. She is diagnosed with a cloacal anomaly. Abdominal ultrasound reveals hydrocolpos and bilateral hydroureteronephrosis. She develops progressive respiratory distress and increasing respiratory support is required. Because of her respiratory distress a percutaneous vaginostomy tube is placed at the bedside to decompress her hydrocolpos. As clear urine drains from the hydrocolpos her respiratory distress improves. Her abdominal distention improves mildly but is still present. She is taken to the operating room for diverting colostomy and vaginostomy. Her vaginostomy drains urine during the postoperative period but her abdominal distention persists. A follow-up ultrasound reveals persistent hydrocolpos and bilateral hydroureteronephrosis.

**What is the next step in her management?**

  A. Bilateral nephrostomy tubes
  B. Vesicostomy
  C. Revision of vaginostomy and evaluation of vaginal septum
  D. Revision of colostomy

*Answer:* C

She is taken back to the operating room where her vaginostomy is revised and a longitudinal vaginal septum is identified and resected. Postoperatively her vaginostomy drains urine and her abdominal distention improves. A follow-up renal ultrasound shows complete resolution of her hydroureteronephrosis.

## 18.1.1  Learning points

Draining hydrocolpos in a child with cloacal malformation can be critical, particularly in the setting of hydronephrosis or respiratory compromise. Percutaneous drainage via a vaginostomy is often adequate initially, but it may not adequately drain the vagina if there is a longitudinal vaginal septum present and the drain is placed only on one side of the septum. Similarly, if a formal vaginostomy is created without evaluating for and removing the vaginal septum, the vaginostomy may not drain the hydrocolpos and additional procedures may be necessary. It is less common that a vesicostomy is necessary on initial drainage but sometimes may be performed. Having experienced surgeons and a multidisciplinary team is important in the initial management of such children to ensure the appropriate intervention is performed and it is carried out in a successful manner in order to prevent unnecessary additional procedures.

# 18.2  Case study 2

A 3-year-old male with rectourethral fistula is diapered for urine. He is doing well with rectal enemas and starting to toilet train for urine. He voids on the toilet but does not have a good stream. He has accidents while sitting on the toilet. His video urodynamics shows a 130-cc capacity bladder with mild detrusor overactivity, a closed bladder neck, and 30 cc PVR. His family is interested in doing antegrade enemas. His current flush regimen is 350 cc saline and 30 mg glycerine. He sits for 45 minutes and does not have accidents between enemas.

**What is the next step in managing this child?**

  A. Proceed with Malone antegrade continent enema
  B. Proceed with Malone and Mitrofanoff using split appendix technique
  C. Continue with rectal enemas and continue to work on toilet training until it is clear this patient will not need a Mitrofanoff, then proceed with Malone

*Answer:* C

## 18.2.1  Learning points

Often, children are ready for a Malone before we know the status of urinary outcomes. The decision to create a Malone should not be made without considering the possible future urologic needs. It is important to wait to use the appendix for a Malone channel until one is sure that the child will not require a Mitrofanoff channel for catheterization of the bladder. Tissue sharing is critical in the surgical planning of complex patients. The appendix should be preferentially used for a Mitrofanoff channel because the alternative to a Mitrofanoff, a Monti channel, requires a bowel resection, bowel anastomosis, and has higher complication rates than Mitrofanoff creation. Additionally, a Malone has other viable alternatives such as cecal flap neo-Malone, cecostomy tube, or continued rectal enemas. If it is not yet known if a child will require a Mitrofanoff, rectal enemas should be continued until that decision can be made. If an antegrade option is required or a child is not tolerating rectal enemas, a temporary cecostomy tube is also an option until the plan for urinary reconstruction can be clarified. Typically by 4 or 5 years of age, the urologic plan can be determined after toilet training efforts have been exhausted. It is critical to fully evaluate both the urologic and gastrointestinal needs of a patient prior to committing the child to an intervention. Frequently these procedures can be done in combination and can allow for tissue sharing [1].

## 18.3  Case study 3

A 15-year-old female with a history of cloacal malformation who underwent primary repair with urogenital separation (leaving the common channel as the urethra and a distal vaginal replacement with small bowel anastomosed to her native upper vagina) presents to urology clinic complaining of urinary incontinence. She previously underwent a bladder neck reconstruction and sling with Mitrofanoff, but recently has developed severe side effects with her anticholinergic medications and has stopped taking them. She now has some leakage per urethra if she does not catheterize her channel every 3 hours. She undergoes urodynamic testing and she has significant detrusor overactivity resulting in leakage per urethra. She was offered intra-detrusor injection of Botox to her bladder for her detrusor overactivity to be done in the operating room. During this visit she was asked about menstruation. She states that she has not yet had a period, but she has had breast development and has developed pubic hair. She is not sexually active. On exam she was found to have severe vaginal stenosis. When she awakes from her urology procedure and is questioned about the vaginal stenosis, she does confirm inability to insert a tampon for menses. She has never been sexually active. She reports her menses are monthly with mild dysmenorrhea, and no heavy menstrual bleeding.

**What is the next step in managing this adolescent?**

    **A.** Introitoplasty
    **B.** Pelvic ultrasound
    **C.** Pelvic ultrasound and introitoplasty
    **D.** Vaginal dilations

*Answer:* C

## 18.3.1  Learning points

When caring for patients with multiorgan system concerns, it is important to systematically assess for any concerns at each visit. Collaborative care across specialties may allow for combination cases, which in the end reduce the patient's total number of trips to the operating room and exposure to anesthesia. In this case, the vaginal stenosis may have been addressed at the time of her urologic procedure. In women who have had a cloacal malformation repair, the assessment of the vaginal introitus diameter (and patency) should be performed at puberty. This ensures distal patency for menstrual egress, ability to use tampons, and the ability to have vaginal intercourse. Of note, an assessment of the patient's pubertal status/stage, with attention to thelarche (breast development) and menarche (first menses), is crucial. Providers should inquire about the patient's menses (menarche, frequency, length and volume of flow, and presence of any dysmenorrhea). Adolescents with anorectal malformations may have associated Müllerian anomalies—some of which may be obstructive. A pelvic ultrasound, and in some cases, a pelvic MRI, is helpful to delineate Müllerian anatomy and evaluate for menstrual outflow obstruction. If introital stenosis is noted, the patient may benefit from an introitoplasty to enlarge the diameter of the introitus. It may be reasonable to attempt dilation of the introitus via patient-directed vaginal dilator use; however, if the tissue is not supple, this may not be adequate and the patient may benefit from an introitoplasty. If there is a narrowing of the introitus, but not complete obstruction, this is not emergent and therefore could be combined with other procedures for the patient's convenience.

## 18.4 Case study 4

A 32-year-old G1P0 presents for her initial prenatal care visit. She has a history of a repaired cloacal malformation. She has a Mitrofanoff for urinary continence. She is continent of stool with an oral bowel management regimen. She has a didelphic uterus and native vagina anastomosed to a colonic neovagina. The longitudinal vaginal septum was resected at the time of her repair. Her renal function is normal. She questions her high-risk obstetrician about the recommended mode of delivery for her baby.

**How would you counsel the patient regarding mode of delivery?**

   **A.** Attempt vaginal delivery
   **B.** Planned cesarean section
   **C.** Cesarean section at onset of labor or rupture of membranes

*Answer:* B

### 18.4.1 Learning points

Fortunately, pregnancy is possible for women with repaired anorectal malformations—including those with cloacal malformations. However, pregnancy outcome data is limited. Ideally women with cloacal malformations should have a preconception counseling visit with a high-risk obstetrician. This allows the obstetrician to evaluate the patient's medical comorbidities, assess the risk of pregnancy, and optimize the patient's health prior to pregnancy. Prenatal care with a high-risk obstetrician is preferred. Women with Müllerian anomalies do have an increased risk of miscarriage, preterm labor, preterm birth, and fetal malpresentation. Monitoring for signs and symptoms of preterm labor is important. Furthermore, coordination and collaboration with the patient's other medical/surgical teams is ideal. Given the rarity of cloacal malformations, not all obstetrician–gynecologists may be familiar with prior surgical procedures—such as a Mitrofanoff or Malone. Coordination with adult urologists and colorectal or general surgeons is paramount. The patient should be encouraged to obtain any available surgical records so that her care team is aware of reconstructed anatomy and all prior procedures. In women with a repaired cloacal malformation, the typically recommended mode of delivery is via cesarean section. This is particularly the case in women with a neovagina. When possible, the cesarean section should be planned—to ensure all available surgical teams are available and have a planned approach. Depending on the patient's reconstructed anatomy typical skin and/or uterine incisions may not be feasible. Care must be taken to avoid any injury to urinary channels. Lastly, given the possibility of associated spinal malformations in women with cloacal malformations, consultation and planning with the obstetric anesthesia team is encouraged.

## 18.5 Overall teaching points

The multidisciplinary model for colorectal care can be a challenge but it is clear that it provides patients with a high level of care in a single setting. Not only does it allow for surgical procedures to be done simultaneously, but also allows for tissue sharing and reduced number of anesthetics. It has been shown that in a multidisciplinary center for colorectal and pelvic reconstruction, the number of procedures a patient undergoes has significantly reduced, the hospital stay has reduced, and the number of postoperative visits has reduced compared to when each procedure was to be performed independently [2]. This multidisciplinary, collaborative approach should begin at the time of birth and continue through adulthood. A systematic evaluation of these complex children should be performed at initial evaluation as in these authors' institution [3]. Children with anorectal malformation have complex colorectal, urologic, and gynecologic systems that require attention from each specialty throughout their lives. If the collaboration between these specialties is achieved, it is possible to streamline the patient's care, consolidate their hospital visit and reduce hospital length of stay, reduce number of procedures, and prevent unnecessary interventions. The importance of this multidisciplinary approach cannot be overemphasized and it is paramount in the success of caring for these complex conditions.

## References

1. Halleran DR, Wood RJ, Vilanova-Sanchez A et al. Simultaneous robotic-assisted laparoscopy for bladder and bowel reconstruction. *J Laparoendosc Adv Surg Tech A*. 2018;28(12):1513–6.
2. Vilanova-Sanchez A, Reck CA, Wood RJ et al. Impact on patient care of a multidisciplinary center specializing in colorectal and pelvic reconstruction. *Front Surg*. 2018;5:68.
3. Vilanova-Sanchez A, Halleran DR, Reck-Burneo CA et al. A descriptive model for a multidisciplinary unit for colorectal and pelvic malformations. *J Pediatr Surg*. 2019;54(3):479–85.

# 19 Bowel management

Michael D. Rollins and Onnalisa Nash

Children who have undergone surgery for Hirschsprung disease, anorectal malformations, and sacrococcygeal teratomas or who have severe medically refractive functional constipation or spine or spinal cord abnormalities may suffer from fecal incontinence or constipation. An individualized and comprehensive bowel management program (BMP) is often required in order to keep the patient clean and in normal underwear. The goal of the program is to find a regimen that achieves social continence and allows the patient to resume daily activities, and get into normal underwear.

The initial question to be determined prior to initiating a BMP is whether the patient suffers from severe constipation with pseudoincontinence or has true fecal incontinence. The BMP will differ based on whether or not the patient has anatomic and physiologic ability to have voluntary bowel control (i.e., normal anal canal, pelvic floor musculature, sphincter function, colonic motility) or if these are congenitally absent, have been damaged during surgery, or have been affected by trauma/tumor. The need for reoperation to address a postoperative complication must be ruled out prior to beginning a BMP. Factors that help predict continence are illustrated in Table 19.1.

Bowel management may take many different forms depending on the clinical setting and available resources. Also, the utility of routine abdominal radiographs to assess stool burden has been debated. However, the patient populations previously mentioned are unique and require more intense involvement by the provider. We also feel that routine abdominal radiographs are necessary in these populations to ensure effective emptying of the colon and rectum in order to avoid complications from severe constipation and fecal impaction such as the development of a megarectum and sigmoid. Follow-up is critical as many patients require frequent minor adjustments to their regimen in order to remain clean. The bowel management strategy described next is used at several specialty centers that have many resources but serves as a guide to any provider caring for patients in need of bowel management.

*Table 19.1* Predictors of continence

| Anorectal malformation | Hirschsprung disease | Functional constipation |
| --- | --- | --- |
| Type of malformation | Quality of sphincters | Normal anal canal, sphincters |
| Quality of sacrum | Intact dentate line | Normal spine |
| Quality of spinal cord | Colonic motility | Colonic dilation |

## 19.1  Bowel management program

The BMP is a week-long outpatient program to treat constipation, hypermotility, or fecal incontinence. The treatment plan is individualized to the patient based on diagnosis, age, current symptoms, previous therapies attempted, and patient/caregiver goals. Patients are placed on either a medical regimen (high-dose stimulant laxatives) or a mechanical regimen (retrograde enemas or antegrade flushes).

A contrast enema precedes the initial clinic visit and an abdominal x-ray is performed the following day prior to the clinic evaluation. These studies provide information regarding the diameter and length of the colon, stool burden, assessment of any potential postoperative problems, and also provide catharsis. Motility can be assessed based on the amount of retained contrast on the x-ray obtained the day after the contrast enema. Treatment plans are determined based on patient history in combination with the findings of these studies. The goal of treatment is for patients to empty their colon daily and to be free of soiling.

Management plans consist of either high-dose senna-based laxatives or a daily large-volume enema. In older patients who have been toilet trained in the past but have soiling from pseudoincontinence or severe constipation without soiling, high-dose laxatives are initiated once the patient has been disimpacted. In patients who have never been toilet trained and have a history of constipation with soiling, patients with a megarectum, or patients with true fecal incontinence, we start with daily large-volume enemas. We feel that it is important for a child to have been previously toilet trained prior to initiating a laxative program. This may be more easily accomplished with the initial use of enemas. Infrequently, children who do not tolerate retrograde enemas or laxatives, such as children with severe autism, undergo appendicostomy as initial therapy.

Laxatives are senna-based and started at a dose of 2 mg/kg (Figure 19.1). If the child does not have a bowel movement within 24 hours a Fleet® enema is administered to evacuate the distal stool and the laxative dose is increased. This process is repeated until the child has one to two soft bowel movements per day. Pectin or water-soluble fiber is administered to patients receiving laxatives if the stool is loose in order to add bulk and increase the efficiency of the laxative. If a child is laxative intolerant, usually due to abdominal cramping, they are switched to enemas.

Initially the patients who are placed on enemas are started on 20 mL/kg of normal saline if ≤30 kg and irritants (soap) are added as needed. For patients >30 kg we start at 600 mL saline

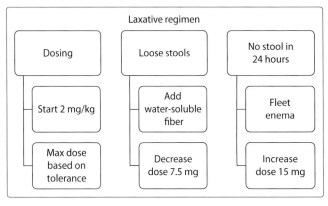

Figure 19.1  Laxative regimen.

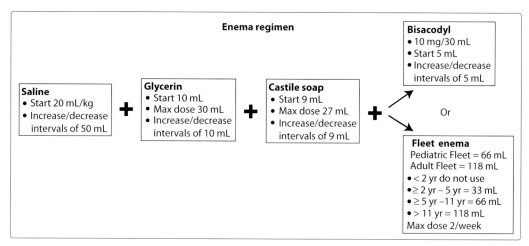

Figure 19.2  Enema regimen.

(Figure 19.2). It is unusual for a patient to need an enema volume >700 mL. If normal saline alone is ineffective the following irritants are added in succession: glycerin (10–30 mL), castile soap (1–3 packets, 9–27 mL), bisacodyl enema (10 mg/30 mL, 15–90 mL), and phosphate (Fleet enema) (30–120 mL). The patients are taught to hold the enema for 10 minutes, and then sit on the toilet for 30–45 minutes. If the patient has a clean distal colon and rectum on abdominal x-ray and a stool accident within several hours of the enema, the enema volume may be too large or the enema might be too strong (irritating). If the abdominal x-ray reveals stool in the rectum and a stool accident occurs within several hours of the enema, the child may not have stayed on the toilet long enough. If the abdominal x-ray reveals stool in the rectum and/or descending colon and accidents happen 12–24 hours after the enema this suggests that the colon was not adequately cleaned. The volume or strength of the enema should be increased. When making changes to enema regimens only one change should be made at a time and the effect is observed.

During the initial week of bowel management, a daily outpatient abdominal x-ray is obtained and the patients/parents are contacted by phone or seen in clinic to evaluate the treatment effect. Treatment regimens are adjusted based on the child's clinical and radiographic response. The treatment plan is considered successful when the abdominal radiograph is clear of stool in the rectum and left colon and the child has had no soiling.

Patients with fecal incontinence and a tendency toward loose stools represent a small and unique group. This clinical scenario most often occurs in patients with long segment Hirschsprung disease who have undergone an endorectal pull-through. These patients have multiple daily stools and a non-dilated colon seen on a contrast enema. Bowel management in this group entails a constipating diet, water-soluble fiber or pectin, anti-diarrheal agents such as loperamide, Lomotil, and/or Levsin, and a daily small-volume saline enema.

## 19.1.1  Follow-up

After the initiation of a successful regimen, children are followed closely for symptomatic changes. Follow-up is performed either by telephone or in clinic at 1 month, 3–6 months, and yearly. Regardless of the type of follow-up visit (in-person or telephone), the families obtain an abdominal x-ray image and any other appropriate testing in preparation for the visit. Follow-up is critical as many patients need minor adjustments to their regimen periodically. After a child has been successful on enemas for 3–6 months we attempt a laxative trial. The week-long laxative trial is performed as described previously. Patients who are repeatedly unsuccessful with laxatives are given the option to continue retrograde enemas and try laxatives again in 6–12 months or undergo an antegrade continence enema (ACE) procedure (appendicostomy or cecostomy). Patients are also encouraged to undergo laxative trials periodically following appendicostomy if they have a diagnosis which would allow them to have voluntary bowel movements.

While segmental colon resection is not our preferred management practice, occasionally children with high laxative requirements or substantial enema needs are offered sigmoidectomy with or without an appendicostomy/cecostomy in an attempt to reduce the laxative dose or enema volume. Approximately 30% of patients do require surgical intervention after bowel management to improve their bowel regimen with either an antegrade option for flushes and/or a colon resection based on colonic manometry studies. Surgical options and indications for bowel management are discussed elsewhere.

## 19.2 Case study 1

A 4-year-old female with a history of Hirschsprung disease (rectosigmoid transition zone, Soave endorectal pull-through) presents for help with bowel management. She wears diapers, has not been toilet trained, stools every 3 days following a Fleet enema, has had two episodes of Hirschsprung-associated enterocolitis post pull-through and is not on regular rectal irrigations. Her PMH is remarkable for developmental delay, deafness, and impaired vision. Other current symptoms include non-bilious vomiting, early satiety, and UTIs. On rectal exam she has good sphincter tone, no anastomotic stricture, and firm stool without fecal impaction. The contrast enema is shown in Figure 19.3a,b. A rectal EUA reveals an intact dentate line and no evidence of a retained muscular Soave cuff. On rectal biopsy, the patient has normal ganglion cells and no hypertrophic nerves.

**What are your recommendations for this patient?**

    **A.** Bowel management with laxatives
    **B.** Bowel management with enemas
    **C.** Redo pull-through
    **D.** Ileostomy

*Answer:* B

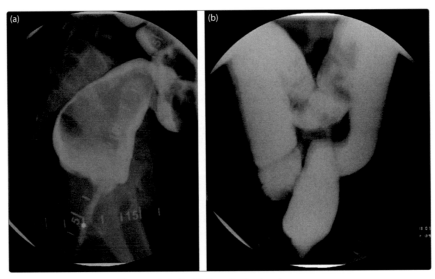

Figure 19.3 (a, b) Case 1: Contrast enema.

### 19.2.1 Key points

- Answer A is not the best choice as this patient has never been toilet trained and has a history of developmental delay which will likely result in unsuccessful bowel management initially.
- Answer C is incorrect because the patient does not have an anatomic or pathologic cause of constipation which is surgically correctable and therefore does not need a redo pull-through.
- Answer D is incorrect as there is moderate rectal dilation on CE with more normal caliber colon proximally suggesting preserved colonic motility. Thus, ileostomy or colostomy would be overly aggressive.

## 19.3  Case study 2

A 10-year-old boy with a lifelong history of constipation. He has an abnormal sacrum and a history of tethered cord release and resection of an anterior meningocele. He has had a rectal biopsy which was normal. Patient is toilet trained for urine and currently has approximately 1 stool per week which is sometimes in the toilet. On rectal exam, he has a skin lined, funnel-type anus but no stenosis, and slightly decreased sphincter tone. His current bowel regimen is 1 capful Miralax daily and 1–2 squares of Ex-Lax daily and has daily stool accidents. Contrast enema is shown in Figure 19.4a–c. The patient refused to try retrograde enemas and underwent a high-dose laxative trial but continued to have accidents.

**What is your next recommendation?**

- **A.** Sigmoid resection
- **B.** Laparoscopic-assisted Malone appendicostomy
- **C.** Ileostomy
- **D.** I don't have enough information

*Answer:* B

### 19.3.1  Key points

- The patient has failed laxatives and has a dilated rectum with redundant sigmoid colon on contrast enema. This suggests chronic fecal impaction and likely dysfunctional sigmoid colon. He also has other anatomical defects which make his potential for bowel control questionable. He would be a good candidate for bowel management with large-volume enemas but refuses the enema. Thus, answer B is the best next step.

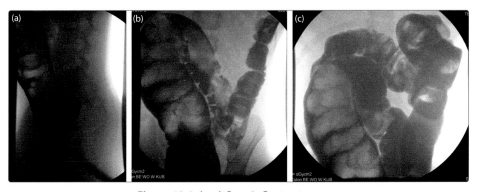

Figure 19.4  (a–c) Case 2: Contrast enema.

- Answers A and C would not be appropriate as initial management strategies without motility studies which demonstrate either focal dysfunction of the sigmoid colon or severe dysfunction of the entire colon. Also, in this patient with sacral and spinal cord abnormalities, mechanical cleansing of the colon with a daily enema will likely be needed for a longer period. Therefore, if a sigmoid resection is performed, an appendicostomy would also be recommended for antegrade enemas.
- Answer D may be appropriate if colonic motility testing is immediately available to guide further recommendations.

An appendicostomy is performed and large volume antegrade enemas initiated with 400 mL of saline + 20 mL of glycerin. He has a good response to the flush but has an accident approximately 6 hours prior to the next flush. Abdominal x-ray the morning after his evening flush shows stool in the rectum and sigmoid.

**How would you adjust the antegrade flush?**

    **A.** Decrease the volume of saline
    **B.** Decrease the amount of glycerin
    **C.** Increase the volume of saline
    **D.** Add a Fleet enema to the enema solution daily

*Answer:* C

## 19.3.2 Key points

- The patient has a good initial response to the flush but has an accident many hours later. This history and the findings on abdominal x-ray suggest incomplete emptying of the colon. In this setting, increasing the volume of saline in the enema is the next best step.
- Addition of a Fleet enema to the bag of enema solution may rarely be indicated if other additives such as glycerin and castile soap have been added and the patient needs a stronger enema. However, the addition of a Fleet enema should not be used in a patient with renal insufficiency as it may result in hyperphosphatemia. Also, Fleet enema should not be added more than twice per week due to the risk of colitis.

## 19.4 Case study 3

A 7-year-old, 42 kg, girl born with a rectovestibular fistula and absent vagina repaired by PSARP and sigmoid colon neovagina presents with nighttime urinary incontinence and constipation with soiling. Her sacrum and spinal cord are normal and she has not had any urinary tract infections. She is toilet trained but has daily smears of stool in her underwear and daily abdominal pain. Her mother gives her 1 square of Ex-Lax intermittently if she does not stool for 2 days. She recently completed first grade and otherwise has had no other complaints. On exam, the abdomen is somewhat full, the sigmoid neovagina is well healed without mucosal prolapse, and the neoanus is appropriately positioned without stricture or prolapse. She has a good gluteal crease and good sphincter tone. An abdominal x-ray is shown in Figure 19.5.

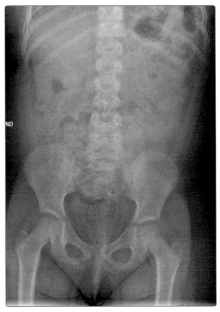

**Figure 19.5** Case 3: Abdominal radiograph.

**What is your treatment recommendation?**

A. 1 Square (15 mg) of Ex-Lax daily
B. Daily large volume enema
C. Intermittent catheterization to manage her urinary incontinence
D. Daily high-dose stimulant laxatives (1–2 mg/kg/day of Ex-Lax) with daily water-soluble fiber (1 tbsp. pectin t.i.d.)

*Answer:* D

### 19.4.1 Key points

- Answer D is the best answer for this patient with good potential for bowel control due to the favorable anorectal malformation, normal sacrum, normal spine, good gluteal musculature (good gluteal crease) and sphincter tone, and uncomplicated, well-performed PSARP. She is also able to sense that she needs to have a bowel movement and go to the toilet. Water-soluble fiber is frequently added to the laxative regimen to add stool bulk and increase the effectiveness.
- Answer A is incorrect as patients born with anorectal malformations usually have some degree of colonic dysmotility and need larger doses of stimulant laxative than generally recommended. While many parents worry about potential side effects of such high laxative doses, no serious adverse effects have been reported.
- Answer C is incorrect because this patient has no history to suggest neurogenic bladder or abnormal urinary continence mechanism. Enuresis is common with severe constipation and usually resolves when bowel management is optimized.

## 19.5 Case study 4

An 8-year-old boy was referred for constipation with soiling. His mother reports that he passed meconium in the first day of life and stooled regularly as an infant. He was toilet trained for stool and urine between 3 and 4 years of age but has had constipation for several years and attends regular school without difficulty. He is on 1 capful of Miralax twice a day and has at least one small bowel movement in the toilet daily. He has stool leakage multiple times per day and occasional nighttime bedwetting. No urinary accidents during the day. He has a good appetite and denies abdominal pain. On exam, the abdomen is soft, non-tender, and non-distended, rectal exam is normal. Anorectal manometry and spinal MRI have previously been performed and are normal. Contrast enema performed the day before his clinic visit (Figure 19.6a,b) and his abdominal radiograph the following day (Figure 19.7).

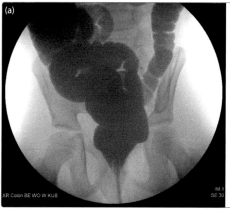 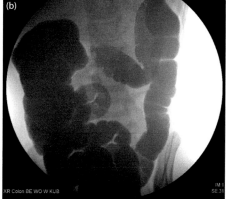

Figure 19.6 (a, b) Case 4: Contrast enema.

**The most effective initial treatment for this patient's soiling would be:**

**A.** Referral to a psychiatrist
**B.** Biofeedback
**C.** Bowel management with high-dose stimulant laxatives
**D.** Placement of a cecostomy for antegrade enemas

*Answer:* C

## 19.5.1  Key points

- Answer C is the best initial management. This patient has functional constipation but has a history of good stooling patterns. He has no history, physical exam, or manometric findings concerning Hirschsprung disease and no radiographic evidence of an occult spinal dysraphism.
- Patients who present with constipation and pseudoincontinence (overflow incontinence) frequently have been labeled with a psychiatric diagnosis or the parents will report that they are "too lazy" to go to the toilet or are "distracted" while playing and forget to go to the toilet. It is not normal for a child to soil themselves and is usually the result of a hypomotile colon rather than a behavioral issue. Therefore answer A would be incorrect.
- Biofeedback may be helpful as an adjunct to stimulant laxative therapy but takes many sessions over a period of time and would not be the most effective initial treatment.

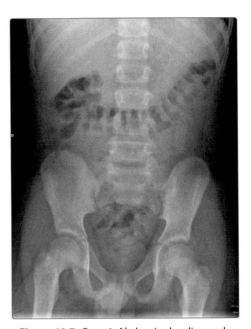

Figure 19.7  Case 4: Abdominal radiograph.

- A conduit for antegrade enemas, such as a cecostomy, would not be indicated as initial treatment for a neurodevelopmentally normal patient with normal anatomy who has not undergone a laxative trial.
- Although not listed as an answer option, starting daily retrograde enemas would also be a reasonable approach initially given the history of daily soiling.

## Further reading

1. Bischoff A, Levitt MA, Bauer C, Jackson L, Holder M, Pena A. Treatment of fecal incontinence with a comprehensive bowel management program. *J Pediatr Surg.* 2009;44(6):1278–83.
2. Levitt MA, Kant A, Pena A. The morbidity of constipation in patients with anorectal malformations. *J Pediatr Surg.* 2010;45(6):1228–33.
3. Levitt MA, Pena A. Pediatric fecal incontinence: A surgeon's perspective. *Pediatr Rev.* 2010;31(3):91–101.
4. Gasior A, Reck C, Vilanova-Sanchez A et al. Surgical management of functional constipation: An intermediate report of a new approach using a laparoscopic sigmoid resection combined with Malone appendicostomy. *J Pediatr Surg.* 2018;53(6):1160–2.
5. Huber J, Barnhart DC, Liechty S, Zobell S, Rollins MD. Characteristics of the contrast enema do not predict an effective bowel management regimen for patients with constipation or fecal incontinence. *Cureus.* 2016;8(8):e745.
6. Russell KW, Barnhart DC, Zobell S, Scaife ER, Rollins MD. Effectiveness of an organized bowel management program in the management of severe chronic constipation in children. *J Pediatr Surg.* 2015;50(3):444–7.
7. Levitt MA, Dickie B, Pena A. The Hirschsprungs patient who is soiling after what was considered a "successful" pull-through. *Semin Pediatr Surg.* 2012;21(4):344–53.

# 20 Evaluation of continence in children with Hirschsprung disease and anorectal malformation

Michael D. Rollins, Richard J. Wood, and Victoria Lane

## 20.1 Case study 1

A 5-year-old boy with a history of Hirschsprung disease and a previous Duhamel pull-through at the age of 3 months presents for evaluation. He initially did well following his surgery, was continent of stool, and potty trained without difficulty. In the last 12 months he has been having recurrent episodes of abdominal distension and fecal incontinence. These intermittent episodes have been managed with rectal washouts.

**What is the next step in your management?**

    **A.** Medical management of his constipation and overflow incontinence
    **B.** Appendicostomy to avoid the need for rectal washouts
    **C.** Contrast enema
    **D.** Examination under anesthesia to assess the dentate line

*Answer:* C

### 20.1.1 Learning points

1. The fact that the child initially did well following the Duhamel pull-through would suggest that the symptoms are unlikely to be related to an operative complication. The patient's symptoms have developed over the last 12 months, which should raise the suspicion for a Duhamel pouch problem. This patient may have a rectal spur, which is intermittently filling with stool, causing compression and a degree of obstruction. Another possible etiology is a dysfunctional pouch which has become dilated leading to abdominal distension and enterocolitis symptoms. This can be managed with a rectal washout, but the rectal spur or dilated pouch is likely to refill causing the cyclical pattern of abdominal distension and overflow incontinence. A contrast enema will demonstrate a dysfunctional pouch, a rectal spur, and help to exclude a twisted pull-through, which should also be in the differential diagnosis.
2. Once the contrast enema has been performed and a rectal spur has been identified an examination under anesthesia should be performed. It is important to ensure that the dentate line is intact and where indicated a transition zone pull-through should be excluded with a repeat rectal biopsy; however, in this case a problematic Duhamel pouch is more likely.

## 20.2 Case study 2

A 10-year-old boy comes to your center for evaluation. He has had previous surgery for Hirschsprung disease, but the procedure is not known. There are no visible scars on the abdomen.

    He complains of fecal incontinence, and the parents report that he has never been potty trained and is still in diapers.

**What is the next step in your management?**

    **A.** Rectal biopsy as this is most likely a transition zone pull-through
    **B.** Contrast enema to assess for a Duhamel pouch
    **C.** Examination under anesthesia to assess the dentate line and sphincters
    **D.** Rectal examination in the office to assess for a Soave cuff

*Answer:* C

### 20.2.1 Learning points

1. Patients with a transition zone pull-through or a Soave cuff are more likely to present with features of obstruction, rather than incontinence.
2. A Duhamel pull-through requires an abdominal approach (laparoscopic assisted or open). The fact that this patient has no abdominal wall scars excludes this particular procedure.
3. This patient is presenting with life-long features of true fecal incontinence. This raises the concern of damage to the dentate line, anal sphincters, or both during his pull-through operation. The first steps in his evaluation should be an examination under anesthesia to assess the presence or absence of the dentate line and quality of the sphincters.

## 20.3  Case study 3

A 5-year-old boy with a history of Hirschsprung disease who underwent a Swenson pull-through at the age of 3 months presents for evaluation. He initially did well and potty trained successfully, but recently has been having problems with fecal incontinence. He has multiple liquid stools daily and often has trouble getting to the toilet in time to avoid an accident. The referring physician felt that he was suffering from constipation with overflow pseudo-incontinence and has started a low-dose stimulant laxative. This has resulted in abdominal cramping and worsening diarrhea.

His workup at the referring center has included an examination under anesthesia which was normal and a rectal biopsy which was reported as normal. The rectal biopsy findings have been confirmed by your histopathologist.

You decide to perform a contrast enema to assess the colon. The contrast enema shows an empty, non-dilated, foreshortened colon.

**What is your next step in medical management?**

A.  Stool softening laxatives
B.  Increased the stimulant laxatives
C.  Loperamide
D.  Rectal enemas
E.  Appendicostomy

*Answer:* C

### 20.3.1  Learning points

1. Stool softeners and stimulant laxatives are not indicated for this patient. He is not constipated. The contrast enema findings and clinical symptoms would be consistent with a hypermotile colon, which explains the exacerbation of symptoms with the introduction of low-dose stimulant laxatives.
2. The first step in management should be daily loperamide and a constipating diet to slow the colonic transit time.
3. If the constipating diet and loperamide fail to resolve the incontinence, more aggressive bowel management with a daily small volume enema would be indicated.

## 20.4  Summary (Cases 1–3)

To accurately evaluate a child following corrective surgery for Hirschsprung disease, it is important to understand the fundamental differences between the most common operations (Swenson, Duhamel, and Soave procedures). The objective of all of these procedures is to remove aganglionic bowel and pull-through normal ganglionic bowel, with the preservation of the anal canal and dentate line. A good understanding of the complications associated with the different procedures is necessary in order to be able to evaluate a child in a systematic and comprehensive way.

Functional problems following pull-through surgery can include constipation, enterocolitis, and fecal incontinence. Children with HD are born with an intact sphincter mechanism and dentate line and therefore should be continent. Fecal incontinence may be due to overflow pseudo-incontinence from severe constipation, loose stools from rapid colonic transit time following an extensive resection, or due to an intraoperative complication resulting in damage to the dentate line and/or sphincters.

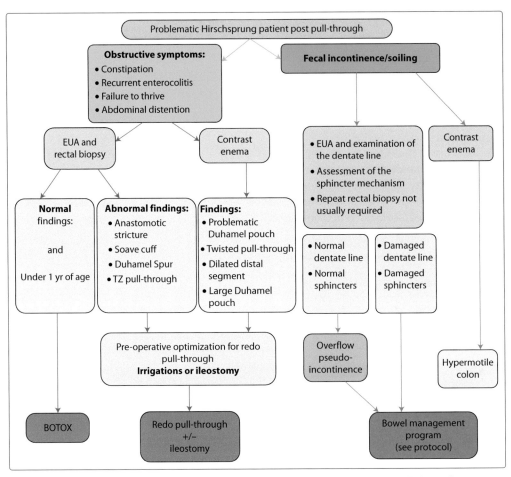

**Figure 20.1** Evaluation of the problematic Hirschsprung patient post pull-through.

It is important to have an investigative algorithm when assessing patients with problems post pull-through procedure. A careful history and physical examination can exclude certain pathologies, but ultimately many will require a contrast enema and examination under anesthesia±repeat rectal biopsy. A suggested algorithm is shown in Figure 20.1.

## 20.5  Case study 4

A 5-year-old girl with a history of a rectovestibular fistula and underwent corrective surgery in the first year of life presents with fecal incontinence. She has been toilet trained for urine.

**What additional information is most useful in predicting her likelihood of fecal continence?**

   A.  Current medication
   B.  Sacral and spinal anatomy
   C.  Position of neo-anus within the sphincter mechanism, presence of rectal prolapse, and quality of sphincters
   D.  Additional VACTERL associations

*Answers:* B, C

On physical exam, she has no evidence of rectal prolapse or stricture of the anoplasty and the position of the neo-anus appears appropriate. On review of her imaging, she has a sacral ratio of 0.68 and no evidence of a tethered cord/spinal dysraphism on the MRI.

**What would be your next step in the management of this child?**

A. Contrast enema
B. Examination under anesthesia with the evaluation of sphincter mechanism
C. Anorectal manometry

*Answer:* A

## 20.5.1 Learning points

1. There are numerous factors that contribute to the continence potential of a child with an anorectal malformation. It can be difficult to predict which has the most influence; however, an understanding of these factors can help in the evaluation of a child with soiling postoperatively. In a girl with a rectovestibular fistula and normal spine/spinal cord, severe constipation is common. This may result in overflow pseudo-incontinence. A contrast enema will help make this diagnosis by demonstrating findings such as a dilated rectum and large stool burden.

2. The type of anorectal malformation and the relative severity on the spectrum of defects is helpful in predicting fecal continence. More severe defects are often associated with a sacral or spinal cord anomaly, poor muscle development, and poor sphincters. This is likely to result in true fecal incontinence.

3. Complications following PSARP need to be understood. Often in a child with good potential for bowel control, such as this patient (rectovestibular fistula, normal spine and sacrum), there may be an anatomical problem contributing to incontinence. Examples include a mislocated neo-anus with or without rectal prolapse. If one suspects that the anoplasty is mislocated, an exam under anesthesia with stimulation of the anal sphincters is necessary.

## 20.6 Case study 5

A 10-year-old boy presents with fecal incontinence following a PSARP for a rectoprostatic fistula. He has previously undergone surgery for a tethered spinal cord and has an abnormal sacrum with a sacral ratio of 0.4. In the last 6 months he has developed daytime and nighttime enuresis. On physical exam, he has a relatively flat bottom and poor sphincter tone.

**What would be your next step in management?**

A. Given the severe anorectal malformation and spinal abnormalities, I would not expect this boy to be continent and I would manage conservatively
B. Examination under anesthesia, MRI spine, and renal ultrasound
C. Contrast enema to evaluate the colon
D. MRI spine
E. Examination under anesthesia

*Answer:* B

## 20.6.1 Learning points

1. This patient has the potential to have a number of complications and requires a systematic workup. The history of 'new onset' enuresis in the last 6 months requires

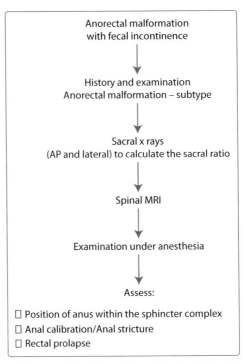

**Figure 20.2** Assessment of anorectal malformation patient with fecal incontinence post repair.

urgent assessment with spinal MRI and renal US with (post void residual measurement) as this may be indicative of:

- Re-tethering of the spinal cord
- Urinary tract dysfunction with poor bladder emptying with secondary urinary tract infection or dilatation of the upper tracts due to a neuropathic bladder

2. In any patient with an anorectal malformation, it is important to assess the anatomy post PSARP to ensure that the neo-anus is appropriately sited within the sphincter mechanism, calibrate the anus to ensure there is no anal stricture and assess for rectal prolapse (Figure 20.2).

## Further reading

1. Chatoorgoon K, Pena A, Lawal TA, Levitt M. The problematic Duhamel pouch in Hirschsprung's disease: Manifestations and treatment. *Eur J Pediatr Surg.* 2011 Dec;21(6):366–9.
2. Levitt MA, Dickie B, Pena A. The Hirschsprung patient who is soiling after what was considered a "successful" pull-through. *Semin Pediatr Surg.* 2012;21:344–53.
3. Dasgupta R, Langer JC. Evaluation and management of persistent problems after surgery for Hirschsprung disease in a child. *J Pediatr Gastroenterol Nutr.* 2008;46(1):13–9.
4. Lane et al. A standardized approach for the assessment and treatment of internationally adopted children with a previously repaired anorectal malformation (ARM). *J Pediatr Surg.* 2016;51:1864–70.
5. Kaul A, Garza JM, Connor FL et al. Colonic hyperactivity results in frequent fecal soiling in a subset of children after surgery for Hirschsprung disease. *J Pediatr Gastroenterol Nutr.* 2011;52(4):433–6.
6. Saadai P, Trappey AF, Goldstein AM et al. American Pediatric Surgical Association Hirschsprung Disease Interest Group. Guidelines for the management of postoperative soiling in children with Hirschsprung disease. *Pediatr Surg Int.* 2019 Aug;35(8):829–34.

**21** 

# Minor anal pathology: Rectal prolapse, perianal abscesses, hemorrhoids, anal fissures, and pilonidal disease

Caitlin A. Smith, Alessandra C. Gasior, and Devin R. Halleran

## 21.1  Case study 1

A 5-year-old girl is referred to your clinic for rectal prolapse. She had several episodes at home that spontaneously reduced. However, in the last week she was brought to the emergency department for an episode of rectal prolapse that required manual reduction. As per the parents, she has a bowel movement approximately once every 10 days and strains significantly with each episode.

**What is the next best step in management?**

  A. MRI of the pelvis
  B. Surgical rectopexy
  C. Constipation management
  D. Injection sclerotherapy

*Answer:* C

### 21.1.1 Learning points

- Rectal prolapse is not uncommon in children. The maximal incidence usually coincides with the toilet training age group [1]. In this age group, gender incidence is almost equivalent between males and females. However, in adults, women have approximately six times the incidence when compared to men [2]. The management of these patients should be primarily geared toward determining the underlying diagnosis that predisposes the child to this condition. A thorough history and physical exam should be performed geared toward determining the potential cause of rectal prolapse.
- Chronic constipation is the main cause of rectal prolapse in this age group. If constipation is determined to be the underlying etiology, conservative management with stool softeners is usually all that is needed for treatment. Other causes of rectal prolapse included in the differential diagnosis include ileocolic intussusception [3], chronic diarrhea conditions that increase bowel motility such as Salmonella, Shigella, and *Escherichia coli* [1] and congenital conditions such as cystic fibrosis, myelomeningocele, spina bifida, and Hirschsprung disease [4]. In a review of 54 pediatric patients with rectal prolapse, chronic constipation was the underlying cause in 28%, followed by chronic diarrheal illness in 20%, cystic fibrosis in 11%, and neurologic or anatomic cause in 24% [5]. Other more rare causes of rectal prolapse in children include prolapsing rectal polyp or duplication cyst and rectal hemorrhoids [6,7].

## 21.2 Case study 2

A 10-year-old girl presents to the emergency department for her fifth episode of protrusion of full thickness extrusion of tissue per rectum. On physical exam she has concentric folds in the prolapsed mucosa. She has been on constipation management with stool softeners for the past year with improvement in stool consistency and no further straining with bowel movements. The family is frustrated with these frequent hospital visits and is interested in procedural information.

**What next step would you recommend?**

  A. Posterior sagittal rectopexy
  B. Laparoscopic rectopexy
  C. Thiersch's anal cerclage
  D. Sclerotherapy

*Answer:* D

### 21.2.1 Learning points

- While medical management geared toward treating the underlying comorbidity is the mainstay of treatment for rectal prolapse in children, there are patients who fail this treatment strategy and will need procedural intervention. While a multitude of surgical procedures have been described for this condition, the main surgical options include sclerotherapy, Thiersch's anal cerclage, laparoscopic suture rectopexy, and posterior sagittal rectopexy.

- Sclerotherapy is the recommended first-line therapy for recalcitrant rectal prolapse for several reasons. The benefits of sclerotherapy include short procedural time, relatively painless for the patient, and few associated complications [8]. Sclerotherapy is performed by injecting a sclerosant, such as saline, submucosally and above the dentate line [9]. This injection results in an inflammatory response in the perirectal tissue. With increased inflammation in this area, the rectal wall becomes adherent to the perirectal tissue and prevents recurrence of prolapse. Multiple other sclerosants have been described such as ethyl alcohol, phenol, and dextrose at various strengths [9,10]. These agents have varying success and complication rates. Repeat sclerotherapy is also sometimes required.
- Thiersch's anal cerclage is a procedure in which a circumferential suture is placed at the anal opening. Electrocautery is used to create a small opening at the posterior aspect of the skin and anal mucosa. An absorbable suture is tied over a Hegar dilator. This procedure can also be combined with sclerotherapy [11]. The overall success rate has been described as 90%, however, repeat procedures are often required [12].
- Laparoscopic suture rectopexy is performed by suturing the perirectal tissues to the presacral region. This ensures correct anatomic position of the rectum, thereby decreasing rectal prolapse. This procedure can also be performed in an open manner. The benefits of a laparoscopic approach are same as those for all laparoscopic procedures including decreased pain and earlier return of bowel function [13].
- The posterior sagittal rectopexy is initiated through a posterior sagittal midline incision. The rectum is identified and the rectal wall is sutured to the cartilage of the coccyx and sacrum. The advantages of this procedure include elimination of the intra-abdominal surgical component, and the ability to reconstruct the sphincter muscles if they are stretched or attenuated [14]. The recurrence rate of posterior sagittal rectopexy has been reported anywhere from 35% to 70% and the success rate is likely related to the underlying anatomical cause [15].

## 21.3  Case study 3

An 8-month-old otherwise healthy infant presented to the emergency department for the evaluation of a swelling near the anus noted by the parents during a diaper change. On physical exam the swelling was found to be approximately 1 cm in diameter and fluctuant on palpation. An incision and drainage procedure is performed at the bedside. Approximately 2 months later the family returns to the emergency department for the evaluation of swelling in the identical location as the previous episode. The next best step in management is:

A. Antibiotics
B. Repeat incision and drainage with planned rectal exam under anesthesia for evaluation with fistula-in-ano
C. Colonoscopy
D. Observation

*Answer:* B

### 21.3.1  Learning points

- Perianal abscesses are common in infants. These are usually superficial and small and originate immediately around the anus. The perianal abscess originates from the anal glands located at the dentate line [16]. Many perianal abscesses in infants can be managed nonoperatively with warm compresses to encourage drainage and oral antibiotics. There is an increased risk of development of fistula-in-ano with initial surgical drainage of perianal abscesses [17,18]. In a study of 140 patients by Christison-Lagay et al., 83 patients underwent abscess drainage procedures. Of those 83 patients, 50 developed fistula-in-ano. Of the 57 who did not have a drainage procedure, only 9 developed fistula-in-ano [18].

- Most pediatric perianal abscesses will not demonstrate fistula-in-ano on initial presentation. If a fistula is suspected due to recurrent symptoms or abscesses in the same location, an exam under anesthesia should be performed in order to rule out a fistula as an underlying cause. While performing a fistulotomy in the setting of incision and drainage for a recurrent abscess does decrease the risk of further recurrent abscess [20], it also carries the increased risk of sphincter injury and incontinence and therefore is recommended to be performed under a separate procedure once the infection has been successfully treated.

## 21.4  Case study 4

A 16-year-old male presents with painless blood per rectum. He states that this has been happening for the past 3 months. The blood stains the toilet paper when he wipes. He states he has a history of hard stools and he has a bowel movement every 5–7 days.

**What is your next best step in management?**

- **A.** Colonoscopy
- **B.** Trial of stimulant laxatives and fiber
- **C.** Anoscopy in the clinic
- **D.** Endorectal ultrasound under anesthesia

*Answer:* C

### 21.4.1  Learning points

- Evaluation for hemorrhoids is a common anorectal complaint in the pediatric population. Oftentimes the surgeon will need to evaluate rectal polyps, skin tags, and anal condyloma that may be misinterpreted for hemorrhoids. Therefore, correct diagnosis after a thorough history and physical examination is key. An examination under anesthesia may be necessary to achieve a proper anoscopy exam if this cannot be done in the office setting.
- Chronic constipation may lead to hemorrhoids in the adolescent populations. This is due to chronic straining or sitting on the toilet for prolonged periods of time. The common symptom from a hemorrhoid is painless bleeding with wiping or stooling. Hemorrhoids are graded from I to IV. Grade I hemorrhoids are inflamed but do not prolapse. Grade II hemorrhoids prolapse but reduce on their own. Grade III hemorrhoids prolapse but only reduce with manual reduction. Finally, grade IV hemorrhoids do not reduce.
- Most pediatric hemorrhoids will resolve with lifestyle modification. The primary treatment of hemorrhoids is lifestyle and behavior modifications to avoid constipation, avoid straining, and avoid prolonged periods of sitting on the toilet. Additionally, 64 oz. of water per day, and 25–35 g of water-soluble fiber should be recommended. Liver failure is another less common etiology of hemorrhoids. In this setting, treatment of the elevated portal pressures is necessary as rectal varices may be confused with rectal hemorrhoids.
- For patients with symptoms that are refractory to a trial of conservative medical management, traditional excision technique with open or closed hemorrhoidectomy may be employed. Hemorrhoidectomy is very painful in the adult population and typically has even worse tolerance in the pediatric population. Hemorrhoidectomy carries risk of

anal stenosis if more than 1 column is removed at a time [21]. Postoperatively, patients with increasing rectal pain, fevers, urinary retention, and bleeding must be taken back to the operating room immediately for an exam under anesthesia to rule out pelvic sepsis.

## 21.5 Case study 5

A 16-year-old female presents to your clinic with a 2-week history of rectal pain. She noticed some blood on the toilet paper with wiping. Her rectal exam is limited due to pain, but you are able to see a tear in the posterior midline of the rectum with underlying muscle fibers exposed.

**What is your treatment plan?**

A. Incision and drainage
B. Sphincterotomy
C. Fistulectomy
D. 2% nifedipine ointment

*Answer:* D

### 21.5.1 Learning points

- Perianal disease includes inflammation at or near the anus with skin tags, fissures, fistula, abscesses, or stenosis. This can cause symptoms such as pain, bleeding, itching, pus drainage as well as fecal incontinence [22]. The spectrum of these disease processes includes a wide range of mild disease for some and debilitating for others with sepsis, compromise of sexual function, and loss of fecal continence leading to a poor quality of life. The severe conditions may require a temporary or even permanent fecal diversion with ostomy.
- Skin tags are fleshy appendages from the anus that are associated with anal fissures. Generally the skin tags range from small to large fleshy "elephant ears." It is generally recommended that these be left alone as surgical excision can lead to poor wound healing and the skin tag will likely recur [23]. Fissures are common in children with constipation after the passage of a hard, firm stool that causes the anoderm to tear, resulting in a fissure. These typically occur in the posterior or anterior midline. The atypical presentation of a fissure in the lateral position should trigger an investigation of atypical causes of fissures including Crohn's disease, tuberculosis, HIV, leukemia, anal neoplasm, and trauma. Fissures are very painful and the patients have pain with subsequent defecation. This anal pain can cause a detrimental cycle of pain followed by stool withholding, worsening constipation with bulky dry stools that reinjure the fissure after passage. Anal fissures occur in 20%–30% of patients with Crohn's disease and are often located posteriorly. Symptoms include pain, bleeding, itching, and drainage. The first-line treatment in the management of fissures includes avoiding constipation by increasing water intake, sitz baths, and the addition of supplemental fiber. The second-line therapy is the treatment of the fissure with topical agents. Fissures generally respond to calcium channel blockers or botulinum toxin injection and sitz baths [24]. In a review of 106 patients, 93.4% had resolution of symptoms after a 4-week treatment course of nifedipine gel with lidocaine. Recurrence rate was 6.6% [25]. Fissures that are nonresponsive to conservative measures or recurrent after treatment with calcium channel blockers should then be treated with an intersphincteric botulinum toxin injection. Rarely would these measures fail, negating the need for a lateral internal sphincterotomy. This procedure is not recommended in the pediatric population as their sphincter complex is very thin and the risk for permanent fecal incontinence is prohibitively high [21]. Additionally, the presence of multiple fissures should prompt an investigation for a non-accidental trauma.

## 21.6 Case study 6

A 17-year-old male presents to his pediatrician with 2 weeks of pain located in the sacrococcygeal area. The pain is worse with sitting, and he has noticed drainage on the back of his underwear. On gluteal examination, he is hirsute and has a fluctuant, tender mass located at the superior aspect of the gluteal cleft.

**What is the next step in management?**

- **A.** Incision and drainage
- **B.** Excision with primary off-midline closure
- **C.** Excision with flap closure
- **D.** Hair depilation (e.g., shaving or laser hair removal)

*Answer:* A

### 21.6.1 Learning points

- Pilonidal disease is a chronic infectious disease that commonly affects young adults with an estimated incidence of 26 per 100,000 people [26]. The etiology is believed to be the result of a chronic foreign body reaction to loose hairs that insert in the superior aspect of the gluteal cleft, resulting in epithelialized tracts and midline pits [27].
- The disease is characterized by acute episodes of abscess, cyst, or painful, inflamed sinuses, followed by periods of quiescence that may last years. When present, a pilonidal abscess should be treated with an incision and drainage. After the resolution of the acute episode of disease, the decision to proceed with an excision should be individualized for each patient, but is generally not indicated after a single episode [28].

## 21.7 Case study 7

A 25-year-old female presents with 2 months of pain and drainage from the area. She has had several similar episodes over the past 10 years that have resolved without intervention. The episodes severely impact her lifestyle and she wishes to pursue an intervention that decreases her risk of future episodes of disease.

**What would you recommend?**

- **A.** Incision and drainage
- **B.** Long-term antibiotics
- **C.** Topical antibiotic ointment
- **D.** Wide surgical excision

*Answer:* D

### 21.7.1 Learning points

- At present, there are no formal guidelines regarding the surgical management of pilonidal disease, however, it is generally believed that patients with multiple previous episodes of disease are more likely to experience subsequent recurrence [28]. The decision to perform an excision should be made taking into consideration the patient's history of disease, their tolerance of their pilonidal symptoms, and their willingness to accept the risk of postoperative wound complications [29]. Patients with mild symptoms and infrequent disease episodes might be more amenable to conservative management compared to those with severe, frequent disease recurrence.

- The patient in the question has a history of several disease episodes, thus making future episodes of disease likely. Furthermore, she reports that the morbidity of her disease significantly impairs her daily functioning. This patient therefore would be a good candidate for an excision.
- There are several techniques available (e.g., midline primary closure, off-midline primary closure, secondary closure, flap closure, etc.) and little good evidence exists to support one technique over another [30–33].

## 21.8 Case study 8

The patient in the aforementioned case returns for routine 3-month follow-up after surgery. She had an uncomplicated postoperative course and her incision has healed well. The patient asks about strategies to prevent future disease recurrence.

**What would you recommend?**

- **A.** Prophylactic antibiotics
- **B.** Hair depilation (e.g., shaving or laser hair removal)
- **C.** Expectant management
- **D.** Sitz baths

*Answer:* B

### 21.8.1 Learning points

- Multiple studies demonstrate that hair depilation of the pilonidal area is associated with a decreased risk of pilonidal disease recurrence. Depilation decreases the amount of free hairs in the region which are believed to insert underneath the skin and causes the foreign body reaction believed to have caused episodes of pilonidal disease [34]. This practice is recommended by the American Society of Colon and Rectal Surgeons to decrease the risk of future recurrence [35].
- Small studies suggest a benefit of laser hair removal, although whether this offers benefit over traditional techniques such as shaving has not been proven but is currently being studied [19,36].

## References

1. Rentea RM, St Peter SD. Pediatric rectal prolapse. *Clin Colon Rectal Surg*. 2018 Mar;31(2):108–16.
2. Corman ML. Rectal prolapse in children. *Dis Colon Rectum*. 1985;28(07):535–9.
3. Chen R, Zhao H, Sang X, Mao Y, Lu X, Yang Y. Severe adult ileosigmoid intussusception prolapsing from the rectum: A case report. *Cases J*. 2008;1(01):198.
4. Jacobs LK, Lin YJ, Orkin BA. The best operation for rectal prolapse. *Surg Clin North Am*. 1997;77(01):49–70.
5. Zempsky WT, Rosenstein BJ. The cause of rectal prolapse in children. *Am J Dis Child*. 1988 Mar;142(3):338–9.
6. Khushbakht S, ul Haq A. Rectal duplication cyst: A rare cause of rectal prolapse in a toddler. *J Coll Physicians Surg Pak*. 2015;25(12):909–10.
7. Mönig SP, Selzner M, Schmitz-Rixen T. Peutz-Jeghers syndrome in a child. Prolapse of a large colonic polyp through the anus. *J Clin Gastroenterol*. 1997;25(04):703–4.
8. Green D. Mechanism of action of sclerotherapy. *Semin Dermatol*. 1993;12(02):88–97.
9. Abeş M, Sarihan H. Injection sclerotherapy of rectal prolapse in children with 15 percent saline solution. *Eur J Pediatr Surg*. 2004 Apr;14(2):100–2.

10. Chan WK, Kay SM, Laberge JM, Gallucci JG, Bensoussan AL, Yazbeck S. Injection sclerotherapy in the treatment of rectal prolapse in infants and children. *J Pediatr Surg.* 1998;33(02):255–8.

11. Gabriel WB. Thiersch's operation for anal incontinence and minor degrees of rectal prolapse. *Am J Surg.* 1953;86(05):583–90.

12. Flum AS, Golladay ES, Teitelbaum DH. Recurrent rectal prolapse following primary surgical treatment. *Pediatr Surg Int.* 2010;26(04):427–31.

13. Senagore AJ. Management of rectal prolapse: The role of laparoscopic approaches. *Semin Laparosc Surg.* 2003;10(04):197–202.

14. Peña A, Hong A. The posterior sagittal trans-sphincteric and trans-rectal approaches. *Tech Coloproctol.* 2003;7(01):35–44.

15. Laituri CA, Garey CL, Fraser JD et al. 15-Year experience in the treatment of rectal prolapse in children. *J Pediatr Surg.* 2010;45(08):1607–9.

16. Serour F, Somekh E, Gorenstein A. Perianal abscess and fistula-in-ano in infants: A different entity? *Dis Colon Rectum.* 2005;48(02):359–64.

17. Afşarlar CE, Karaman A, Tanır G et al. Perianal abscess and fistula-in-ano in children: Clinical characteristic, management and outcome. *Pediatr Surg Int.* 2011;27(10):1063–8.

18. Christison-Lagay ER, Hall JF, Wales PW et al. Nonoperative management of perianal abscess in infants is associated with decreased risk for fistula formation. *Pediatrics.* 2007;120(03):e548–52.

19. Minneci PC, Halleran DR, Lawrence AE et al. Laser hair depilation for the prevention of disease recurrence in adolescents and young adults with pilonidal disease: Study protocol for a randomized controlled trial. *Trials.* 2018;19(1):599.

20. Murthi GV, Okoye BO, Spicer RD, Cusick EL, Noblett HR. Perianal abscess in childhood. *Pediatr Surg Int.* 2002;18(08):689–91.

21. Jamshidi R. Anorectal complaints: Hemorrhoids, fissures, abscesses, fistulae. *Clin Colon Rectal Surg.* 2018 Mar;31(2):117–20.

22. De Zoeten EF, Pasternak BA, Mattei P et al. Diagnosis and treatment of perianal Crohn disease: NASPGAN clinical report and consensus statement. *J Pediatr Gastroenterol Nutr.* 2013 Sep;57(3):401–12.

23. Bonheur JL, Braunstein J, Korelitz BI et al. Anal skin tags in inflammatory bowel disease: New observations and a clinical review. *Inflamm Bowel Dis.* 2008;14:1236–9.

24. Nelson RL, Thomas K, Morgan J et al. Non-surgical therapy for anal fissure. *Cochrane Database Syst Rev.* 2012;5(2).

25. Klin B, Efrati Y, Berkovitch M et al. Anal fissure in children: A 10-year clinical experience with nifedipine gel with lidocaine. *Minerva Pediatr.* 2016 June;68(3):196–200.

26. Sondenaa K, Andersen E, Nesvik I et al. Patient characteristics and symptoms in chronic pilonidal sinus disease. *Int J Colorectal Dis.* 1995;10(1):39–42.

27. Karydakis GE. Easy and successful treatment of pilonidal sinus after explanation of its causative process. *Aust N Z J Surg.* 1992;62(5):385–9.

28. Halleran DR, Lopez JJ, Lawrence AE et al. Recurrence of pilonidal disease: Our best is not good enough. *J Surg Res.* 2018;232:430–6.

29. Lopez JJ, Cooper JN, Halleran DR et al. High rate of major morbidity after surgical excision for pilonidal disease. *Surg Infect (Larchmt).* 2018;19(6):603–7.

30. Anderson JH, Yip CO, Nagabhushan JS et al. Day-case Karydakis flap for pilonidal sinus. *Dis Colon Rectum.* 2008;51(1):134–8.

31. Mentes O, Bagci M, Bilgin T et al. Limberg flap procedure for pilonidal sinus disease: Results of 353 patients. *Langenbecks Arch Surg.* 2008;393(2):185–9.

32. Milito G, Gargiani M, Gallinela MM et al. Modified Limberg's transposition flap for pilonidal sinus. Long term follow up of 216 cases. *Ann Ital Chir.* 2007;78(3):227–31.

33. Matter I, Kunin J, Schein M et al. Total excision versus non-resectional methods in the treatment of acute and chronic pilonidal disease. *Br J Surg.* 1995;82(6):752–3.

34. Armstrong JH, Barcia PJ. Pilonidal sinus disease. The conservative approach. *Arch Surg.* 1994;129(9):914–7; discussion 7–9.

35. Steele SR, Perry WB, Mills S et al. Practice parameters for the management of pilonidal disease. *Dis Colon Rectum.* 2013;56(9):1021–7.

36. Halleran DR, Onwuka AJ, Lawrence AE et al. Laser hair depilation in the treatment of pilonidal disease: A systematic review. *Surg Infect (Larchmt).* 2018;19(6):566–72.

# Familial adenomatous polyposis

Alessandra C. Gasior and Mark Arnold

## 22.1  Case study 1

A 16-year-old female presents with a family history of intestinal polyps. Her mother has a history of colon resection for these polyps. She recently had her first colonoscopy due to rectal bleeding. This showed 100+ polyps. She denies symptoms of abdominal pain, diarrhea, or constipation. She has no other medical history. She comes to your clinic after genetic testing reveals APC gene mutation. Her mother has had multiple upper endoscopies as well, which have been normal.

**When should FAP patients start surveillance endoscopy?**

    A. 10 years old
    B. 12–14 years old
    C. 20 years old
    D. 40 years old

**20 years later this patient gives birth to a healthy baby boy. She asks you what is his risk of FAP?**

    A. 100%
    B. 75%
    C. 50%
    D. 25%

**The patient also asks you when should her son be screened for genetic mutations?**

    A. At birth
    B. 2 years old
    C. 10 years old
    D. 12 years old

*Answers:* B, C, D

### 22.1.1  Learning points

- Familial adenomatous polyposis (FAP) is an autosomal dominant inherited condition due to a mutation in *APC*. This occurs in 1:10,000 births. Roughly 22% of FAP patients have no family history of polyp, likely due to a de novo mutation.
- Familial adenomatous polyposis patients start to develop adenomas at the age of 12–14. There have been reports of polyps and even cancers occurring earlier, however this is rare. Genetic mutation testing should also be conducted at the same time the surveillance colonoscopy is performed. There is no need to perform this testing earlier as the disease usually does not manifest clinically before mid-teens. Additionally, the patient should be old enough to participate in the genetic counseling discussion. If the patient does not carry the FAP mutation, she/he can resume general population guidelines for surveillance.
- 60% of the unscreened, asymptomatic patients present with colorectal cancer, usually diagnosed at a mean age of 40 years.
- Extracolonic manifestations must be screened for as well. Upper endoscopy screening for duodenal polyps begins at the age of 20. 90% of patients develop duodenal adenomas. Some mutations include ocular disease. An ophthalmologic exam may demonstrate congenital hypertrophy of the retinal pigmented epithelium (CHRPE) with hypo- or hyperpigmented spots. These spots have no effect on vision but may be markers for FAP in 60%–85% of patients. Duodenal disease and desmoid tumors are the highest risk for morbidity in this patient population. There is a 2% risk of thyroid cancer, primarily papillary carcinoma that develops at an average age of 27. Therefore annual thyroid ultrasound screening should begin in adolescence.

## 22.2  Case study 2

A 23-year-old newly married female underwent a colonoscopy for rectal bleeding. She was found to have >1000 colonic polyps and no rectal polyps. She and her husband wish to have children.

**What procedure would you offer her?**

- **A.** Total proctocolectomy and end ileostomy
- **B.** Colectomy with ileorectal anastomosis
- **C.** Total proctocolectomy with ileal pouch-anal anastomosis (IPAA)
- **D.** Continued surveillance

*Answer:* B

### 22.2.1  Learning points

As pelvic surgery decreases fertility, females who wish to give birth with low rectal polyp burden may consider delaying proctectomy with a strict surveillance program until childbearing is completed. However, patients with >1000 polyps should not delay operation further. A rectum with less than 5 polyps is considered a low-risk rectum and may consider keeping the rectum in place along with annual surveillance proctoscopy.

## 22.3  Case study 3

A 34-year-old male with FAP had a proctocolectomy with J pouch anastomosis 4 years ago. He presents to your office with a non-tender, firm, fixed, enlarging lump underneath one of his laparoscopic port sites. His abdomen is otherwise benign. He has 5–6 bowel movements per day. He has no other symptoms.

**What is your diagnosis?**

A. Port site hernia
B. Scar tissue
C. Desmoid tumor
D. Lipomatous tumor

*Answer:* C

## 22.3.1 Learning points

- Gardner's syndrome describes the association between FAP, epidermoid cysts, desmoid tumors, osteomas, and supranumerary teeth. Desmoid disease affects 5% of patients with FAP. 50% of patients with desmoid disease have a tumor in the bowel mesentery. 40% of desmoids develop in the abdominal wall. They tend to occur within 5 years of the operation due to the inflammatory response. Female gender, family history of desmoids, and APC mutations with 3′ end of codon 1440 are associated with the development of desmoid tumors.
- Turcot's syndrome is the association between FAP and neurologic tumors. Cerebellar medulloblastoma is the most common brain tumor [1,2].
- Preoperative considerations relevant for surgeons:
  - Timing and type of operation should be a high priority for a young asymptomatic patient that takes into consideration the fertility wishes, academic, social, and occupation concerns. Patients who have >1000 polyps, >20 rectal polyps, or are symptomatic should have surgery as soon as possible. For patients with milder polyposis syndrome, surveillance colonoscopy should continue annually until the patient reaches physical and mental maturity.
  - Morbidly obese patients may delay IPAA until adequate weight loss is achieved. Additionally, patients with a history of desmoid disease may delay surgery as most desmoids develop as a result of surgical inflammation.
  - The decision regarding which operation to perform is a complex one. The choices of procedures include: colectomy with ileorectal anastomosis, total proctocolectomy with end ileostomy (with or without continent ileostomy), or total proctocolectomy with IPAA. Quality of life with bowel function and future cancer risk must be weighed by the patient and surgeon. Patients with IPAA will have more frequent bowel movements, more risk of incontinence, and decreased quality of life. The ileorectal anastomosis carries the risk of future rectal cancer, however, it may be ideal for patients with a low rectal polyp burden. Patients with >20 rectal polyps are not candidates for rectal sparing surgery as the future risk of rectal cancer and subsequent proctectomy rate is 56%. However, patients with <20 rectal polyps may be candidates for surveillance [3].
  - Proctectomy is associated with an increased risk of urinary, sexual dysfunction, and infertility complications as well as lower quality of life scores. This can be even more devastating in this young, otherwise healthy patient group [4].
- Intraoperative considerations relevant for surgeons:
  - Intraoperative considerations should include the placement of an omental pedicle flap to occlude the small bowel from the pelvis if a patient is not planned to have an IPAA. This will potentially keep the small bowel out of the radiation field should postoperative radiotherapy be unexpectedly required.
  - Mucosectomy and hand-sewn anastomosis versus using a double-stapled anastomosis remains a controversy in patients undergoing a total abdominal colectomy and IPAA. If a mucosectomy fails to remove all of the mucosa this leaves behind a potential risk for cancer. Up to 21% of patients have been found to have residual islands of mucosa

outside of the ileal pouch or next to the IPAA, after an incomplete mucosectomy was performed. Conversely, a double-stapled anastomosis with a small strip of anal transition zone can be surveilled for cancer. Additionally patients with a double-stapled anastomosis have improved nocturnal incontinence and better resting and squeeze pressures compared to the mucosectomy patients [5,6].

# References

1. Ripa R, Bisgaard ML, Bulow S et al. De novo mutations in familial adenomatous polyposis (FAP). *Eur J Hum Genet.* 2002;10:631–7.
2. Valanzano R, Cama A, Volpe R et al. Congenital hypertrophy of the retinal pigment epithelium in familial adenomatous polyposis. Novel criteria of assessment and correlations with constitutional adenomatous polyposis coli gene mutations. *Cancer.* 1996;78(11):200–10.
3. Gunther K, Braunrieder G, Bittorf BR et al. Patients with familial adenomatous polyposis experience better bowel function and quality of life after ileorectal anastomosis than after ileoanal pouch. *Colorectal Dis.* 2003;5(1):38–44.
4. Olsen KO, Juul S, Bulow S et al. Female fecundity before and after operation for familial adenomatous polyposis. *Br J Surg.* 2003;90(2):227–31.
5. O'Connell PR, Pemberton JH, Weiland LH et al. Does rectal mucosa regenerate after ileoanal anastomosis? *Dis Colon Rectum.* 1987;30(1):1–5.
6. Lovegrove RE, Constantinides VA, Heriot AG et al. A comparison of hand-sewn versus stapled ileal pouch anal anastomosis (IPAA) following proctocolecotmy: A meta-analysis of 4183 patients. *Ann Surg.* 2006;244(1):18–26.

# 23 Ulcerative colitis and indeterminate colitis in children

Alessandra C. Gasior and Ross Maltz

## 23.1 Case study 1

A 9-year-old female with a history of ulcerative colitis is admitted to the GI service. She has a 1-week history of bloody diarrhea, abdominal pain, and abdominal distension. Stool studies were negative for infection. She has been treated with IV steroids; however, she continues to have 8 episodes of bloody diarrhea per day with a PUCAI of 70. Flexible sigmoidoscopy performed which ruled out cytomegalovirus (CMV) colitis. Surgery was consulted at this time. Second-line therapy infliximab started on day 5 of admission with no response.

**What is your next step?**

   **A.** Proctocolectomy with ileal pouch-anal anastomosis (IPAA)
   **B.** Total abdominal colectomy with end ileostomy
   **C.** Proctocolectomy with end ileostomy
   **D.** Total abdominal colectomy with ileoanal anastomosis

*Answer:* B

### 23.1.1 Learning points

- Ulcerative colitis (UC) is a chronic inflammatory condition that is limited to the colon. The endoscopic findings include friable mucosa with the loss of vascular pattern continually from the rectum extending proximally. Ulcerative colitis in the pediatric population tends to have a more severe disease course than in the adult population. Patients may present with acute severe colitis (ASC) and require inpatient hospitalization. However, a subset of patients may be refractory to medical management and may require surgical intervention. Approximately 29% of adults and up to 33% of children may not respond to medical management and will require surgical management of their disease [1]. Patients with poor prognostic factors include deep ulcerations on endoscopy, metabolic alkalosis, and gaseous distension of the small bowel. Patients should also have stool samples sent to rule out *Clostridium difficile* infection as well as colonic biopsies to evaluate CMV colitis.

- Patients are initially treated with IV steroids using 1 mg/kg up to 40 mg/day [1]. Up to 30% of patients with ASC are nonresponders to the first-line therapy medications [2]. Patients who fail steroid treatment will move on to second-line therapy infliximab for anti-TNF naïve patients. Calcineurin inhibitors (tacrolimus and cyclosporine) can be used as an alternative second-line therapy. 71% of patients will respond to second-line therapy [3]. It is recommended to involve the surgical team early on in the care of patients with acute severe colitis. Indications for emergency surgery include toxic megacolon, perforation, severe hemorrhage, significant decline during rescue treatment or failure to respond to aggressive medical rescue therapy [11].
- A bowel prep should be performed as long as the patient is in a stable condition to do so. Patients take a cleansing mechanical prep the day before surgery. Clearly, emergent procedures with peritonitis will proceed straight to surgery without delay and without bowel prep.
- The primary goal of surgery is to remove the diseased colon and construct an ileostomy. The level of transection of the bowel is at the rectosigmoid junction. The rectum is left in place for a potential future restorative procedure with an ileal pouch-anal anastomosis.
- A three-stage procedure should be the mainstay in the pediatric population with a protective ileostomy [4]. This allows the patient a chance to thrive nutritionally and be taken off of immunosuppressant medications prior to a restorative procedure as well as confirm the diagnosis of ulcerative colitis with the pathology specimen of the colon. This is particularly important in younger patients in order to avoid a pouch placement in Crohn's disease or indeterminate colitis patient.
- Indeterminate colitis (IC) is a term reserved for patients with established inflammatory bowel disease that have features that cannot be distinguished between ulcerative colitis and Crohn's disease [5,6]. IC can make up 3%–13% of a centers pediatric IBD population [7–10]. There is a higher incidence of indeterminate colitis in patients less than 2 years old. These patients tend to have a more severe disease pattern with severe colitis at onset. These patients have a higher failure rate of IPAA.

## 23.2  Case study 2

During an ileal pouch-anal anastomosis procedure, you are having difficulty in getting your pouch to reach into the pelvis.

**How do you proceed?**

  A.  Perform perpendicular releasing incisions across the mesentery of the small bowel
  B.  Leave the J-pouch in the pelvis unattached and try attachment months later
  C.  High ligation of the ileocolic vessels
  D.  Mobilize the duodenum
  E.  Perform a hand-sewn anastomosis
  F.  All of the above except E

*Answer:* F

### 23.2.1  Learning points

- Contraindications for performing a J-pouch include fecal incontinence, obesity, Crohn's disease, unreliable patient for surveillance, and presence of rectal mucosa dysplasia.

- Hand-sewn versus double-stapled anastomosis has been widely studied. The level of the anastomosis of the J-pouch in the anal canal is determined by the technique. The double-stapled anastomosis preserves the anal transition zone (ATZ) with the anastomosis just above this area. The hand-sewn anastomosis with mucosectomy removes the ATZ. It is thought that the preservation of the ATZ will give the patient better continence, defecatory function, satisfaction, and quality of life as the ATZ has some sensory ability which allows for the identification of the rectal contents. Additionally, keeping a short rectal cuff intact decreases the tension on the anastomosis. Patients with a hand-sewn anastomosis with mucosectomy are at the same level of risk for dysplasia in the anal transition zone as a double-stapled anastomosis. This is because mucosectomy does not reliably remove the entire rectal mucosa and small islands of rectal mucosa remain [12]. Additionally, the risk of fistula and pouch failure is similar for both techniques as well. Therefore, the surgical technique is at the discretion of the surgeon.
- Adequate reach of the pouch can be technically difficult, especially in obese or tall patients. There are several maneuvers that should be there in the surgeon's toolbox when performing J-pouch surgery. These include high ligation of the ileocolic vessels, mobilization of the duodenum, releasing incisions perpendicular to the mesenteric arcade to gain length, or completely releasing the small bowel from the retroperitoneum. Additionally, an S pouch configuration will lend an additional 2 cm if needed. In rare circumstances, the J-pouch can be left in situ in the pelvis with a diverting ileostomy and the surgeon can return months later, allowing the pouch to gain length over time.
- Pouch surveillance is recommended every 1–3 years with pouchoscopy.

## 23.3  Case study 3

A 12-year-old male with a history of UC has undergone the second stage of surgery of proctectomy and J-pouch creation. You have performed a contrast enema and the pouch appears to have smooth edges without the evidence of pouchitis. There is no evidence of fistula or stricture. A pouchoscopy confirms this as well.

**Assuming he is thriving and doing well, how soon after his second-stage procedure do you close his protective ileostomy?**

A. 4 weeks
B. 8 weeks
C. 12 weeks
D. 16 weeks

*Answer:* C

### 23.3.1  Learning points

- Prior to closing the ileostomy, the J-pouch should be inspected with a contrast enema and/or pouchoscopy to assess for the evidence of severe inflammation of the pouch, fistula, stricture, and adequate healing.
- Typically patients are diverted with a temporary loop ileostomy for 3 months to allow the J-pouch the full opportunity to heal. J-pouches that have not healed well or have subsequent leaks are at high risk for pouch failure.

## References

1. Turner D, Walsh CM, Steinhart AH et al. Response to corticosteroids in severe ulcerative colitis: A systematic review of the literature and a meta-regression. *Clin Gastroenterol Hepatol.* 2007;5(1):103–10.

2. Turner D, Levine A, Escher JC et al. European Crohn's and Colitis Organization; European Society for Paediatric Gastroenterology, Hepatology, and Nutrition. Management of pediatric ulcerative colitis: Joint ECCO and ESPGHAN evidence-based consensus guidelines. *J Pediatr Gastroenterol Nutr.* 2012;55(3):340–61.

3. Jarnerot G, Hertervig E, Friis-Liby I et al. Infliximab as rescue therapy in severe to moderately severe ulcerative colitis: A randomized, placebo-controlled study. *Gastroenterology.* 2005 Jun;128(7):1805–11.

4. Romano C, Syed S, Kugathasan S. Management of acute severe colitis in children with ulcerative colitis in the biologics era. *Pediatrics.* 2016 May;137(5).

5. Carvalho RS, Abadom V, Dilworth HP et al. Indeterminate colitis: A significant subgroup of pediatric IBD. *Inflamm Bowel Dis.* 2006 Apr;12(4):258–62.

6. Romano C, Famiani A, Gallizzi R et al. Indeterminate colitis: A distinctive clinical pattern of inflammatory bowel disease in children. *Pediatrics.* 2008 Dec;122(6): e1278–81.

7. Winter DA, Karolewska-Bochenek K, Lazowska-Przeorek I et al. Pediatric IBD-unclassified is less common than previously reported; results of an 8-year audit of the EUROKIDS registry. *Inflamm Bowel Dis.* 2015 Sep;21(9):2145–53.

8. Bequet E, Sarter H, Fumery M, Vasseur F et al. Incidence and phenotype at diagnosis of very-early onset compared with later-onset paediatric inflammatory bowel disease: A population-based study [1988–2011]. *J Crohns Colitis.* 2017 May;11(5):519–26.

9. Vernier-Massouille G, Balde M, Salleron J et al. Natural history of pediatric Crohn's disease: A population-based cohort study. *Gastroenterology.* 2008 Oct;135(4):11106–13.

10. Prenzel F, Uhlig HH. Frequency of indeterminate colitis in children and adults with IBD-a metaanalysis. *J Crohns Colitis.* 2009 Dec;3(4):277–81.

11. Turner D, Ruemmele FM, Orlansk-Meyer E et al. Management of paediatric ulcerative colitis, part 2: Acute severe colitis—An evidence based consensus guideline from the European Crohn's and Colitis Organization and European Society of Paediatric Gastroenterology, Hepatology and Nutrition. *J Pediatr Gastroenterol Nutr.* 2018 Aug;67(2):292–310.

12. Schaus BJ, Fazio VW, Remzi FH et al. Clinical features of ileal pouch polyps in patients with underlying ulcerative colitis. *Dis Colon Rectum.* 2007;50:832–8.

# 24 Crohn's disease in children

Alessandra C. Gasior and Jennifer L. Dotson

## 24.1 Case study 1

A 12-year-old female presents to the emergency room for the evaluation of chronic diarrhea and abdominal pain. She had a known history of Crohn's disease. This has been ongoing for several months. She also has a prior history of a perirectal abscess drained at a local hospital. She was subsequently referred to your hospital for further workup. She is a pale, thin, frail appearing girl. Infectious diarrhea workup is negative. A CT scan performed in the ED demonstrates the evidence of colonic strictures. She is admitted to the hospital. A colonoscopy is performed which demonstrates transmural thickening and inflammation with a tight and narrowed portion in the colon.

**What is next step in her acute management?**

A. Exploratory laparotomy for resection of strictured bowel
B. Covered stent placement
C. Exploratory laparotomy for stricturoplasty

*Answer:* B

### 24.1.1 Learning points

- Crohn's disease is characterized by transmural inflammation involving any portion of the gastrointestinal tract from the mouth to the anus and can present with a wide variety of gastrointestinal or extraintestinal symptoms. Patients often present with abdominal pain, diarrhea, and weight loss [1]. Evidence of perianal disease, failure to thrive, pubertal delay, anemia and pallor should be suggestive of an inflammatory bowel disease. Additionally, patients with joint disease or mucocutaneous disease should be considered for IBD [2]. Pediatric Crohn's disease is oftentimes more extensive and severe with more atypical presentations compared to patients diagnosed as adults.
- The worldwide incidence of Crohn's disease is increasing, particularly in children aged 10–19 with at least 25% of all new Crohn's cases being diagnosed in childhood or adolescence [3–6]. 30% of the children require a surgical intervention within the first 5 years of Crohn's diagnosis for complicated disease such as fistula, perianal disease, stricture, or obstruction [7].

### 24.1.2 Crohn's strictures

- Crohn's strictures can be categorized as inflammatory, fibrotic, or mixed. Categorization of strictures becomes important for determining the best treatment strategy. Patients with mainly inflammatory strictures will benefit from anti-inflammatory medical management whereas patients with fibrotic strictures are best served with either endoscopic or surgical intervention [8]. 30% of patients with Crohn's disease will develop symptomatic intestinal strictures [9]. Chronic inflammatory bowel damage leads to abscess, strictures, or fistula through cumulative deposits of extracellular matrix protein (ECM) [10]. Some factors that may aid in the prediction that a patient may develop small bowel stricturing disease include perianal disease, age of Crohn's disease onset less than 40 years old, and usage of steroids as therapy during the first flare [11]. If a patient carries two of these three factors, the chance of having severe Crohn's disease in the future is 90% [12].

### 24.1.3 Diagnosis

- Imaging modalities for diagnosis include upper gastrointestinal with small bowel follow-through to determine the extent and the severity of the strictures. Additionally, upper endoscopy, colonoscopy, and double-lumen endoscopy can assess the severity of the stricture with severe luminal narrowing or the inability to pass the endoscope through the stricture. However, the extent of the transmural and extraintestinal disease cannot be measured through endoscopy. CT and MRI cross-sectional imaging has become more prevalent in recent years. CT enterography (CTE) is replacing small bowel follow-through imaging due to the ease of usage with decreased radiation exposure, improved imaging quality, and rapidity of the study. CTE has a sensitivity for small bowel stenosis of 85%–93% and specificity of 100% [13]. However, CTE will either overcall or undercall strictures in 31% of patients with Crohn's disease [14]. Comparatively, MRI eliminates radiation exposure, however, has increased cost and decreased availability. MRI has a sensitivity of 78% and specificity of 85% for the diagnosis of Crohn's disease. The usage of MRI for the detection of strictures has a sensitivity of 75%–100% and a specificity of 91%–100%. A direct comparison of MRI with CTE for the detection of strictures showed a comparable sensitivity of 92% versus 85% and specificity of 90% versus 100%[13].

### 24.1.4 Medical therapy

- Medical therapy for inflammatory Crohn's strictures include corticosteroids, immuno-modulators, and biologic agents, in addition to bowel rest in the setting of high-grade strictures or if obstructive symptoms are present. Biologic agents (i.e., anti-TNF alpha) have emerged as first-line therapy for medical management of moderate-to-severe CD, including those with stricturing disease [15,16]. Despite this medical progress, the use of these agents has not been shown to consistently prevent stricture formation. If the patient fails to improve then endoscopic or surgical intervention is necessary. Kids with strictures are at high risk and we usually treat with biologics as first line of treatment.
- If concerns for obstruction from the surgical end of things, bowel rest would be indicated, otherwise feeding (oral diet, low residue if concerns for strictures, enteral therapy either orally or via a feeding tube, etc.) would be promoted.
- No current medical therapy exists to treat fibrotic strictures.

### 24.1.5 Endoscopic intervention

- Strictured bowel segments without concern for possible fistulous disease may be treated with endoscopic balloon dilation if the bowel segment is less than 5 cm [17].

Endoscopic balloon dilation may act as a bridge to surgery. The most common area that is dilated is the distal ileum or an area of a previous ileocolonic anastomosis; however, any region of the bowel can be affected by Crohn's disease including the upper gastrointestinal tract, colon, and rectum. The chance of developing a stricture at the site of a previous anastomosis in a Crohn's patient is 50% [18]. In a systematic review of 1463 patients, 89% had clinical improvement of symptoms in a systematic analysis after endoscopic balloon dilation. However, long-term data with a follow-up of 5 years showed that 80% of the patients required repeat interventions of dilations and even surgery in 75% [9].

## 24.1.6 Surgical management

- If the stricture cannot to be treated with dilations, then surgical intervention becomes necessary. Intraoperative decisions for bowel strictures include resection with primary anastomosis or stricturoplasty. Resection with anastomosis becomes problematic as many patients with Crohn's disease will have recurrent disease and multiple resections will place the patient at risk for loss of gastrointestinal function and short bowel syndrome [10]. Therefore, surgical resection should be thoughtful and as limited as possible. The margins for resection are chosen based on gross examination of the bowel. The operator must examine the bowel for tissue thickening and reanastomose normal bowel to normal bowel.
- Stricturoplasty is a procedure that can be performed to preserve bowel length in that it allows for widening of the bowel. Stricturoplasty was first used for pyloric strictures in 1886 and first described for Crohn's disease in 1982 [19,20]. Stricturoplasty can be used for multiple small strictures over a long length of bowel, anastomotic strictures, or duodenal strictures. Heineke-Mikulicz stricturoplasty is used in over 80% of cases and therefore is the most commonly performed stricturoplasty. Heineke-Mikulicz stricturoplasty is used for strictures less than 10 cm. It involves a single enterotomy with transverse closure. A Finney procedure can be used for strictures greater than 10 cm but less than 25 cm. This is done by folding the strictured segment into a U shape thus forming a longitudinal enterotomy and anastomosing adjacent bowel edges to form a blind pouch [21]. For longer strictures (>20 cm) a Michelassi stricturoplasty may be used [22]. This is side-to-side isoperistaltic strictureplasty. Strictureplasty should not be used when the involved strictured bowel has an associated abscess, fistula, peritonitis associated with perforation, stricture due to cancer or poor nutritional status of the patient [23]. A Heineke−Mikulicz stricturoplasty has a lower morbidity but higher risk of recurrence and reoperation than a Finney stricturoplasty [24].

# 24.2 Case study 2

An 18-year-old male presents to the emergency department with a 4-day history of fever, chill, abdominal pain, nausea, and vomiting. He was diagnosed with Crohn's disease 4 years ago. On exam he is mildly tender in the right lower quadrant. A CT scan is performed which demonstrates a rim-enhancing fluid collection that is 2×3 cm in the right lower quadrant with associated bowel wall thickening.

**What is your next step in management?**

- **A.** NPO, IV antibiotics, interventional radiology for percutaneous drainage
- **B.** Ileocolic resection
- **C.** Appendectomy

*Answer:* A

### 24.2.1 Learning points

#### 24.2.1.1 Interloop fistula

- Entero-entero fistulas are commonly seen in Crohn's disease. The inflammatory process triggers the release of inflammatory mediators which in turn causes a full-thickness injury and local perforation in the intestinal wall with the formation of a fistula and/or abscess. Interloop fistulas occur in 17%–50% of patients with Crohn's disease [25]. Abdominal fistula can be categorized into fistula between bowel segments and those between bowel and other organs (rectovaginal, entero-vesical, or abdominal wall). Mortality rate of Crohn's fistula ranges from 6% to 25% due to sepsis, dehydration, or other metabolic abnormality related to the fistula [26].

- The diagnosis of interloop fistula is made by CT or MRI which identifies the anatomy and extent of the disease. Patients with an intestinal stricture on imaging with proximally dilated bowel are more likely to require surgical intervention [27]. The treatment of interloop fistula is medical and/or surgical. If the fistula is controlled locally then medical management is appropriate. However, septic individuals with peritonitis would require emergent surgical intervention. Medical management to treat the underlying Crohn's disease includes anti-TNF agents with or without adjunctive thiopurines [28]. Patients with an associated abscess may be treated with intravenous antibiotics and percutaneous drainage if they do not have systemic signs of infection [29]. Additionally, patients treated initially with medical management may fail and have a poor quality of life ultimately leading to surgical resection.

- Preoperative considerations for surgical resection include the patient's nutrition status and history of previous bowel resections with consideration to avoid short bowel syndrome and optimization of current medical therapy. As there is a high rate of recurrence of disease, the surgeon must consider the ultimate possibility of short bowel syndrome with the associated metabolic and nutritional morbidity. Total parenteral nutrition (TPN) and bowel rest may be necessary as the metabolic derangements are corrected. TPN and bowel rest has been associated with spontaneous closure in 60%–75% of fistula [30].

- The most common surgical procedure is an ileocolic resection. The fistula tract must be routinely excised along with the involved bowel segments. Patients with poor nutritional status or severe disease may require a temporary diverting ostomy proximal to the diverting stoma. Postoperatively recurrence rates are high, particularly in patients with severe Crohn's disease, due to the recurring nature of the inflammation. Therefore, medical management should continue. Patients typically undergo repeat colonoscopy approximately 6 months after resection to assess for disease recurrence.

- Complex patients with Crohn's disease must have a multidisciplinary team using a comanagement approach with pediatric surgery, gastroenterology, radiology, nutrition, and stoma therapy nurses.

## 24.3 Case study 3

A 21-year-old male with a 3-year history of Crohn's disease presents to your office with 1 week of constant rectal pain. He denies diarrhea or blood per rectum. On exam you see a firm, red mass 3 cm from his rectum on the right that measures 4×3 cm. He does not allow you to perform a digital rectal exam due to pain. You take him to the operating room later that day for an exam under anesthesia with incision and drainage. Purulent fluid drains from the mass upon insertion of a scalpel. Upon insertion of an anoscope into the rectum you are able to place a lacrimal duct probe through an internal opening 1.5 cm proximal to the sphincter complex that communicates with the abscess.

**How do you proceed?**

A. Pack the abscess cavity after a good washout
B. Place a cutting seton through the fistula tract
C. Perform an endorectal advancement flap over the internal opening of the fistula
D. Place a non-cutting seton through the fistula tract

*Answer:* D

## 24.3.1 Perianal fistula and abscesses

- A fistula can be categorized as either simple or complex. A simple fistula is one with a low intersphincteric or transphincteric location, single short tract, an anal opening close to the anal verge, or a cutaneous opening near the anal verge without an associated abscess. A complex fistula is one that involves the sphincter muscle, has multiple fistula branches with or without an abscess, an anal opening of the fistula above the sphincters, or a cutaneous opening further way from the anal opening [31].

## 24.3.2 Diagnosis

- In the absence of clear external signs of perianal disease, most children tolerate a gentle and succinct digital rectal exam. If the exam is restricted due to pain then imaging modalities or an exam under anesthesia may be necessary and less traumatizing to the child. MRI and CT scans may be used to help define the anatomy. CT scans are better for locating strictures and abscesses, but may be limited when examining soft tissues and fistulous tracts. However, MRI is more useful for soft tissue delineating and identifying fistula and abscesses with the benefit of avoiding exposure to radiation. Compared to an exam under anesthesia (EUA), MRI has a specificity of 76%–100% for identifying the fistulous tract [32]. An EUA is the diagnostic procedure of choice if a perineal abscess is suspected as it allows for the opportunity to treat the disease as well.

## 24.3.3 Treatment

- Medical management includes the treatment of active Crohn's disease to increase the chance of the fistula healing. Patients treated with corticosteroids in the setting of active proctitis have been shown to have a decreased rate of fistula healing [33]. Despite the lack of evidence, antibiotics have been a mainstay of treatment for fistula or abscess and remain the first-line therapy recommendation from the adult clinical practice guidelines published in 2003 [34]. Whether ciprofloxacin and/or metronidazole is the most effective therapy remains a matter of debate. Antibiotics, immunomodulators and infliximab remain the main therapeutic recommendations for perianal fistula with response rates of fistula healing at high as 75% [35]. Perianal abscesses are treated with incision and drainage alone unless deep abdominal abscess is present which requires an additional treatment of the intestinal disease with infliximab.
- An EUA will include external examination for erythema, induration, and fluctuance which may represent an abscess. Any area of dimpling or fistula should be probed to identify the fistulous tract. Methylene blue or hydrogen peroxide can also be used to identify the internal fistulous tract if it is not obviously identifiable. Abscesses should

be incised and drained without the placement of packing as packing actually impedes adequate drainage and is extremely painful for the patient when changed. A cruciate incision can be made to allow all the effluent to drain with debridement of granulation tissue. A mushroom catheter or a silastic drain can be placed to maintain drainage of the cavity. Any connecting fistulous tracts should be identified with an internal and external opening. Simple fistula can be opened with a fistulotomy or excised with an open or closed fistulectomy.

- Complex fistula can be treated with the placement of a non-cutting seton, which can include a silastic vessel loop. The placement of a seton is helpful as it allows the abscess cavity to fully drain and can allow the patient to be treated until medically optimized and the active Crohn's disease is treated. Subsequently if there are no signs of inflammation or infection, the seton can be removed in the office with the continuation of medical therapy. Setons can be left in place indefinitely as a treatment strategy and usually fall out on their own at about 1 year. If the ongoing inflammation and infection is present, the seton may need to be replaced every 6 months.
- Persistent complex fistula that have healed and have no evidence of ongoing infection can be treated with a variety of surgical advancement flaps, however, these all have a high rate of failure in the Crohn's patient. Treatment with fibrin glue or fibrin plug also has questionable longevity.
- Generally, any active inflammation in the tissues may create large wounds with poor healing ability. Therefore a combination of acute management of abscess and infection should be undertaken with concomitant medical optimization prior to definitive surgical repair of any fistula-in-ano. Patients with severe perianal Crohn's disease may require fecal diversion with an ostomy. The risk of this ostomy becoming permanent is significant. Typically consideration for closure of the ostomy occurs after an extended period of time for the tissues to completely heal, usually 6–12 months. There is a high likelihood of recurrence and need for repeat diversion [31].

### 24.3.4 Rectal strictures

Strictures occur in a much smaller proportion of pediatric patients compared to adult patients with Crohn's disease. Rectal strictures are a poor predictor of outcome and occur in 7%–9% of adult IBD patients [36]. Typically these strictures occur with a varying degree of narrowing of the anal opening, length, and response to therapy. They are caused by chronic circumferential rectal inflammation or after response to a medical therapy that has healed the inflammation. These strictures may appear to be skin-level only fibrosis or extend to the entire length of the rectum. Treatment includes anal dilatation under general anesthesia with frequent intervals starting at the smallest allowed caliper dilator progressing in a stepwise manner to a minimum of 18 mm or 24–26 mm in teenagers or young adults. Gentle stretching of the fibrotic ring will cause bleeding but excessive stretching may cause more inflammation and scar which may worsen the stricture. Patients who have a tight, long, refractory stricture may require ostomy diversion and proctectomy [31].

## References

1. Sawczenko A, Sandhu BK. Presenting features of inflammatory bowel disease in Great Britain and Ireland. *Arch Dis Child.* 2003;88(11):995–1000.
2. Yu YR, Rodriguez JR. Clinical presentation of Crohn's ulcerative colitis and indeterminate colitis: Symptoms, extraintestinal manifestations and disease phenotypes. *Semin Pediatr Surg.* 2017 Dec;26(6):349–55.

3. Stewart D. Surgical care of the pediatric Crohn's disease patient. *Semin Pediatr Surg.* 2017 Dec;26(6):373–8.

4. Benchimol EI, Kaplan GG, Otley AR et al. Rural and urban residence during early life is associated with risk of inflammatory bowel disease: A population-based inception and birth cohort study. *Am J Gastroenterol.* 2017 Sep;112(9):1412–22.

5. Henderson P, Hansen R, Cameron FL et al. The rising incidence of paediatric inflammatory bowel disease in Scotland. *Inflamm Bowel Dis.* 2012;18(6):999–1005.

6. Martin-de-Carpi J, Rodriguez A, Ramos E et al. Increasing incidence of pediatric inflammatory bowel disease in Spain (1996–2009): The SPIRIT registry. *Inflamm Bowel Dis.* 2013;19(1):73–80.

7. Vernier-Massouille G, Balde M, Salleron J et al. Natural history of pediatric Crohn's disease: A population-based cohort study. *Gastroenterology.* 2008;135(4):1106–113.

8. Bettenworth D, Nowacki TM, Cordes F et al. Assessment of stricturing Crohn's disease: Current clinical practice and future avenues. *World J Gastroenterol.* 2016 Jan 21;22(3):1008–16.

9. Bessissow T, Reinglas J, Arujothy A et al. Endoscopic management of Crohn's strictures. *World J Gastroenterol.* 2018 May;24(17):1859–67.

10. Rieder F, Zimmermann E, Remzi FH et al. Crohn's disease complicated by strictures: A systematic review. *Gut.* 2013;62:1072–84.

11. Rieder F, Lawrance IC, Leite A et al. Predictors of fibrostenotic Crohn's disease. *Inflamm Bowel Dis.* 2011 Sep;17(9):2000–7.

12. Lakatos PL, Czegledi Z, Szamosi T et al. Perianal disease, small bowel disease, smoking, prior steroid or early azathioprine/biological therapy are predictors of disease behavior change in patients with Crohn's disease. *World J Gastroenterol.* 2009;15:3504–10.

13. Fiorino G, Bonifacio C, Peyrin-Biroulet L et al. Prospective comparison of computed tomography enterography and magnetic resonance enterography for assessment of disease activity and complications of ileocolonic Crohn's disease. *Inflamm Bowel Dis.* 2011;17(5):1073–80.

14. Vogel J, da Luz Moreira A, Baker M et al. CT enterography for Crohn's disease: Accurate preoperative diagnostic imaging. *Dis Colon Rectum.* 2007;50:1761–9.

15. Mark G. Biological therapies improve inflammatory bowel disease symptoms, national audit finds. *BMJ* 2013;347:f5340.

16. Vahabnezhad E, Rabizadeh S, Dubinsky MC. A 10-year, single tertiary care center experience on the durability of infliximab in pediatric inflammatory bowel disease. *Inflamm Bowel Dis.* 2014;20(4):606–13.

17. Taida T, Nakagawa T, Ohta Y et al. Long-term outcome of endoscopic balloon dilation for strictures in patients with Crohn's disease. *Digestion.* 2018;98(1):26–32.

18. Rutgeerts P, Geboes K, Vantrappen G et al. Natural history of recurrent Crohn's disease at the ileocolonic anastomosis after curative surgery. *Gut.* 1984;25:665–72.

19. Heineke Operation de Pylorusstenose. Inaug. Dissert., Furth, 1886.

20. Lee EC, Papaioannou N. Minimal surgery for chronic obstruction in patients with extensive or universal Crohn's disease. *Ann R Coll Surg Engl.* 1982;64:229–33.

21. Brown C. Heineke-Mikulicz and Finney strictureplasty in Crohn's disease. *Oper Tech Gen Surg.* 2007;9:3–7.

22. Limmer AM, Koh HC, Gilmore A. Stricturoplasty-a bowel-sparing option for long segment small bowel Crohn's disease. *J Surg Case Rep.* 2017 Aug;2017(8):1–5.

23. Schlussel A, Steele S, Alvai K. Current challenges in the surgical management of Crohn's disease: A systematic review. *Am J Surg.* 2016;212:345–51.

24. Tichansky D, Cagir B, Yoo E et al. Strictureplasty for Crohn's disease: Meta-analysis. *Dis Colon Rectum.* 2000;43:911–19.

25. Bell SJ, Williams AB, Wiesel P et al. The clinical course of fistulating Crohn's disease. *Aliment Pharmacol Ther.* 2003 May;17(9):1145–51.

26. Tassiopoulos AK, Baum G, Halverson JD. Small bowel fistulas. *Surg Clin North Am.* 1996;76(5):1175–81.

27. Yaari S, Benson A, Aviaran E et al. Factors associated with surgery in patients with intra-abdominal fistulizing Crohn's disease. *World J Gastroenterol.* 2016 Dec;22(47):10380–7.

28. Present DH, Rutgeerts P, Targan S et al. Infliximab for the treatment of fistulas in patients with Crohn's disease. *N Engl J Med.* 1999;340:1398–405.

29. Feagins LA, Holubar SD, Kane SV et al. Current strategies in the management of intraabdominal abscesses in Crohn's disease. *Clin Gastroenterol Hepatol.* 2001;9:842–50.

30. O'Dwyer ST. Enterocutaneous fistula: Conservative and surgical management. In: Allan RN, Rhodes JM, Hanauer SB et al., eds. *Inflammatory Bowel Diseases*. 3rd ed. Churchill Livingstone, New York, pp. 883–93.
31. de Zoeten EF, Pasternak BA, Mattei P, Kramer RE, Kader HA. *J Pediatr Gastroenterol Nutr*. 2013 Sep;57(3):401–12
32. Dagia C, Ditchfield M, Kean M et al. Feasibility of 3-T MRI for the evaluation of Crohn disease in children. *Pediatr Radiol*. 2010;40:1615–24.
33. Malchow H, Ewe K, Brandes JW et al. European Cooperative Crohn's Disease Study (ECCDS): Results of drug treatment. *Gastroenterology*. 1984;6:249–66.
34. Sandborn WJ, Fazio VW, Feagan BG et al. AGA technical review on perianal Crohn's disease. *Gastroenterology*. 2003;125:1508–30.
35. Crandall W, Hyams J, Kugathasan S et al. Infliximab therapy in children with concurrent perianal Crohn disease: Observations from REACH. *J Pediatr Gastroenterol Nutr*. 2009; 49(2):183–190.
36. Fields S. Rosainz L, Korelitz BI et al. Rectal strictures in Crohn's disease and coexisting perirectal complications. *Inflamm Bowel Dis*. 2008;14:29–31.

# 25 Pediatric colorectal surgery in low- and middle-income settings: Adaptation to the resources available

Chris Westgarth-Taylor and Marion Arnold

## 25.1 Case study 1

A previously well 5-year-old male presents with an acute abdomen and severe septic shock after 5 days of diarrhea and vomiting. At laparotomy, **total colonic necrosis** is found, extending up to the peritoneal reflection. Traditional hot-water enema administration is denied by caregivers but is suspected by the clinicians. After a damage control laparotomy at which a total colectomy is done with ligation of the terminal ileum and the abdomen is closed with a Bogota bag, an end-ileostomy is created at a relook laparotomy 48 hours later. The rectum is necrotic to the dentate line at the time of relook laparotomy. Histology of the resected necrotic bowel demonstrates ganglionated bowel, and an infectious agent is not identified. (Serological tests for *Salmonella typhi* and stool samples for *Campylobacter*, *Yersinia*, *Shigella*, hemorrhagic *Escherichia coli*, and amoebiasis are negative.)

**What surgical alternatives for anorectal reconstruction should be considered?**

A. Immediate resection of necrotic rectum, pull-through of end-ileostomy and ileo-anal anastomosis
B. Debridement of necrotic rectum, with review under anesthesia every 2–3 days until all sepsis is controlled, followed by ileal pull-through with ileo-anal anastomosis and covering proximal ileostomy
C. No further surgical intervention
D. Delayed surgical reconstruction after 6 months, depending on the condition

*Answer:* C

Due to the poor general condition of the patient, further surgery is deferred. The anal opening is completely **stenosed closed at the mucocutaneous junction** on examination under anesthetic 3 months later.

**What is your advice to his caregivers regarding future prognosis now?**

A. A permanent ileostomy is the only option
B. Full continence is likely after reconstructive surgery to dilate open the rectum and pull-through the ileum
C. An ileo-cutaneous neo-anus can be created through a posterior sagittal approach, but a bowel management program will be required to limit soiling
D. A permanent ileostomy is advisable if formed stools cannot be achieved through medical management
E. C and D are correct

*Answer:* E

### 25.1.1 Learning points

- Formed stools are required before considering the creation of a perineal stoma, to avoid severe excoriation of perineal skin. Stoma reversal should not be considered before the child is over 3 years of age and continent for urine.
- In rural and informal settlements, it can be very dangerous to send a child home with an ileostomy. Due to poor nutrition, hygiene issues, unclean water, and no access to emergency medical care, gastroenteritis, especially with an ileostomy can be fatal. Caregivers must be thoroughly educated on this problem.
- The use of a "bananogram or porridge test" can be helpful in assessing the adequacy of continence mechanism: mashed banana or porridge is instilled into a mucous fistula to see if the patient can control the passage of this "stool" or not.

- An additional way to assess the ability of continence is to perform bowel management through the stoma. If this is successful, in conjunction with medical management, the stoma can be closed.
- A trial of medical management with loperamide (0.1–0.4 mg/kg/day in 2 or 3 divided doses) ± clonidine (1 mcg/kg/day in 2–4 divided doses) and possibly codeine phosphate (1 mg/kg/dose, up to 3 times a day), together with a constipating diet, should be performed to improve the consistency of stools before considering reconstructive surgery and closure of the ileostomy.
- If surgery is deemed appropriate, a posterior sagittal approach as for an anorectal malformation can be utilized to ensure the placement of the terminal ileum within the sphincter complex. A covering ileostomy is recommended until the ileo-perineal anastomosis has healed.
- Counsel the caregiver and the patient that bowel irrigations will be required on a once- to twice-daily basis after stoma closure to manage incontinence, in conjunction with medications to slow transit.

Common complications of a perineal stoma include perineal excoriation, anal stenosis, and social ostracization when bowel management cannot optimize control of incontinence.

### 25.1.2  Follow-up: Perineal stoma

Regular follow-up to optimize the medical management of stool consistency is important for a chance of success. A permanent stoma is preferable when this is not likely.

## 25.2  Case study 2

A 1-year-old male presents with a history of recurrent intermittent abdominal distension, diarrhea, and failure to thrive associated with a peri-anal fistula after an endo-anal pull-through for Hirschsprung disease performed at another institution, for which a diverting end sigmoid colostomy was performed. A full-thickness rectal biopsy confirms ganglionated bowel with no thickened nerves present. A narrow fistula draining pus at the anastomotic site 1 cm above the dentate line is noted to exit 1 cm lateral to the anal mucocutaneous junction at 5 o'clock. Curettage of the tract is performed, and tuberculosis is excluded. However, **the colostomy is now significantly prolapsed** by about 30 cm, and engorged, although viable. Stoma closure is only planned after the confirmation of a healed fistula at examination under anesthesia in 3 months' time.

**What is your next step in management?**

A. Leave the prolapsed stoma until a repeat examination under anesthetic to assess whether the fistula has healed in 3 months, as it is a temporary fistula.
B. Reduce the stoma and transfix the side of the stoma through the abdominal wall to prevent further prolapse under local anesthetic, using silicone tubing to prevent the erosion of the external suture through the anterior abdominal wall.
C. Reduce the stoma under general anesthetic, mobilize half the circumference of the stoma, pexy the serosa of the bowel to the abdominal wall at multiple points and narrow the diameter of the sheath around the stoma prior to maturation of the revised stoma. Care should be taken to avoid full-thickness sutures in the bowel to limit the risk of perforation at subsequent mobilization and closure as well as fistulization.
D. Resect the prolapsed bowel and refashion stoma.

*Answer:* C

### 25.2.1 Learning points: Management of stoma prolapse

- Stomal prolapse can be prevented by siting the stoma close to a site of retroperitoneal fixation where possible, and by pexying the serosa to the abdominal wall several centimeters proximal to the stoma site and also to the sheath edges at the stoma site if it is in mobile bowel.
- A covering ileostomy rather than a colostomy should be considered to preserve the colonic vascular arcades for revision surgery.
- Transmural pexy predisposes to disfiguring enterocutaneous fistulae and should be avoided if facilities for general anesthetic are available.
- Significant prolapse predisposes to partial obstruction and ulceration of bowel and prolapse should be addressed expeditiously. However, simple excision can lead to significant loss of bowel.
- Stoma closure in the event of resolution of distal pathology, or resiting of a stoma more proximally (e.g., terminal ileum), should be considered.
- A loop stoma is particularly prone to distal segment prolapse, and revision with a proximal end stoma and narrow distal mucous fistula (flush with the skin to allow easy stoma appliance application) is preferred.

## 25.3 Case study 3

A 6-month-old girl presents with feces passing from the vagina for the past month. Past medical history includes a few episodes of diarrhea and poor weight gain. Her mother has HIV/AIDS but defaulted highly active antiretroviral therapy (HAART) due to financial constraints. A normal anus and vagina is visualized. Examination under anesthesia confirms a 3-mm wide fistula at the level of the anal crypts on the dentate line to the posterior fourchette of the vagina (rectovestibular fistula). The tract is not mucosa-lined, but friable with slight bleeding on probing. Serological and PCR tests confirm that the child is HIV positive. Histology of a biopsy of the fistula fails to demonstrate cytomegalovirus or herpes inclusion bodies on H&E staining, or mycobacterium tuberculosis on Ziehl–Nielsen staining.

**What is the most important next step for this girl in the management of the fistula?**

- A. Commence HAART
- B. Fashion a divided sigmoid colostomy
- C. Perform layered repair of fistula, covering defect with mobilized full-thickness rectal flap

*Answer:* A

### 25.3.1 Learning points: HIV-associated rectovestibular, recto-vaginal and recto-urethral fistulae

- HIV-associated rectal fistulae can occur in both sexes. Tuberculosis and cytomegalovirus infections should be actively investigated for, while Crohn disease remains a less likely consideration in older children [1–4,10].
- A small fistula may close spontaneously with nutritional support and HAART, with or without a covering stoma. A large fistula is unlikely to close spontaneously, even with a covering colostomy.
- Surgical repair, using hemi-circumferential mobilization of the healthy proximal rectal wall to cover a layered repair, should only be considered once virological HIV control and good nutritional status is achieved as there is a high failure rate (Figure 25.1).

## 25.4 Case study 4

An 11-year-old male patient presents to your pediatric surgical outpatients department with a 3-year history of gradual abdominal distension, failure to thrive, and anorexia. Abdominal x-ray demonstrates massive dilatation of the entire colon with gas trapping. On digital rectal examination, there is soft stool in a capacious rectum with no release of gas or stool on the removal of the finger. He is started on irrigations that have some effect to make him more comfortable. A full-thickness rectal biopsy is done which demonstrates smooth muscle degeneration and necrosis with replacement by fibrous tissue and ganglion cells are present. With this, the diagnosis of degenerative leiomyopathy is made.

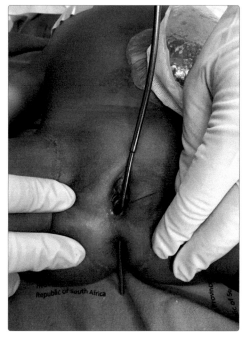

Figure 25.1 HIV-associated rectovagal fistula.

**What does your further medical management include?**

A. Colonic irrigations
B. Prokinetic agents
C. Low-residue diet
D. Antibiotics for bacterial overgrowth
E. All of the above

*Answer:* E

**What are your possible further surgical options for the child?**

A. Surgery is usually only indicated for complications of the disease (i.e., volvulus)
B. Colonic resection with ileostomy formation
C. Colostomy formation
D. Venting continent stoma (MACE, Mic-Key button)
E. A and D are correct

*Answer:* E

### 25.4.1 Learning points: Degenerative leiomyopathy

- Degenerative leiomyopathy is an acquired visceral myopathy of unknown etiology. It is predominantly identified in Southern and Southeastern Africa. It results in chronic intestinal pseudo-obstruction that is uniformly fatal. Patients usually present in the first or second decade of life and demise in the late second or early third decade. The presentation is usually colonic, but progresses to involve the entire gastrointestinal tract [5,6].
- Patients uniformly present with chronic episodes of abdominal distension, abdominal pain, vomiting, anorexia, and malnutrition. The x-ray picture is that of a megacolon with massive gaseous distension.
- The diagnosis is made histologically with smooth muscle degeneration with vacuolated cytoplasm, extracellular edema, and replacement of the muscle fibers by fibrous tissue.

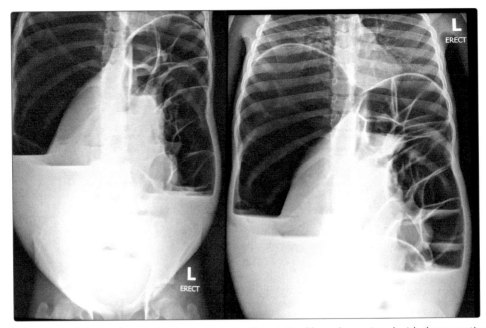

Figure 25.2 Abdominal x-ray showing massively dilated distal bowel associated with degenerative leiomyopathy.

- Treatment is primarily medical with intestinal irrigations, broad-spectrum antibiotics to curb bacterial overgrowth, nutritional support with low-residue diet, and prokinetic agents.
- Surgery such as colonic resection is universally unsatisfactory as the disease progresses to involve the entire gastrointestinal tract. It has thus been reserved for complications such as volvulus or adhesional obstruction. Decompression of the gas trapping via a Malone or Mic-Key button has been described to give symptomatic relief and improve quality of life. (Figure 25.2).

## 25.5 Application of general colorectal surgery principles to challenging cases prevalent in the developing world

### 25.5.1 Operative techniques

#### 25.5.1.1 Technical aspects: Reduction of wound infection and dehiscence

Higher incidence of wound infection and wound breakdown has been reported in low- and middle-income countries. This may be due to sepsis associated with late presentation, poor nutritional status, human immunodeficiency virus (HIV) infection or exposure to maternal HIV infection, infrastructure factors affecting adherence to aseptic technique and sterility during surgery and inadequate postoperative care due to limited availability of trained nursing staff and lack of education on the part of caregivers [7–9].

The following is recommended (in addition to routine strict aseptic technique and careful tissue handling, preservation of anatomical blood supply, and hemostasis):

- *All patients preoperatively*: In theater prior to surgical skin preparation, wash the surgical site and surrounding area with soap (e.g., chlorhexidine in water is used for surgical hand washing). The whole child may be washed similarly on the preceding morning or evening in the ward.

- Colostomy formation:
  - *All patients*: Ensure snug approximation of sheath and skin to bowel serosa. Interrupted sutures are preferred. Avoid excessive use of sutures to minimize foreign body reaction and tissue necrosis. Adhesive tape skin closure (which may be in lieu of skin sutures except directly adjacent to the stoma) covered by an adhesive clear film dressing for the first 5 days protects the wound from stoma effluent.
  - *Hirschsprung disease*: On-table rectal irrigation [10] until effluent is clear via large-bore round-tipped tubes (e.g., Foley's catheter, chest drain tube), massaging the abdomen until well decompressed and all irrigation fluid is evacuated.
  - Anorectal malformation:
    - *Intraoperatively*: Evacuate all proximal and distal stool with saline irrigation via a large-bore Foley's catheter to minimize effluent from the stoma during the first 48 hours, particularly if commercial stoma bags are not available to protect the wound postoperatively.
    - Separate incisions for the functional stoma and mucous fistula have been used in some settings, to minimize the risk of wound dehiscence, although not widely practiced for cosmetic reasons. The proximal stoma may be brought out through an additional small incision above the left iliac fossa oblique incision, with the tapered mucous fistula in the caudal aspect of the wound, leaving a bridge of tissue between the two wounds (see Figure 25.1). A transverse left iliac fossa incision with the proximal and distal stoma above and below the wound respectively has also been utilized (Figure 25.3).
    - Topical tissue glue applied to the skin bridge may help to reduce wound dehiscence by acting as a barrier, with a cost similar to sutures, although evidence is very limited [11,12]. Care should be taken to apply the glue over approximated skin (which should not be under any tension) and not within the wound.
- Colostomy closure:
  - Preoperatively:
    - Consider delaying closure until skin is healthy if significant peristomal excoriation.

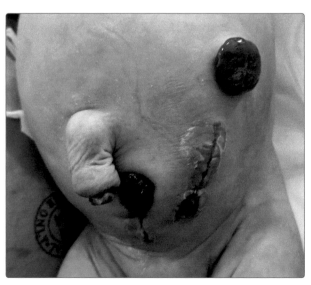

Figure 25.3 Bridge between matured proximal sigmoid stoma and separate left iliac fossa wound containing distal mucous fistula (flush with level of skin). (Subsequent control of stoma effluent was poor due to difficulty in the placement of stoma appliances over the proximal stoma.)

- Mechanical bowel preparation is not routinely practiced, but may be considered using polyethylene glycol or even saline [14]. Oral antibiotics during the preceding 24 hours, in conjunction with mechanical bowel preparation, previously has been shown in meta-analysis of adult randomized trials to reduce surgical site infections [13]. Oral formulations of aminoglycosides such as neomycin and kanamycin are not registered for human use in some countries, but erythromycin, metronidazole, and ciprofloxacin have been used in addition. Adult randomized trial meta-analysis shows no evidence of reduced surgical site infection with mechanical bowel preparation alone [15].
- Intraoperatively:
  - On-table lavage of the proximal and distal stomas (prior to sterile skin preparation) is not routinely practiced but may reduce the risk of intraoperative soiling. Note: care should be taken to completely aspirate all fluid once effluent is clear, as liquid spillage is more difficult to prevent and control than formed stool.
  - Suture the functional stoma closed at the start of the procedure.
  - Excise an ellipse of skin around the stoma, more so if skin is excoriated.
  - Occlude the lumen of the bowel about 5 cm proximal to the proposed site of division with a non-crushing bowel clamp or silicone vascular ribbon/large caliber braided suture material (slung through a small puncture in the mesentery directly adjacent to the bowel) to avoid soiling prior to distal clamping and transection.
- Postoperatively:
  - 24–48 hours of broad-spectrum antibiotic prophylaxis; consider extending to 5 days if skin surrounding stoma was significantly excoriated.
  - Consider perioperative nutritional support with zinc sulfate (10–20 mg daily) and Vitamin C (50–100 mg daily) to optimize wound healing for 2–4 weeks in malnourished patients.

## 25.6 Technical aspects: Performing neonatal colostomy under local anesthesia

### 25.6.1 Patient selection

- Distal neonatal bowel obstruction AND [10][16]
  - Delayed presentation (>48 hours after birth) with no referral hospital within reasonable distance AND
  - No experienced neonatal anesthetist capabilities ± postoperative neonatal intensive care AND
  - Unable to decompress bowel via rectal irrigation (if normal anus) or perineal/vestibular fistula (if anorectal malformation) AND/OR
  - Severe sepsis including septic shock not responding to 40 mL/kg intravenous crystalloid bolus, abdominal wall erythema, and edema AND/OR
  - Associated conditions that make general anesthesia high risk, including prematurity, low birth weight (<2.5 kg) [11], cardiac condition, etc.

### 25.6.2 Preoperative considerations

- Decompress stomach with nasogastric tube
- Intravenous rehydration with isotonic crystalloids in 10 mL/kg aliquots as needed, followed by 10% dextrose-containing intravenous maintenance fluid
- Intravenous Vitamin K and broad-spectrum antibiotic administration

- Intramuscular tetanus toxoid administration if mother was not immunized during pregnancy
- Analgesia, e.g., intravenous acetaminophen/paracetamol 15 mg/kg OR ketamine 0.5 mg/kg IVI
- Even though the procedure is performed under local anesthesia, oxygen saturation and heart rate monitoring should be continued throughout the procedure, preferably by a health-care member other than the one performing the surgery
- Nasal cannula or face mask oxygen may be administered especially if there is respiratory distress
- Strap the supine infant in a crucifix position under a radiant heater or over a warm-air blanket
- Insert a urine catheter (e.g., 6-French Foley catheter or 5-French infant feeding tube)
- Plastic can be taped over the sides and legs for added warmth
- Nonnutritive sucking in alert infants can help to calm the infant during the procedure (e.g., pacifier dipped in 10% dextrose solution)
- Draw up 7 mg/kg of 2% lignocaine with adrenaline in a sterile fashion

## 25.6.3 Operative technique

- Sterile skin preparation and draping of abdomen.
- It is helpful to indicate incision site (3-cm hockey-stick or transverse incision midway between umbilicus and anterior superior iliac spine) in left iliac fossa with skin marker.
- Infiltrate skin and subcutaneous tissue with local anesthetic. Allow 2–5 minutes for effect. Incise and infiltrate underlying muscle and incise.
- Place 3/0 polydiaxonone or polyglactic acid holding sutures midway along muscle and fascial sheath on either side of wound.
- A moist cotton swab should be held in preparation at the opening of the peritoneum to limit evisceration of the small bowel and may be used to gently pack the small bowel back into the abdomen.
- Sweep fingers or forceps such as Babcock or Dennis Browne from lateral abdominal wall medially to grasp sigmoid colon, which can be identified by its thickened, striated, edematous appearance. Confirm anatomy by digital palpation proximally along lateral abdominal wall to retroperitoneal attachment of descending colon, as well as distally toward rectum, and excluding attached omentum indicating that it is actually low-lying transverse colon.
- A purse-string 5/0 suture or two stay sutures can be placed in the most proximal aspect of the sigmoid accessible within the wound, and a large-bore (e.g., 12–16 French) Foley's catheter or similar round-tipped hollow tube is inserted within a hole incised inside the purse-string or between the stay sutures. Meconium is aspirated via the catheter until the bowel is decompressed sufficiently to mobilize it out of the wound. Warm saline lavage via the catheter can be helpful to evacuate thick viscous meconium.
- Once it is decompressed, proximally and distally, proximal and distal palpation again confirms anatomy. Ideally, the purse-string suture will be at the preferred site of colostomy, a few centimeters below the junction of the peritoneally fixed descending colon and mobile sigmoid colon. If not, this hole can be oversewed. The colon is also inspected for any signs of necrosis or perforation, which once again may be suitable as a site for colostomy or may be repaired if distal to the desired proximal sigmoid colostomy site.
- A curved artery forceps is used to create a defect in the mesentery adjacent to the preferred colostomy site, and the mesentery is divided at this level, preserving the marginal vessels if possible.

- The holding sutures previously placed on the sheath are drawn on one side through the mesenteric defect and tied to the sutures on the opposite side to approximate the fascial sheath underneath the loop of bowel.
- The serosa of the proximal and distal bowel is sutured in at least four quadrants to the sheath.
- The bowel is now transected (ideally at the level of the previously made purse-string enclosed hole) a few millimeters above skin level on the distal aspect of the exposed loop of bowel, after placing a clamp across the lumen. This can also be done prior to sheath closure.
- The distal (mucous fistula) stoma defect is made as small as possible, closing the sheath edges snugly after suturing it to the corner of the sheath, and then suturing the edges flush to the skin. It may also be left long initially and then trimmed a few days later to be more flush with the skin once the skin bridge has settled.
- The proximal stoma should allow a small fingertip or 14-French Foley's catheter to pass, and Brooks maturation should be done after closing the subcutaneous tissue and skin between the stomas.
- Further irrigation to decompress the proximal bowel and fully evacuate the distal bowel can be done after skin closure, provided the wound is protected with plastic film dressing or cotton swabs.

Transverse loop colostomy under local anesthesia is also an option which may be lifesaving for babies in extremis [17], but has much higher complication rates (e.g., prolapse, retraction, stenosis) compared to a divided sigmoid stoma.

### 25.6.4  Postoperative considerations

Monitor for signs of raised intra-abdominal pressure and sepsis suggesting bowel necrosis or wound infection. Feeds may be started once the stoma is functioning and the infant is no longer showing signs of sepsis. Continue broad-spectrum antibiotics for 5 days or according to clinical picture.

## 25.7  Technical aspects: Periumbilical/umbilical approach as alternative to laparoscopic colonic biopsy and proximal colon mobilization for long-segment Hirschsprung disease

### 25.7.1  Patient selection

Patients with Hirschsprung disease confirmed histologically on rectal biopsy with radiologic suggestion of a transition zone above mid-sigmoid level, who have well-decompressed proximal bowel on rectal irrigations. Use may be considered at all one-stage trans-anal pull-through procedures in order to obtain confirmation of correct pull-through level [18] early during the procedure depending on turnaround time for intraoperative frozen section results.

### 25.7.2  Preoperative consideration

Availability of reliable intraoperative frozen section to confirm histologically normal bowel at the level of pull-through will determine whether a staged approach (with initial biopsies only followed by subsequent pull-through within the next few weeks) or one-stage leveling biopsies with pull-through is considered.

### 25.7.3 Intraoperative considerations

A 2-cm incision (through the umbilicus or an inferior circum-umbilical incision between 180° to a maximum of 270° of the circumference of the umbilicus) is made. Umbilical vessels and urachal remnant are divided. An instrument passed trans-rectally such as a Hegar dilator, Poole suction tip guard, or urethral sound guides the sigmoid into the wound, permitting stay-suture placement and biopsy [19]. Serial biopsies can be taken along the colon, using Denis Browne or Babcock forceps to "walk" proximally along the bowel. In neonates in whom the abdominal wall is pliable, retraction of the wound gives ready access to the entire colon, allowing mobilization as required for biopsy and subsequent pull-through. Colectomy in older patients using this technique has also been described.

The same wound may be used to site a stoma in Hirschsprung disease where necessary [19].

## 25.8 Technical aspects: Ano(recto)plasty

The following have been described to reduce morbidity in regions where postoperative care and follow-up are inadequate, but are not universally appropriate:

1. Large anastomosis to reduce anal stenosis and need for dilations
   - *Indications*: Poor follow-up or difficulty with home dilations (e.g., older child) likely.
   - *Operative technique*: Anorectoplasty: The neo-anus is created slightly wider than usual (at the extremes of the muscle sphincter complex) to limit or avoid subsequent need for anal dilations [10].
   - *Hirschsprung disease pull-through*: Similarly, a wide anastomosis may be created through an oblique incision above the dentate line, 3–5 mm posteriorly and 10 mm anteriorly, taking care to preserve the dentate line when suturing.
2. Long closed rectal stump with subsequent trimming to reduce perineal wound infection [20]
   - *Indication*: Shortage of nursing staff and resources for hygiene to manage mucous extravasation post-PSARP.
   - *Operative technique*: Anchor a 3-cm long rectal stump at skin level with 8 sutures to the skin within the sphincter complex. Suture the tip of the rectum closed (ligate and then close with purse-string) to prevent mucous extravasation. Trim to skin level after 2 weeks once posterior sagittal wound has healed (described using thermal cautery device under sedation [13]).

## 25.9 Perioperative care considerations

### 25.9.1 Technical aspects: Early Recovery After Surgery (ERAS) principles

Early postoperative feeding reduces intravenous fluid requirements and permits early discharge [21].

#### 25.9.1.1 Immediate postoperative feeding

Patient selection:

- Colostomy for anorectal malformations presenting within 48 hours of birth without signs of sepsis, uncomplicated stoma closure, distal recto-sigmoid trans-anal pull-through, posterior sagittal anorectoplasty with covering stoma.

Notes:

- Breastfed babies tend to tolerate full feeds sooner and may be weaned off intravenous fluids within 8–24 hours.

- Consider delaying feeds until after 12–24 hours postoperatively in formula-fed infants and older children; however, clear fluids may be given per os on demand.
- Reduce or halt oral intake in case of vomiting or abdominal distension, and reintroduce after 12–24 hours.
- Discharge is possible within 48 hours provided that the patient is apyrexial and has had no vomits for at least 24 hours, stool has been passed, and there is no redness around the wound, with clear follow-up instructions.

# 25.10 Equipment

## 25.10.1 Technical aspects: Alternatives to stoma appliances

Protection of skin from excoriation by stool in the absence of commercially available stoma bags can be achieved by:

- Regular (3–5-hourly) changing of overlying cloth napkins or commercially available diapers, protecting surrounding skin with ointment such as petroleum jelly, zinc oxide paste [22], or sucrulfate paste [23].
- Betel leaves [23,24] and other broad, nontoxic leaves have been used, after protecting the surrounding skin with an emollient as described previously.
- Commercially available Karaya gum-based barrier pastes.
- "Home-made" stoma bag fashioned from plastic bag and adhesive tape (older children) [25].

## 25.10.2 Technical aspects: Alternatives to the pena muscle stimulator

### 25.10.2.1 Patient selection

- All patients with **anorectal malformations** require accurate placement of the neo-anus within the sphincter complex at anorectoplasty.
- Patients undergoing **investigation for incontinence** after previous surgery (including pull-through for Hirschsprung disease and ano(recto)plasty for anorectal malformations) or trauma to the anal canal.

### 25.10.2.2 Preoperative consideration

General anesthesia is required, including for examinations for continence. Muscle relaxant and caudal anesthesia should not affect the sphincter contraction significantly provided that the nerve stimulator is applied directly to the sphincter muscle or overlying skin.

### 25.10.2.3 Intraoperative considerations

The ideal nerve stimulator for use in anorectoplasties has a fixed distance between the electrode probes to ensure even stimulation (e.g., Pena muscle stimulator), is safely insulated, and has probes and leads that can be sterilized. However, adequate evaluation of sphincter muscle contractions can be assessed using one of the following attachments applied to an anesthetic nerve stimulator, at up to 75 times lower cost [26]:

a. Bipolar forceps (Figure 25.4).
b. Electrocardiogram "crocodile/alligator" clips applied to hypodermic needles.
c. Copper wire bent in half, preferably covered in an insulating plastic tube except at the tips.

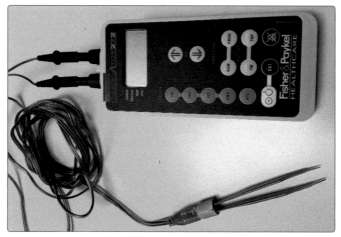

**Figure 25.4** Example of anesthetic nerve stimulator (Fisher and Pykel Healthcare, REF 233201586C, New Zealand) connected to bipolar diathermy forceps to assess location of anal sphincter complex. The preferred setting on this device is "external" "tetany" at 80 Hz.

### 25.10.3 Technical aspects: Dilator alternatives

#### 25.10.3.1 Patient selection

Anorectal malformation:

- *Neo-anus (mucocutaneous junction)*: Starting routinely ~2 weeks after anorectoplasty
- Stomal stenosis

Hirschsprung disease:

- Anastomotic (mucosal) stricture post Hirschsprung endorectal pull-through
- Obstructive symptoms despite patency after ganglionated endorectal pull-through

Alternatives to commercially available graded Hegar dilators:

- Caregiver digit (lubricated and protecting area under fingernail with soft soap).
- *Homemade candle dilators*: Parents are given a template of different diameter sizes to guide them in whittling wax taper candles to the correct size.
- Foley's catheters (especially suited in Hirschsprung disease, due to softer mucosal anastomoses).
- Blood specimen collection tubes.
- *Plastic pipes*: A lathe can produce the correct size dilator using a polyethylene or similar plastic rod. *Care needs to be taken to ensure that parents take the angle of insertion into account as these straight dilators need more care negotiating the curve of the anal canal than the already-curved Hegar dilators.*

## References

1. Akhparov NN, Aipov RR, Ormantayev KS. The surgical treatment of H-fistula with normal anus in girls. *Pediatr Surg Int.* 2008;24(11):1207–10.
2. Banieghbal B, Fonseca J. Acquired rectovaginal fistulae in South Africa. *Arch Dis Child.* 1997;77(1):94.

3. Uba AF, Chirdan LB, Ardill W, Ramyil VM, Kidmas AT. Acquired rectal fistula in human immunodeficiency virus-positive children: A causal or casual relationship? *Pediatr Surg Int*. 2004;20(11–12):898–901.

4. Wiersma R. HIV-positive African children with rectal fistulae. *J Pediatr Surg*. 2003;38(1):62–4.

5. Chitnis M, Lazarus C, Simango I, Elsen M, Van rensburg C, Von delft D, Tovell-Trollope L. Laparoscopically inserted button colostomy as a venting stoma and access port for the administration of antegrade enemas in African degenerative leiomyopathy. *S Afr J Surg*. 2011 Febraury;49(1).44–6.

6. Moore SW, Schneider JW, Kaschula RDC. Non-familial visceral myopathy: Clinical and pathologic features of degenerative leiomyopathy. *Pediatr Surg Int*. 2002;18:6–12.

7. Chirdan LB, Uba FA, Ameh EA, Mshelbwala PM. Colostomy for high anorectal malformation: An evaluation of morbidity and mortality in a developing country. *Pediatr Surg Int*. 2008;24(4):407–10.

8. Biccard BM, Madiba TE, Kluyts HL et al. Perioperative patient outcomes in the African Surgical Outcomes Study: A 7-day prospective observational cohort study. *Lancet*. 2018;391(10130):1589–98.

9. Karpelowsky JS, Leva E, Kelley B, Numanoglu A, Rode H, Millar AJ. Outcomes of human immunodeficiency virus-infected and -exposed children undergoing surgery—A prospective study. *J Pediatr Surg*. 2009;44(4):681–7.

10. Poenaru D, Borgstein E, Numanoglu A, Azzie G. Caring for children with colorectal disease in the context of limited resources. *Semin Pediatr Surg*. 2010;19(2):118–27.

11. Machin M, Liu C, Coupland A, Davies AH, Thapar A. Systematic review of the use of cyanoacrylate glue in addition to standard wound closure in the prevention of surgical site infection. *Int Wound J*. 2019 Apr;16(2):387–93.

12. Dumville JC, Gray TA, Walter CJ et al. Dressings for the prevention of surgical site infection. *Cochrane Database Syst Rev*. 2016;12:Cd003091.

13. Toh JWT, Phan K, Ctercteko G et al. The role of mechanical bowel preparation and oral antibiotics for left-sided laparoscopic and open elective restorative colorectal surgery with and without faecal diversion. *Int J Colorectal Dis*. 2018;33(12):1781–91.

14. Ameh EA, Lukong CS, Mshelbwala PM, Anumah MA, Gomna A. One-day bowel preparation in children with colostomy using normal saline. *Afr J Paediatr Surg*. 2011;8(3):291–3.

15. Ohman KA, Wan L, Guthrie T et al. Combination of oral antibiotics and mechanical bowel preparation reduces surgical site infection in colorectal surgery. *J Am Coll Surg*. 2017;225(4):465–71.

16. Lukong CS, Jabo BA, Mfuh AY. Colostomy in neonates under local anaesthesia: Indications, technique and outcome. *Afr J Paediatr Surg*. 2012;9(2):176–80.

17. Chowdhary SK, Chalapathi G, Narasimhan KL et al. An audit of neonatal colostomy for high anorectal malformation: The developing world perspective. *Pediatr Surg Int*. 2004;20(2):111–3.

18. Nasr A, Langer JC. Evolution of the technique in the transanal pull-through for Hirschsprung's disease: Effect on outcome. *J Paediatr Surg*. 2007;42(1):36–9.

19. Raj P, Sarin YK. Umbilicus: A site for stoma in Hirschsprung's disease. *J Neonatal Surg*. 2015;4(2):24.

20. Olivieri C, Belay K, Coletta R, Retrosi G, Molle P, Calisti A. Preventing posterior sagittal anoplasty 'cripples' in areas with limited medical resources: A few modifications to surgical approach in anorectal malformations. *Afr J Paediatr Surg*. 2012;9(3):223–6.

21. Sangkhathat S, Patrapinyokul S, Tadyathikom K. Early enteral feeding after closure of colostomy in pediatric patients. *J Paediatr Surg*. 2003;38(10):1516–9.

22. Ameh EA, Mshelbwala PM, Sabiu L, Chirdan LB. Colostomy in children—An evaluation of acceptance among mothers and caregivers in a developing country. *S Afr J Surg*. 2006;44(4):138–9.

23. Banerjee S, Haque J. An indigenous method of enterostomy management. *J Indian Assoc Pediatr Surg*. 2001;6(3):77–9.

24. Banu T, Talukder R, Chowdhury TK, Hoque M. Betel leaf in stoma care. *J Paediatr Surg*. 2007;42(7):1263–5.

25. Anyanwu LJ, Mohammad A, Oyebanji T. A descriptive study of commonly used postoperative approaches to pediatric stoma care in a developing country. *Ostomy Wound Manage*. 2013;59(12):32–7.

26. Short S, Kimble K, Zhai S, Frykman G, Frykman P. A low-cost improvised nerve stimulator is equivalent to high-cost muscle stimulator for anorectal malformation surgery. *Eur J Pediatr Surg*. 2013;23(1):25–8.

# 26 Transitional care in colorectal and pelvic reconstruction surgery

Alessandra C. Gasior

## 26.1 Case study 1

A 14-year-old female with a history of anorectal malformation presents to your clinic for her annual follow-up. She denies any current complaints. She takes senna daily and has good control of her bowel movements. Her abdominal x-ray is clear of stool today. She denies any history of urinary tract infections. She has started her period and is able to insert a tampon without difficulty. The patient's mother asks you what will her medical follow-up look like in 10 years.

**Will she continue to be seen by her pediatric surgeon?**

    A. She no longer needs to be seen by a physician and can be discharged from colorectal care for her anorectal malformation
    B. She can continue to be seen by her pediatric surgeon indefinitely
    C. She will need to be transitioned to an adult colorectal surgeon who specializes in the needs of adults living with anorectal malformations

*Answer:* C

### 26.1.1 Learning points

- Transitional care for pediatric patients with chronic diseases is a topic that has been recognized as a priority in our health-care system. However, the practice of transitioning patients, particularly congenital colorectal patients, has not been implemented. Only 22% of adolescents and young adults receive planning for health-care transition [1].
- The complexity of the original malformation and associated anomalies will affect the patient's fecal and urinary continence throughout adolescents and adulthood [2].

- There is no international consensus for long-term follow-up or transition of care to adulthood.
- The psychosocial needs of a patient will also need to be addressed by health-care providers [3].
- The process for transitional care should begin around 12–14 years of age [4]. A general health knowledge tool should be used to assess the patient's own understanding of their medical condition including surgical history, medications, and recent imaging. An annual readiness to transition worksheet should be completed by the caregiver and patient starting at the age of 12 years.
- The most common reason that a patient does not transition from a pediatric surgeon is the fear that the adult surgeon will not understand the treatment and specific needs of the anorectal malformation patient [5]. An appropriate adult surgical provider should be identified early in the process. The patient should transfer to an adult surgical provider when they are at a stable period in their medical care and not during an acute intervention if at all possible.
- A multidisciplinary approach should be used for transition. The stakeholders include: urologist, gynecologist, fertility specialist, colorectal surgeons, gastroenterologist, social workers, and psychiatrist.

## 26.2  Case study 2

A 32-year-old male presents with a history of pull-through for Hirschsprung disease (HD). He complains of fecal incontinence. Unfortunately the patient does not have any medical records from his childhood. He does not recall episodes of enterocolitis during his postsurgical childhood or adolescence. He denies a history of abdominal distension, fever, or emesis. He does not take any enemas, or antimotility agents. On abdominal examination, he has a left transverse scar, presumably from a colostomy site.

**What studies would you like to obtain?**

A. Water-soluble contrast enema
B. Anorectal manometry
C. Rectal biopsy
D. Exam under anesthesia
E. All of the above

*Answer:* E

### 26.2.1  Learning points

- Hirschsprung-associated enterocolitis (HAEC) occurs in 5% of adult patients and has the potential to be life threatening if unrecognized by adult providers, therefore this should be a consideration in any HD patient presenting with distension or obstructive symptoms, even for adults that are postsurgical repair.
- The majority of HD patients have life-long GI complications with constipation occurring in up to 44% of patients.
- Fecal incontinence occurs in up to 76% of patients due to damage to the sphincters during dissection [6,7].
- Evaluation of the Hirschsprung patient who is not doing well should include: an exam under anesthesia to examine the anatomy which includes evaluating the dentate line, inspection for the type of surgery performed which may include a palpable soave cuff, Duhamel spur, or stricture [8].

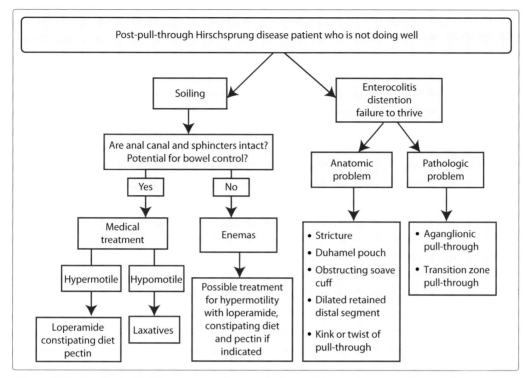

**Figure 26.1** A patient with Hirschsprung disease who is not doing well post a pull-through procedure.

- Patients with obstructive symptoms will benefit from a full-thickness rectal biopsy to evaluate for a transition zone pull-through or aganglionic pull-through [9].
- A contrast enema will demonstrate if the patient has hypermotility or hypomotility, which will require different treatments. Hypermotile bowel will require antidiarrheal medications to slow transit that may be contributing to fecal incontinence. Hypomotility occurs more commonly in HD patients affected with constipation requiring a bowel regimen with laxatives that may require periodic adjustments. The contrast enema will also identify a possible retained distal segment as well as a kink or twist of the pull-through (Figure 26.1).

## 26.3  Case study 3

A 19-year-old female with a history of an imperforate anus (unknown type) s/p repair presents to your clinic for the evaluation of fecal incontinence. She does not have any records from her previous surgeries. You are able to see a left-side scar that appears to be a colostomy closure site. She has a history of urinary tract infections and urinary retention. She performs a straight catheterization 4–6 times per day. She does not take any medications for a bowel regimen, although she remembers doing enemas when she was younger but she has stopped now because she did not like them. She also says she would like to have children of her own one day and asks you what her chances of conceiving are.

**What is your next step?**

A. Water-soluble contrast enema
B. Rectal exam either under anesthesia or in the office
C. Pelvic exam

    **D.** MRI spine and MRI pelvis
    **E.** All of the above

*Answer:* E

### 26.3.1 Learning points

- 73% of anorectal malformation patients are followed by a multidisciplinary team from birth. Additionally during adolescence, 73% of these patients develop significant new problems including fecal incontinence, chronic constipation, urinary incontinence, ejaculatory dysfunction, erectile dysfunction, psychosocial issues, and quality of life that require a multidisciplinary team. However, 33% of pediatric surgeons discharge patients from care before 10 years old [10]. This occurs despite the patient having ongoing unaddressed issues. This underscores the importance of maintaining a multidisciplinary team for anorectal malformation patients through adulthood, as their needs evolve and change over time.
- Pelvic exam and rectal exam should be performed to evaluate the surgical site for stricture, prolapse, vaginal introital stenosis, quality of perineal body, and residual vaginal septum. This may have implications for menstrual hygiene, intercourse, obstetric indications as well as can affect bowel regimen. A pelvic MRI may be necessary to determine the presence of Müllerian structures.
- Pelvic anatomy is also important for reproductive potential. Preconception counseling should be offered by a high-risk obstetrician. Pregnancy is possible in patients with anorectal malformations and cloacal malformations. Mode of delivery must be individually addressed with a risk versus benefit especially for increased risk of fecal and urinary incontinence with vaginal delivery [11].

## References

1. Chu PY, Maslow GR, von Isenburg M et al. Systematic review of the impact of transition interventions for adolescents with chronic illness on transfer from pediatric to adult healthcare. *J Pediatr Nur.* 2015;30:e19–e27.
2. Cairo SB, Gasior A, Rollins MD, Rothstein DH. Delivery of Surgical Care Committee of the American Academy of Pediatrics Section on Surgery. Challenges in transition of care for patients with anorectal malformations: A systematic review and recommendations for comprehensive care. *Dis Colon Rectum.* 2018 Mar;61(3):390–9.
3. Schwartz LA, Brumley LD, Tuchman LK et al. Stakeholder validation of a model of readiness for transition to adult care. *JAMA Pediatr.* 2013;167(10):939–46.
4. Giuliani S, Grano C, Aminoff D et al. Transition of care in patients with anorectal malformations: Consensus by the ARM-net consortium. *J Pediatr Surg.* 2017 Nov;52(11):1866–72.
5. Cairo SB, Chiu PP, Dasgupta R et al. Transitions in care from pediatric to adult general surgery: Evaluating an unmet need for patients with anorectal malformation and Hirschsprung disease. *J Pediatr Surg.* 2018 Aug;53(8):1566–72.
6. Yanchar NL, Soucy P. Long-term outcome after Hirschsprung's disease: Patients' perspectives. *J Pediatr Surg.* 1999;34:1152–60.
7. Scott AE, Jay JG. Long-term results of treatment of Hirschsprung's disease. *Semin Pediatr Surg.* 2004;13:273–85.
8. Levitt MA, Dickie B, Pena A. Evaluation and treatment of the patient with Hirschsprung disease who is not doing well after a pull-through procedure. *Semin Pediatr Surg.* 2010 May;19(2):146–53.
9. Peña A, Elicevik M, Levitt MA. Reoperations in Hirschsprung's disease. *J Pediatr Surg.* 2007;42:1008–14.
10. Giuliani S, Decker E, Leva E et al. Long term follow-up and transition of care in anorectal malformations: An international survey. *J Pediatr Surg.* 2016 Sep;51(9):1450–7.
11. Breech L. Gynecologic concerns in patients with cloacal anomaly. *Semin Pediatr Surg.* 2016 Apr;25(2):90–5.

# 27 Operative reports of the most common procedures in pediatric colorectal surgery: Key steps

Alejandra Vilanova-Sánchez, Giulia Brisighelli, and Carlos A. Reck-Burneo

## 27.1 Laparoscopic-assisted Swenson pull-through for Hirschsprung disease

### 27.1.1 Equipment

- Four (4 mm) trocars
- One (3 mm) 30° laparoscope
- Two or three atraumatic graspers
- One (3 mm) Maryland dissector
- One (3 mm) Hook monopolar cautery
- 4 or 5/0 Absorbable braided suture for the coloanal anastomosis
- Lone star ring
- Eight lone star pins
- Foley catheter
- Forceps and needle driver for open surgery

### 27.1.2 Operative report

Patient was placed supine in the middle of the table. General endotracheal anesthesia was administered and a total body preparation was performed (see Section 2.3). During the procedure the surgeon stands at the right upper side of the patient at the shoulder in front of the monitor, which is at the foot and end of the bed. The assistant is on the left upper side holding the camera and graspers during the sigmoid dissection. The scrub nurse is on the left lower side of the table in line with the surgeon.

We started with the laparoscopic portion of the case inserting a 4 mm trocar in the umbilicus and another 4 mm in the right upper quadrant. The peritoneum was insufflated using pressure of 8–10 mm Hg and a flow of 1–2 L/min. We selected the biopsy site at the level of the transition zone suspected in the contrast enema (proximal sigmoid) and pulled it out through the umbilical port with a grasper. Once the full-thickness biopsy was taken we closed the defect with interrupted extracorporeal stitches and put the bowel back into the abdomen.

After receiving the pathologist's report we then inserted a left upper quadrant and right lower quadrant 4 mm ports to start the sigmoid arcade dissection. The right upper quadrant port is for the camera and the right lower quadrant port is for the surgeon's right hand. The umbilical port is for the surgeon's left hand and the left upper quadrant is the assisting port. We first open a mesenteric window at the level of our previous biopsy and start the dissection with thermal energy. The IMA arcade to the sigmoid is carefully preserved.

Once we reach the rectum we start the dissection in a Swenson-type fashion, right on the rectal wall. When the dissection of the distal rectum completed from the abdomen, we removed the laparoscopic ports and place the patient's legs up to begin the transanal dissection. We placed the lone start ring and pins. We identified the dentate line and hid it with the lone star pens. We created circumferential traction with silk stitches placed 1 cm proximal to the dentate line and begin the dissection.

Once we were able to enter the peritoneum from below, we could see the branches of the sigmoid mesentery ligated from our previous dissection and the biopsy site. We select the segment for our first layer anastomosis 3–5 cm proximal to the biopsy. The first layer was performed from anal canal muscle to colonic serosa. We then replaced the lone star pins to show the previously hidden mucosal edge and then completed our second layer of the anastomosis at the level of the previous resection utilizing 16 well-placed interrupted Vicryl sutures, from mucosa to mucosa. Sterile dressing was applied.

## 27.2 Open sigmoid resection for segmental colonic dysmotility

### 27.2.1 Equipment

- Regular laparotomy set
- Foley catheter (size according to the size of the patient)
- Catheter tip syringe
- Ligasure (optional)
- GIA linear stapler (optional)
- 4 or 5/0 Braided sutures for the stay sutures
- 4 or 5/0 Absorbable braided suture for the coloanal anastomosis
- Diathermy/monopolar with needle tip and standard tip

### 27.2.2 Operative report

The patient was placed supine on the operating table. General endotracheal anesthesia was administered. The abdomen was prepped and draped in the usual sterile fashion. The abdomen was entered through a PfannenStiel incision, with a vertical split of the fascia to the level of the umbilicus. We identified the sigmoid colon. The rectosigmoid had the typical dilation with a more normal caliber proximal sigmoid and left colon. We released the left retroperitoneal attachments so the left colon was loose. We dissected clean to the location of the planned transaction at the upper rectum, several centimeters above the peritoneal reflection. We ligated several mesenteric vessels between clamps and ties, and then placed bowel clamps across the rectum and the upper sigmoid. The two ends of the planned anastomosis reached each other without tension. We then transected across the bowel and took the intervening mesentery between clamps and ties. We sutured closed the right side of the large rectal opening so that the remaining lumen matched the proximal sigmoid lumen. This was performed in two layers, running and interrupted with long-term absorbable suture. We aligned the mesentery, and then performed a primary anastomosis in two layers with Vicryl. We closed the small mesenteric defect. Hemostasis was ensured, and the abdomen was irrigated. The bowel was returned to its normal anatomic position. The peritoneum and posterior fascia were closed with interrupted absorbable suture, as was Scarpa's fascia and a subdermal layer. The skin was closed with a subcuticular closure. Sterile dressing was applied.

## 27.3 Laparoscopic sigmoid resection plus Malone

### 27.3.1 Equipment

- Two (5 mm) trocars
- One 12 mm trocars
- One (5 mm) 30° laparoscope
- Two atraumatic graspers
- One (5 mm) ligasure Maryland dissector
- One endo-GIA stapler (purple load)
- One EEA stapler 28, 31, or 33
- One Alexis wound protector
- Foley catheter

### 27.3.2 Operative report

The patient was placed supine on the operating room table. General endotracheal anesthesia was administered and the abdomen was prepped and draped in the usual sterile fashion. The rectum caliber was checked to select the right EEA size according to the size of the patient. The legs are placed in stirrups to elevate the legs and place the patient in lithotomy position during EEA insertion.

A V-plasty skin incision was made and a 5-mm incision was made through the fascia of the umbilicus and blunt dissection carried down into the peritoneum. A 5 mm port was placed through this incision and the abdomen insufflated to a pressure of 15 mm Hg. On visual inspection, the sigmoid colon was redundant and dilated. A 12-mm incision was then made in the right lower quadrant and a 12-mm port was placed through this incision under direct visualization. A 5-mm incision was then made in the left lower quadrant just below the level of the umbilicus. A 5-mm port was then placed under direct visualization. The surgeon stands on the right at the level of the shoulder of the patient. The right hand is for the right lower quadrant port and the left hand for the left lower quadrant. The assistant is placed in the left side of the patient. The umbilical port is for the camera. The sigmoid colon was then retracted and a window made through the mesentery adjacent to the wall of the colon using the Ligasure sealing device. The mesentery of the sigmoid and rectum was then divided in a similar manner down to the peritoneal reflection. The peritoneal reflection was then circumferentially dissected to mobilize the rectum and dissection carried down to approximately 6 cm above the dentate line.

The white line of Toldt was then divided to mobilize the descending colon. The point of mesenteric division allowed adequate length for the descending colon to reach the pelvis for the anastomosis. The right colon and cecum were also mobilized by taking down the retroperitoneal attachments so that the cecum was freely mobile. The cecum and the appendix were also mobilized to facilitate the laparoscopic Malone.

The colon was then divided using an EndoGIA endoscopic stapler (purple load) through the 12-mm port in the right lower quadrant. The stapled end was then grasped with a blunt grasper. The right lower quadrant port was then removed and extended by 1.5 cm opening the fascia. The wound protector was placed and the stapled end of the distal rectum was brought out through this incision. The colon was divided at the margin of viability and the anvil of the EEA stapler is inserted into the proximal colon which will be anastomosed distally with the dissected rectum. A 2-0 Prolene suture was used to run the edge of the colon in a pursestring fashion and then tied securely. The colon with the anvil was then returned to the abdominal cavity. A sterile glove was placed around the wound protector to allow pneumoperitoneum. The abdomen was re-insufflated. A hole was made in one of the "glove finger" to place the 12-mm port without losing the pneumoperitoneum.

The anvil was grasped using the anvil grasper being careful to maintain the proper alignment of the colon to avoid twisting the mesentery. At this moment the legs of the patient were elevated. The assistant surgeon (outside the sterile field) introduced the circular 28 mm EEA stapler through the anus. The 31 or 33 mm EEA stapler was then brought in through the rectum and its trocar deployed until the marker was visible. The anvil was then attached securely and the stapler fired without difficulty. Once the anastomosis was completed it was checked to make sure there were two complete circles of tissue. The anastomosis was airtight on submersion test with saline introducing air through the anus with a 60-cc syringe.

The cecum was brought up through the right lower quadrant incision and then plicated around the appendix without interfering with the blood supply in four positions with #3-0 silk, creating a valve-like mechanism for the base of the appendix. The appendix was transected at an appropriate length to reach the fascia and brought up through the V-plasty incision at the umbilicus. A Y to V anastomosis from the appendix to the umbilical skin was performed. This recreated the umbilical ring and the orifice was hidden nicely within it. A #10 French tube was placed through the appendix. It passed easily and was sutured in place with a 3/0 silk. A sterile dressing was applied.

The right lower quadrant port site was closed with interrupted 0-Vicryl and the skin with a 5-0 Monocryl running subcuticular. The left lower quadrant incision was closed using a 3-0 Vicryl suture at the fascia and a 5-0 Monocryl subcuticular suture was used to close the skin. Sterile dressing was applied.

## 27.4 Laparoscopic Malone

### 27.4.1 Equipment

- Three (4–5 mm) trocars
- One (3 mm) 30° laparoscope
- One laparoscopic atraumatic graspers
- 5/0 Absorbable braided suture for the anastomosis to the skin
- 5/0 Silk suture for the cecal valve
- Forceps and needle driver for open surgery
- A #10 feeding tube

### 27.4.2 Operative report

The patient was placed supine on the operating room table. General endotracheal anesthesia was administered and the abdomen was prepped and draped in the usual sterile fashion. We insufflated the abdomen with $CO_2$ through a 5-mm trocar, taking care to make a V incision on the umbilicus for the Y to V appendix to skin anastomosis. We insufflated with $CO_2$. We placed a 5-mm trocar in the left upper quadrant and another 5-mm trocar in the left lower quadrant for our dissection. The surgeon stands on the left side of the patient and the assistant to the left. The surgeon's right hand is for the left lower quadrant port and the left hand for the right lower quadrant port. We mobilized the right colon taking down its retroperitoneal attachments so that the cecum was freely mobile. We placed a stitch in the cecum through the umbilicus removing the umbilical port so that we could elevate it out of the umbilicus. We then extended our umbilical incision down for approximately 4.5 cm and then brought the cecum out of the incision. We plicated the cecum around the appendix without interfering with the blood supply in three positions with #5-0 silk, creating a valve-like mechanism for the base of the appendix. The appendix reached comfortably to the umbilicus. We then began closure of the fascia, taking bites of fascia and the cecum so that the tip of the appendix lay just at the prepared umbilical skin. We then performed a Y to V anastomosis from the appendix to the umbilical skin and then closed the umbilical dermis to itself, making the appendiceal mucosa hidden. We completed the closure of the incision at the Scarpa's and dermal layers and ran subcuticular for the skin. A #10 French tube was placed through the appendix. It passed easily and was left in place. A sterile dressing was applied.

## 27.5 Neoappendicostomy

### 27.5.1 Equipment

- Three (4–5 mm) trocars
- One (3 mm) 30° laparoscope
- One laparoscopic atraumatic graspers
- 5/0 Absorbable braided suture for the anastomosis to the skin
- 5/0 Silk suture for the cecal valve
- Forceps and needle driver for open surgery
- A #10 feeding tube

### 27.5.2 Operative report

The patient was placed supine on the operating room table. General anesthesia was administered. The abdomen was prepped and draped in a sterile fashion. We insufflated the abdomen with $CO_2$ through a 5-mm trocar placed in the umbilicus, cutting the umbilical skin in a V for the planned appendiceal-to-umbilical anastomosis. We placed two 5-mm trocars into his previous laparoscopy trocar sites. We mobilized the cecum until it comfortably reached the midline and then extended the infraumbilical incision approximately 4 cm and elevated the cecum through this incision. We then planned a cecal flap using two vessels and incised a U, rolled it out, and then tubularized over a #10 feeding tube, closing the cecal wall. We did this in two layers. This, thus, created a neo-appendix. We plicated the cecal wall around the base of the appendix to form a valve mechanism. We then lay the cecum with the appendix oriented toward the umbilicus, closed the fascia, taking bites of cecal wall to incorporate it and then performed a Y to V anastomosis from the umbilical skin to the neo-appendix with multiple 6-0 Vicryl sutures. We closed the Scarpa's fascia subdermal and used DermaBond for the skin. Hemostasis was ensured prior to closure and we closed the two-trocar sites with interrupted 5-0 Vicryl. Sterile dressing was applied.

## 27.6 Laparoscopic-assisted posterior sagittal anorectoplasty for anorectal malformation

### 27.6.1 Equipment

- Three (4-mm) trocars
- One (5-mm) 30° laparoscope
- Two atraumatic graspers
- Three (3-mm) endosealer
- One (3-mm) hook monopolar cautery
- 2/0 Monofilament non-absorbable suture for the bladder stay suture
- 2/0 Monofilament absorbable preloaded endoloop
- 4 or 5/0 Absorbable braided suture for the coloanal anastomosis
- Coude tip urethral catheter
- Peripheral nerve stimulator
- Hegar dilators
- Marking pen for the sphincter complex

### 27.6.2 Operative report

The patient was placed supine in the middle of the table and a total body preparation was performed. The surgeon stands to the right upper part of the patient at the patient right shoulder. The assistant stands to the left upper side of the patient. The scrub nurse is positioned on the right lower side of the patient, in line with the surgeon. We used a 5-mm 30° scope and 4-mm trocars (two or three) were utilized for the instruments (5-mm trocars are also accepted). Hook electrocautery and a 3-mm endosealer were utilized to avoid thermal spread when approaching the bladder/vagina.

The right upper quadrant port is for the camera access. The right lower quadrant port is for the surgeon's right hand and the umbilicus is for the surgeon's left hand. A 3-mm port in the mid-left abdomen is to help with the fistula ligation and is useful to retract the rectosigmoid.

The first step was to fix the bladder to the anterior abdominal wall with a transcutaneous stay suture to have a better exposure of the pelvis. Once we had a better exposure of the pelvis with the bladder fixed we started the rectal dissection using thermal dissection in a circumferential fashion. We identified both ureters and vas.

Once the fistula is dissected circumferentially, at the point of maximal tapering near the bladder/vagina, the fistula was divided. The bladder/vagina side is secured with a grasper and a 2/0 preloaded endoloop closes the fistula site. Once there is enough rectal length the patient's legs were elevated. The muscle complex was defined with the nerve stimulator, and a limited posterior sagittal incision was made.

The incision was opened with electrocautery and blunt dissection in order to reach the peritoneal reflection. We then tacked the muscles to the pull-through rectum to avoid prolapse and performed an anoplasty with 16 interrupted stitches. The posterior sagittal incision was closed in two layers with 4/0 non-absorbable suture. The skin was closed with 4/0 interrupted stitches. Sterile dressing was applied.

## 27.7 Heineke–Mikulicz plasty for skin level stricture after anoplasty

### 27.7.1 Equipment

- Regular herniorrhaphy set
- Foley catheter (size according to the size of the patient)
- Catheter tip syringe
- Ligasure (optional)
- GIA linear stapler (optional)
- 4 or 5/0 Braided sutures for the stay sutures
- 4 or 5/0 Absorbable braided suture for the coloanal anastomosis
- Diathermy/monopolar with needle tip and standard tip

### 27.7.2 Operative report

The patient was placed supine on the operating room table. The patient was sedated. A caudal block was given. The patient was then placed in lithotomy position allowing a good exposure of the anus. The perineal area was prepped and draped in the usual sterile fashion. A Hegar dilator was used to calibrate the anal size. Four-quadrant 4/0 silk stay suture stitches were placed and referred with mosquitoes. Pulling up and out two mosquitoes a longitudinal incision was made in the middle incising the scarred mucocutaneal junction. The defect was closed with transversal interrupted stitches in a Heineke–Mikulicz plasty manner making the circumference wider. This technique was done in 1, 2, 3, or 4 quadrants (as needed). We checked the increase in the anal circumference by introducing a Hegar dilator at the end of the procedure. No dressing was applied.

## 27.8 PSARP recto-vestibular fistula (female)

### 27.8.1 Equipment

- Regular laparotomy set
- Foley catheter (size according to the size of the patient)
- Catheter tip syringe
- Peripheral nerve stimulator
- 4 or 5/0 Braided sutures for the stay sutures
- 4 or 5/0 Absorbable braided suture for the coloanal anastomosis
- Diathermy/monopolar with needle tip and standard tip
- Hegar dilators

### 27.8.2 Operative report

The patient was placed supine on the operating table. The perineum was prepped and draped. We used cystoscope to delineate the urethra. She had a normal bladder neck that contracted well and a normal bladder mucosa. Inspection of the vagina revealed it to be normal. The distal rectum was in the vestibule. After the completion of the cystoscopy, we placed the patient prone and began our repair. We placed multiple silk stitches in the mucocutaneous junction of the rectum which was in the vestibule of the vagina and then made a posterior sagittal incision through the skin and subcutaneous tissue. The sphincter mechanism was easily delineated with a pink ellipse and we went directly through this and delineated the entire posterior wall of the rectum, noting a whitish fascia surrounding it. We dissected laterally to define the lateral plane and then began to come circumferentially around our sutures. We then carefully lifted the rectum superiorly and dissected the common wall between the rectum and the vagina. We completely separated the rectum from the posterior wall of the vagina reaching the areolar tissue that defines the two separate walls. We then began dissection of the attachments to the rectum so that we could gain adequate length for our anoplasty and it reached easily to the perineum without any tension. We then closed the perineal body with multiple long-term absorbable sutures including interrupted sutures at the skin level, up to the anterior limit of the sphincter mechanism which we delineated with the electrical stimulator. We then placed tension on the rectum and tacked the rectum to the posterior edge of the muscle complex, all the way to the level of the levator and up to the level of the skin. We then completed our reconstruction of the posterior sagittal incision, reapproximated the ischiorectal fat and parasagittal fibers, and used interrupted 5-0 Vicryl for the skin. We performed an anoplasty with 16 interrupted Vicryl sutures. The patient tolerated the procedure well, with no complications.

## 27.9 PSARP perineal fistula (male)

### 27.9.1 Equipment

- Regular laparotomy set
- Foley catheter (size according to the size of the patient)
- Catheter tip syringe
- Peripheral nerve stimulator
- 4 or 5/0 Braided sutures for the stay sutures
- 4 or 5/0 Absorbable braided suture for the coloanal anastomosis
- Diathermy/monopolar with needle tip and standard tip
- Hegar dilators

### 27.9.2 Operative report

The patient was placed supine on the operating table. General endotracheal anesthesia was administered. A Foley catheter was placed. The perineum was prepped and draped. The distal rectum ended as a tiny hole at the anterior aspect of the sphincter mechanism, consistent with a rectoperineal fistula. We placed the patient prone. We placed multiple silk stitches in the mucocutaneous junction of the fistula and then made a small (2–3 cm) posterior sagittal incision through the skin and subcutaneous tissue. The sphincter mechanism was easily delineated with a pink ellipse and we went directly through this and delineated the entire posterior wall of the rectum, noting a whitish fascia surrounding it. We dissected laterally to define the lateral plane and then began to come circumferentially around our sutures. We then carefully lifted the rectum superiorly and dissected the common wall between the rectum and the posterior urethra. We completely separated the rectum from the area of the posterior urethra, never getting so close as to visualize the urethral wall. We reached the areolar tissue that defines the two separate walls. We then began dissection of the attachments to the rectum so that we could gain adequate length for our anoplasty and it reached easily to the perineum without any tension. There was approximately 1–2 cm of fistula distal to the normal rectal tissue. We then closed the perineal body with multiple long-term absorbable sutures including interrupted sutures at the skin level, up to the anterior limit of the sphincter mechanism which we delineated with the electrical stimulator. We then placed tension on the rectum and tacked the rectum to the posterior edge of the muscle complex. We then completed our reconstruction of the posterior sagittal incision, with long-term absorbable suture in the subcutaneous tissue, and at the skin level. We performed an anoplasty with 16 interrupted Vicryl sutures after trimming 1–2 cm of excess tissue which was the fistula. The patient tolerated the procedure well, with no complications.

## 27.10 Cloaca total urogenital mobilization

### 27.10.1 Equipment

- Regular laparotomy set
- Foley catheter (size according to the size of the patient)
- Catheter tip syringe
- Peripheral nerve stimulator
- 4 or 5/0 Braided sutures for the stay sutures
- 4 or 5/0 Absorbable braided suture for the coloanal anastomosis
- 5 and 6/0 Sutures for the total urogenital mobilization (TUM)
- Diathermy/monopolar with needle tip and standard tip
- Hegar dilators

### 27.10.2 Operative report

The patient was placed supine on the operating room table.

The perineum was prepped and draped and then carefully inspected.

We then proceeded with a long posterior sagittal incision staying within the midline. This incision was carried down entirely in the midline splitting the parasagittal fibers, fascial rectal fat, muscle complex, and levator down to the level of the perineum.

We opened the entire common channel until we were able to identify the orifice of the rectum.

We placed multiple silk stitches on the borders of the split common channel to provide uniform traction and began to carefully dissect the rectal wall laterally on the lateral plane and then started our dissection anteriorly, carefully separating the rectum from the posterior wall of the vagina being sure to keep the vaginal and rectal walls intact.

We dissected until the rectum and the vagina were distinct and separate structures. During this dissection, we repeatedly checked the thickness of both the vaginal wall and the rectal wall using a lacrimal duct probe. The rectum was then further mobilized by removing some of its attached fasciae until it reached the perineum comfortably and with no tension for our planned anoplasty. We then lifted the rectum out and retracted it superiorly out of the field so that we could direct our attention toward the total urogenital mobilization. Again, traction sutures were entirely placed around the urogenital tract anteriorly approximately 5 mm posterior to the clitoris and then around the entire vagina. At this point, we visualized and identified the urethra so we cannulated it with the Foley catheter. Mobilization then began circumferentially around the urogenital tract using silk sutures for continuous traction. We were able to divide the suspensory ligament anteriorly to the urethra which allowed proper mobilization. At this point, it still did not appear that the vagina would reach the perineum, and this required further mobilization along the lateral aspect of the vagina being careful to preserve the blood supply to the vagina. Now we split the common channel in the midline. Multiple fine 6-0 Vicryl sutures were then utilized to reapproximate the urethra down to the perineum as well as the now splayed common channel laterally on both sides to recreate the labia. It came down nicely and without tension. We then brought the vagina down, again using 6-0 Vicryl sutures to the perineum circumferentially. Posteriorly, we marked the sites of the sphincter complex which was visible as well as used the muscle stimulator to define our anterior limit of the sphincter. We identified where a perineal body would fit and recreated our perineal body using 5-0 Vicryl sutures to bring soft tissue as well as the skin together posteriorly. The vagina was well perfused and fit nicely without tension at this point. Once our sphincter complex was marked, again using visual identification of the sphincter complex as well as the electrical stimulation we marked both the posterior and anterior limits. We then closed the levator muscle with several stitches and pulled the rectum underneath these stitches so that the muscle complex then lay on either side of the rectum. We held some gentle tension on the rectum and placed stitches from the posterior edge of the muscle complex into the back wall of the rectum and secured these, so the rectum lay entirely within the sphincter mechanism. We completed the closure of the posterior sagittal incision up to the skin in layers. We then performed an anoplasty with 16 interrupted long-term absorbable sutures after trimming off approximately the distal remains of the rectum. The anoplasty was performed under slight tension so that after the stitches were cut the anus retracted slightly with no evidence of prolapse. We completed the closure of the posterior sagittal incision with a combination of interrupted 6-0 Vicryl sutures. The baby was then returned to the supine position, again taking care to do this in coordination with anesthesia.

## 27.11 Cloaca PSARVUP: Posterior sagittal anorectovaginourethroplasty

### 27.11.1 Equipment

- Regular laparotomy set
- Foley catheter (size according to the size of the patient)
- Catheter tip syringe
- Peripheral nerve stimulator
- 4 or 5/0 Braided sutures for the stay sutures
- 4 or 5/0 Absorbable braided suture for the coloanal anastomosis
- Diathermy/monopolar with needle tip and standard tip

### 27.11.2 Operative report

The patient was placed supine on the operating room table.

The perineum was prepped and draped and then carefully inspected.

We then proceeded with a long posterior sagittal incision staying within the midline. This incision was carried down entirely in the midline splitting the parasagittal fibers, fascial rectal fat, muscle complex, and levator down to the level of the perineum.

We opened the entire common channel until we were able to identify the orifice of the rectum.

We placed multiple silk stitches on the borders of the split common channel to provide uniform traction and began to carefully dissect the rectal wall laterally on the lateral plane and then started our dissection anteriorly, carefully separating the rectum from the posterior wall of the vagina being sure to keep the vaginal and rectal walls intact.

We dissected until the rectum and the vagina were distinct and separate structures. During this dissection, we repeatedly checked the thickness of both the vaginal wall and the rectal wall using a lacrimal duct probe. The rectum was then further mobilized by removing some of its attached fasciae until it reached the perineum comfortably and with no tension for our planned anoplasty. We then lifted the rectum out and retracted it superiorly out of the field so we could then direct our attention toward the total urogenital mobilization. Again, traction sutures were entirely placed around the urogenital tract anteriorly approximately 5 mm posterior to the clitoris and then around the entire vagina. At this point, we visualized and identified the urethra so we cannulated it with the Foley catheter. We placed traction sutures around the vagina and carefully separated it from the ureter until fully mobilized. The common channel was then closed as urethra with a PDS 6-0 running suture. At this point, it still did not appear that the vagina would reach the perineum, and this required further mobilization along the lateral aspect of the vagina. We now reapproximated the vagina into the perineum using 6-0 Vicryl sutures making sure no tension was present and that no vagina replacement was needed.

Posteriorly, we marked the sites of the sphincter complex which was visible as well as used the muscle stimulator to define our anterior limit of the sphincter. We identified where a perineal body would fit and recreated our perineal body using 5-0 Vicryl sutures to bring soft tissue as well as the skin together posteriorly. The vagina was well perfused and fit nicely without tension at this point. Once our sphincter complex was marked, again using visual identification of the sphincter complex as well as the electrical stimulation we marked both the posterior and anterior limits. We then closed the levator muscle with several stitches and pulled the rectum underneath these stitches so that the muscle complex lay on either side of the rectum. We held some gentle tension on the rectum and placed stitches from the posterior edge of the muscle complex into the back wall of the rectum and secured these, so the rectum lay entirely within the sphincter mechanism. We completed the closure of the posterior sagittal incision up to the skin in layers. We then performed an anoplasty with 16 interrupted long-term absorbable sutures after trimming off approximately the distal remains of the rectum. The anoplasty was performed under slight tension so that after the stitches were cut the anus retracted slightly with no evidence of prolapse. We completed the closure of the posterior sagittal incision with a combination of interrupted 6-0 Vicryl sutures. The baby was then returned to the supine position, again taking care to do this in coordination with anesthesia.

## 27.12 Transanal Swenson pull-through for Hirschsprung disease

### 27.12.1 Equipment

- Regular laparotomy set
- Foley catheter (size according to the size of the patient)
- Catheter tip syringe
- Lone star ring
- Eight lone star pins
- Denis Browne retractor
- Ligasure (optional)
- GIA linear stapler (optional)
- 4 or 5/0 Braided sutures for the stay sutures
- 4 or 5/0 Absorbable braided suture for the coloanal anastomosis
- Diathermy/monopolar with needle tip and standard tip

### 27.12.2  Operative report

With the patient in supine position a general anesthesia is administered and a cuffed ETT tube is inserted. A caudal block may be given according to the center's protocols and IV antibiotics are started. At the same stage also a Foley catheter is inserted and the balloon inflated with 3–5 mL of normal saline. A rectal irrigation is then performed using the size 22 Foley catheter, until the water is clean.

The patient is then placed prone in the middle of the table with the hips raised in jack knife position. During the procedure the surgeon stands either at the right side of the patient or at the end of the bed, according to the personal preference. The assistant is on the left side of the patient and the scrub nurse is either at the right side of the bed or at the end of the bed.

A lone star is positioned to expose the anal canal and the pins are then positioned deeper on the dentate line, in order to hide it and protect it.

Stay sutures (5/0 Silk or 5/0 Vycril) are then positioned circumferentially 1 cm above the dentate line. Using the needle-tip diathermy a circular incision is performed on the rectal mucosa, 1–2 mm externally to the stay sutures. The dissection is then carried on full thickness, staying right on the rectal wall thus avoiding nerves and pelvic organs. The dissection was started on the posterior aspect of the anal canal and continued with lateral sides. A right angle dissector is used to isolate and cauterize the vessels on the rectal wall. Once the plane was fully defined in the posterior and lateral sides the anterior part was started. Careful attention was made when dissecting the anterior rectal wall to avoid damage to the urethra/vagina. A full-thickness biopsy in the posterior wall of the rectum is performed once the transition zone is visually identified. The defect is then closed with 4/0 Vycril and the dissection is carried on proximally while awaiting the pathologist's report. We dissected at least 5 cm above the site of the biopsy that shows normal ganglion cells and no hypertrophic nerves, trying to also resect as much of the dilated normoganglionic bowel. Extreme caution must be exercised to avoid twisting the pulled-through segment (biopsy taken in the posterior wall). Once the selected bowel is identified we proceed to the anastomosis. Initially the serosal layer of the colon is secured to the anal canal muscles with three interrupted 4/0 Vycril stitches (on the posterior and later walls). Afterwards the lone star pins are moved backward in order to expose the dentate line and the colo-anal anastomosis is started. The normoganglionic colon is opened anteriorly with a diathermy and a full-thickness 5/0 Vycril suture is positioned between the colon and the superior edge of the anal canal, just above the dentate line. The colon is then opened further until four full-thickness stitches are positioned in the four quadrants. The aganglionic colon is then resected and the anastomosis is completed with a single layer of full-thickness 16–5/0 Vycril interrupted stitches. Sterile dressing was applied.

## 27.13  Transanal Soave pull-through for Hirschsprung disease

### 27.13.1  Equipment

- Regular laparotomy set
- Foley catheter (size according to the size of the patient)
- Catheter tip syringe
- Lone star ring
- Eight lone star pins
- Denis Browne retractor
- Ligasure (optional)
- GIA linear stapler (optional)
- 4 or 5/0 Braided sutures for the stay sutures

- 4 or 5/0 Absorbable braided suture for the coloanal anastomosis
- Diathermy/monopolar with needle tip and standard tip

### 27.13.2  Operative report

The contrast enema images and the histology report are reviewed.

With the patient in supine position a general anesthesia is administered and a cuffed ETT tube is inserted. A caudal block may be given according to the center's protocols and IV antibiotics are started. At the same stage also a Foley catheter is inserted and the balloon inflated with 3–5 mL of normal saline. A rectal irrigation is then performed using the size 22 Foley catheter, until the water is clean.

The patient is then placed prone in the middle of the table with the hips raised in jack knife position. During the procedure the surgeon stands either at the right side of the patient or at the end of the bed, according to the personal preference. The assistant is on the left side of the patient and the scrub nurse is either at the right side of the bed or at the end of the bed.

A lone star is positioned to expose the anal canal and the pins are then positioned deeper on the dentate line, in order to hide it and protect it.

The rectal mucosa is circumferentially incised using a needle-tip diathermy 1 cm above the dentate line. 5/0 Silk or 5/0 Vycril stay suture are then positioned circumferentially in the proximal edge of the mucosa. Uniform traction is applied and using the needle-tip diathermy the endorectal submucosal dissection is carried proximally.

The dissection is then carried on full thickness, breaking through onto the full-thickness plane, staying right on the rectal wall thus avoiding nerves and pelvic organs.

A go rounder can be used to isolate and cauterize the vessels on the rectal wall. The assistant can help retracting the anal wall with a Langenbeck, avoiding tension damage to the nerves. We know that we are in the right plane when we work on a white avascular plane and when the dissection is carried out mostly outside of the anus. A fatty plane is encountered if our dissection is performed too deep. Careful attention should be paid when dissecting the anterior rectal wall in both males and females. At this level the dissection should be performed as close as possible to the rectal wall and even going submucosally could be accepted.

A full-thickness biopsy is performed where we visually identify the transition zone. The defect is then closed with 4/0 Vycril and the dissection is carried on proximally while awaiting the pathologist's report. We go at least 5 cm above the site of the biopsy that shows normal ganglion cells and no hypertrophic nerves, trying to also resect as much of the dilated normoganglionic bowel. Extreme caution must be exercised to avoid twisting the pulled-through segment. Once the selected bowel is identified we proceed to the anastomosis. Initially the serosal layer of the colon is secured to the anal canal muscles with three interrupted 4/0 Vycril stitches (on the posterior and later walls). Afterwards the lone star pins are moved backward in order to expose the dentate line and the coloanal anastomosis is started. The normoganglionic colon is opened anteriorly with a diathermy and a full-thickness 5/0 Vycril suture is positioned between the colon and the superior edge of the anal canal, just above the dentate line. The colon is then opened further until four full-thickness stitches are positioned in the four quadrants. The aganglionic colon is then resected and sent for histology and the anastomosis is completed with a single layer of full-thickness 5/0 Vycril interrupted stitches.

## 27.14  Open Swenson for TCHD

### 27.14.1  Equipment

- Regular laparotomy set
- Foley catheter (size according to the size of the patient)

- Catheter tip syringe
- Lone star ring
- Eight lone star pins
- Denis Browne retractor
- Ligasure (optional)
- GIA linear stapler (optional)
- 4 or 5/0 Braided sutures for the stay sutures
- 4 or 5/0 Absorbable braided suture for the coloanal anastomosis
- Diathermy/monopolar with needle tip and standard tip

### 27.14.2  Operative report

The contrast enema images and the histology report are reviewed.

With the patient in supine position, IV access is inserted and secured in the upper limbs, a general anesthesia is administered, and a cuffed ETT tube is inserted. A caudal block may be given according to the center's protocols and IV antibiotics are started. At the same stage also a Foley catheter is inserted and the balloon inflated with 3–5 mL of normal saline. If the patient does not have a stoma, a rectal irrigation can be performed using the size 22 Foley catheter, until the water is clean.

A total body preparation is then performed. A pursestring suture is placed around the ileostomy to avoid stool spillage during the procedure. Sterile stockinets are placed on the child's legs and the patient is positioned supine in the middle of the table. During the procedure the surgeon stands on the right side of the patient, the assistant on the left side of the patient, and the scrub nurse is at the left side of the assistant.

A lower midline laparotomy is performed and the peritoneum is entered with a muscle splitting technique. A Denis Browne retractor is applied and the bladder is emptied with Credè maneuver. The bladder is lifted out of the abdomen with a stay suture. According to the results of the previously performed leveling biopsies the segment to be pulled through is the ileostomy. The ileostomy is dissected from the inside until the ileum is completely free. The colectomy was started from the descending colon making a window in the sigmoid mesentery. The mesocolon is cauterized (using either a diathermy and reabsorbable ties or using a Ligasure or an armonic instrument). The colectomy is done proximally ligating the left colic, middle colic, right colic, and ileocolic vessels. Once we reached the ileostomy the length of the bowel that needs to be pulled through is examined. (If the bowel reaches the inferior aspect of the pubic bone then the length is sufficient to perform a tension-free anastomosis. Otherwise further length needs to be gained. This can be done by further resecting the mesentery, making sure not to compromise the vascularization.)

Once we selected the piece of bowel a resection of the aganglionic colon is performed using a linear stapler. Once adequate length is reached the right and left aspect of the bowel that needs to be pulled through are marked with different sutures. The peritoneal reflection is then opened anteriorly to the rectum and then laterally. A full-thickness dissection right at the bowel wall is started with special attention on not damaging the ureters, the vas deferens, the seminal vesicles/gonads, and fallopian tubes, the dissection is carried on as low as possible.

The child's legs are then elevated and a lone star retractor is applied. The pins are gradually positioned deeper at the dentate line, in order to hide it and protect it.

Stay sutures (5/0 Silk or 5/0 Vycril) are positioned circumferentially 1 cm above the dentate line. Using the needle-tip diathermy a circular incision is performed on the rectal mucosa, 1–2 mm externally to the stay sutures. The dissection is then carried on full thickness, staying right on the rectal wall at the same plane of the dissection done intraabdominally. A right angle is used to isolate and cauterize the vessels on the rectal wall. Giving preference to the posterior and the lateral rectal wall, the full-thickness dissection is carried on at the same plane of dissection done intraabdominally. The aganglionic rectum dissected intraabdominally is reached. The ileum is pulled through by placing a curved clamp inside the anus. Extreme caution must be exercised to avoid twisting the pulled-through segment and the stitches that were placed previously. The mesentery was checked and found to be straight and tension free. The anastomosis is started by securing the pulled-through bowel to the anal canal muscles with three interrupted 4/0 Vycril stitches (on the posterior and later walls). The normoganglionic ileum is then opened anteriorly and a full-thickness 5/0 Vycril suture is positioned between the colon and the superior edge of the anal canal, just above the dentate line. The ileum is then opened further until four full-thickness stitches are positioned in the four quadrants. The anastomosis is completed with a single layer of full-thickness 16–5/0 Vycril interrupted stitches. The lone star is then removed and the child's legs are released. The peritoneal cavity is carefully washed out with normal saline. The peritoneum and posterior fascia were closed with interrupted absorbable suture, as was Scarpa's fascia and a subdermal layer. The skin was closed with a subcuticular closure. Sterile dressing was applied.

## 27.15  Duhamel pull-through for Hirschsprung disease

See Chapter 12.

# 28 Tracking operative results and outcomes

Laura Weaver and Devin R. Halleran

## 28.1 Case study 1

The mother of a patient with an anorectal malformation contacts your center to establish care. You learn that the patient has undergone several operations at another institution.

**What information is needed before seeing this patient in your clinic?**

   A. No information is needed, schedule a clinic appointment and take a thorough history in person
   B. The last operative note only
   C. A letter from the patient's pediatrician
   D. A protocolized new intake form must be filled out that details all the patient's previous operations, all prior testing, and current symptoms

*Answer:* D

### 28.1.1 New intake and long-term follow-up

The goal of the intake process is to obtain as much information regarding the patient's history as possible prior to their initial visit. This allows for the treating physicians to determine which additional information is needed to fully understand the patient's current medical status.

This is best accomplished through new intake forms which are sent to the patient or family prior to their initial visit. These forms assess important demographic, social, surgical, and medical aspects of the patient's history. It is important that these forms are comprehensive to allow for a complete understanding of the patient, yet concise to allow for the forms to be filled out in their entirety with minimal added stress. It may help to explain to the families the importance of these intake documents in order to maximize compliance.

In addition to the social, surgical, and medical history, it is often important to assess a patient using validated surveys. This provides additional, valuable information on the patient's clinical status, and provides a benchmark by which to assess the patient's progress following various interventions. Surveys that are applicable to a pediatric colorectal population include the Baylor Social Continence Scale, the Cleveland Clinic Constipation Scoring System, the Vancouver Dysfunctional Elimination Syndrome Survey, and the Pediatric Quality of Life Inventory.

These assessments should be filled out on a regular basis in order to track a patient's progress longitudinally. Depending on the family's ability to travel and the patient's clinical status, these assessments can be made in person or remotely via telephone or e-mail. Our practice is to follow patients at 1, 3, 6, and 12 months postoperatively, and then annually thereafter. By periodically assessing patients using standardized tools over time, it is possible to track their clinical response to an intervention and compare patients against a similar benchmark.

## 28.2 Case study 2

The patient in the previous scenario comes to your clinic for the evaluation of ongoing soiling. She is planned for an examination under anesthesia.

**Which data points should you record as part of your assessment?**

   **A.** The size of the anal opening
   **B.** The position of the anal opening within the sphincters
   **C.** The appearance of the introitus
   **D.** Whether a stricture or prolapse is present
   **E.** All of the above

*Answer:* E

### 28.2.1 Examination under anesthesia

An examination under anesthesia (EUA) is a commonly performed procedure in pediatric patients with colorectal disease. This provides an opportunity to thoroughly examine the anatomy of the anus and rectum, genitalia, and lower urinary tract, either preoperatively to determine whether corrective surgery is needed or postoperatively to assess for complications of a prior surgery.

The EUA should be tailored to the patient's underlying diagnosis and surgical history. For example, in a patient with an ARM:

- Assess the size of the anal opening with a Hegar dilator
- If a stricture is present, is it:
     **A.** Skin level (e.g., <3 mm)
     **B.** Deeper than skin level (e.g., >3 mm)
- Determine the position of the anus relative to the sphincter complex using electrostimulation
- Identify whether a rectal prolapse is present, and if so, note the degree and whether it is circumferential
- Perform cystoscopy if indicated, commenting on:
  - External anatomy (normal/abnormal)
  - Urethral orifice/meatus
  - Urethral lumen
  - Bladder neck (open/closed)
  - Bladder mucosa
  - Ureteral orifices
  - Estimated bladder volume
  - Actual bladder volume
  - Ureterocele
- In females:
  - Assess the adequacy of the perineal body
  - Assess the size of the introitus
  - Perform vaginoscopy if indicated

For a patient with Hirschsprung disease, it is important to note:

- The size of the anal opening with a Hegar dilator
- Dentate line (intact/partially intact/absent)
- Sphincters (intact/patulous)
- Retained obstructing Soave cuff
- Anastomotic stricture
- Transition zone pull-through
- Twisted pull-through
- Obstructing Duhamel pouch
- Duhamel spur
- Wound dehiscence
- Botox administration needed

## 28.3  Case study 3

A colleague from a nearby institution with an interest in pediatric colorectal surgery asks you if you would be interested in collaborating on a research project.

**What is a potential benefit of multicenter academic collaboration?**

- **A.** Allows for an increased patient population/higher powered studies
- **B.** Minimizes bias associated with single institution studies
- **C.** Permits comparison of the effects of different techniques on outcomes
- **D.** All of the above

*Answer:* D

### 28.3.1  Consortium/database

Research is paramount in improving medical and surgical outcomes. Because many conditions treated by pediatric colorectal surgeons are rare, there are few high-quality studies by which to inform practice. Over recent years, a number of institutions have formed multicenter consortiums in order to aggregate data and perform large-scale research studies. An example of this is the Pediatric Colorectal Pelvic Learning Consortium (PCPLC), which was formed in 2017 to compile and share clinical research data for the purpose of large outcomes studies. Multicenter research consortiums such as these facilitate studies of rare diseases on a large scale, which would otherwise take years to perform at a single institution.

## Further reading

1. Brandt ML, Daigneau C, Graviss EA, Naik-Mathuria B, Fitch ME, Washburn KK. Validation of the Baylor Continence Scale in children with anorectal malformations. *J Pediatr Surg*. 2007 Jun;42(6):1015–21.
2. Afshar K, Mirbagheri A, Scott H, MacNeily AE. Development of a symptom score for dysfunctional elimination syndrome. *J Urol*. 2009 Oct; 182(4 Suppl):1939–43.
3. Agachan F, Chen T, Pfeifer J, Reissman P, Wexner SD. A constipation scoring system to simplify evaluation and management of constipated patients. *Dis Colon Rectum*. 1996 Jun.
4. Reeder RW, Wood RJ, Avansino JR et al. The Pediatric Colorectal and Pelvic Learning Consortium rationale, infrastructure, and initial steps. *Tech Coloproctol*. 2018 May; 22(5):395–99.

# 29 Patient education

Meghan Fisher, Stephanie Vyrostek, and Kristina Booth

## 29.1 Introduction

### 29.1.1 Case 1

A 12-year-old patient presents with a history of anorectal malformation and neurogenic bladder. He is followed by a pediatric urologist, who is recommending the patient to start clean intermittent catheterization (CIC). The colorectal team is also planning to start rectal enemas.

**What is the best option for teaching and educating patients and families about these procedures?**

A. Call the family on the phone to review and explain CIC and rectal enemas
B. Email the family a video with CIC and rectal enema instructions
C. Have the patient and family scheduled for a clinic visit with the nursing team to discuss and return to demonstrate CIC and rectal enemas
D. Send them a booklet with step-by-step instructions on CIC and rectal enemas
E. All of the above could be utilized

*Answer:* E

Various teaching strategies and methods of delivery for patient education can be found in the medical literature. Included in these strategies are computer-based information specific to their own situation, DVDs, audiotapes of the teaching performed for recall of verbal teaching, tailored written materials at appropriate reading level, verbal instruction in conjunction with another teaching method, demonstration of a skill with teach-back approach, and illustrations with text description. The methods of delivery should be patient specific and involve multiple teaching strategies with sensitivity to cultural issues [1].

Patients who have colorectal diagnoses often require tailored education as these diagnoses are often unfamiliar to parents and even medical professionals. These patients and families require general education about the diagnoses and long-term care outcomes including the importance of routine bowel and urological management, and gynecological needs. In addition, patients with colorectal diagnoses may require education about various medical treatments that families will perform in the home setting. These may include treatments such as anal dilations, rectal enemas, rectal irrigations, antegrade enemas, and clean intermittent catheterization.

## 29.2  Anorectal malformation

Every day in hospitals across the world, children are seen with a new diagnosis of an anorectal malformation (ARM). The most common question families have is "Will my child poop normally?" This unknown haunts parents whose babies are born "different." It is the job of the provider to help put the information known about the child into clear explanations of how their malformation equates into continence. This is how the Anorectal Malformation Continence Predictor Index was created (see Figure 15.1). Every patient seen should get one of these as a handout for visual learners and have it reviewed verbally with their provider for auditory learners. The provider should review each section and how it pertains to the specifics of each child's case. This continence predictor helps guide the conversation about what parents can expect as the child grows and their potential for continence. The discussion with family should also focus on the malformation the child has and how that falls into the scoring system of this tool.

### 29.2.1  Handouts

The Anorectal Malformation Continence Predictor Index handout is a good tool to utilize for each patient to review the specifics of their child's anorectal malformation, spine, and sacrum. This allows the families to follow along on a handout during the discussion and they can visually see where the child falls in the spectrum of all children.

The sections discussed in the predictor are: ARM type, quality of spine, and quality of sacrum. These sections are broken down into three subcategories. These subcategories are then distinguished with a scoring system. The scoring system is used to add all three sections together to then predict the potential for continence in the child.

#### 29.2.1.1  ARM type

The ARM type is the largest of the three sections as there are many different variations of malformations. Based on the malformation a score is given. Those with good potential for continence (perineal fistula, anal stenosis, rectal atresia, rectovestibular fistula, rectobulbar fistula, and ARM without fistula) are awarded 1 point. Fair potential (cloaca with <3 cm common channel, rectoprostatic fistula, and rectovaginal fistula) are awarded 2 points. The last subcategory of poor potential for continence (rectobladderneck fistula, cloaca >3 cm common channel, and cloacal exstrophy) are given 3 points. The proper diagnosis of the original malformation is vital in identifying where the child falls on the spectrum and can impact the overall score of the index, and therefore impact the kind of discussion you are having with the family.

#### 29.2.1.2  Spine

Spinal anomalies can impact the potential for continence as well. Many children with anorectal malformations have spinal anomalies, so it is very important to screen all ARM patients for spinal abnormalities. As with ARM type, there is a spectrum of spinal abnormalities that can affect the child's potential for continence. The spine that appears "normal" (termination of conus at L1-L2, and normal filum appearance) has a good potential for continence and is awarded 1 point. Abnormally low termination of the conus (below L3) and abnormal thickening of the fatty filum have been shown to impact the potential for continence and is noted as such with a 2-point notation. Those who have myelomeningocele have the poorest potential for continence in this group of patients and are given 3 points.

### 29.2.1.3 Sacrum

The sacrum is evaluated based on the sacral ratio and any anomalies associated with the formation of the sacral bones. This section is also rated using a scoring system. Sacral ratio equal to or greater than 0.7 is awarded 1 point. Ratio between 0.69 and 0.4, hemisacrum, sacral hemivertebrae, or presacral mass, is given 2 points. Finally, a sacral ratio less than 0.4 gets 3 points.

### 29.2.1.4 Overall score

The goal of the evaluation and interpretation of this data and scoring system is to get them a final number. This is explained to family that it resembles the game of golf, the lower the number the better the potential for continence. The final scores and potential for continence are outlined in Chapter 15 (Figure 15.1).

Once a prediction has been made, it is essential to discuss with families there are always exceptions to every rule, and most children rely on a formalized bowel management regimen, no matter what the index has predicted. Making sure to keep the family informed is critical in the process as we manage their expectations of what they can expect for their child's continence.

## 29.3 Hirschsprung disease

### 29.3.1 Case 1

A 6-year-old patient with Hirschsprung disease is referred to your institution as a new patient due to obstructing symptoms. His family never performed irrigation before, only rectal enemas with glycerin.

**What do you think is the best option for families to understand what experiment their child would be exposed to?**

A. Send them an email with the instructions
B. Have a conversation in a multidisciplinary facility including specialized urology and colorectal nursing team
C. Call them on the phone to explain how they will be doing irrigations and when to perform them
D. Send them a booklet with a step-by-step explanation and differences between rectal enemas and irrigations
E. All the above could be utilized

*Answer:* E

### 29.3.1.1 Learning points

Hirschsprung disease (HD), like many colorectal diagnoses, requires diagnosis education and surgical intervention in a child's early years of life that will need to continue throughout their life span. For many families, this may start within the first few days of life as their child's symptoms prompt testing of the disease process. Key times of education include initial diagnosis, time of their pull-through, postoperative follow-up, and at subsequent follow-up visits. Families and patients need to understand that HD is a disease that requires long-term attention including enterocolitis prevention and bowel management for hyper- or hypomotility.

Throughout all these intervals of care, keep in mind that these materials are written at an appropriate reading level and that discussions are held knowing that the family may have minimal to no medical knowledge. Education for families on the diagnosis itself should be presented in various forms—in-person discussion, written handouts, and if possible video education [2].

### 29.3.2 Diagnosis education

Education and discussion on initial testing to confirm the diagnosis (contrast enema, rectal biopsy) and how that information helps to guide treatment are vital. For patients who require an ostomy placement as their first intervention, it is crucial to provide the family with hands-on ostomy education and management. Families must also start to understand the process and medical concern regarding the heightened risk of enterocolitis. Hands-on teaching on how to perform a rectal irrigation and discussion regarding prevention could be held at the bedside or within the clinical setting. Consider written education with visual images reviewing step by step of how to perform a rectal irrigation at home. This should also include education on the common signs and symptoms of enterocolitis, and when to contact their medical team.

### 29.3.3 Surgery and postoperative education

Between the overwhelming news that their child has Hirschsprung disease and will require surgery, it may be hard for families to absorb the information and education you are trying to deliver. While the patient and parent are in the hospital for their pull-through operation, take advantage of the opportunity to teach them key post pull-through concepts like enterocolitis prevention, when to do a rectal irrigation, and what their long-term follow-up plan will include.

For those who are not diverted with a stoma or who have just had their ostomy taken down, skin care prevention education is vital. Provide handouts or written instructions on what products to use for routine prevention, mild, and severe skin breakdown. Include pictures of the products and where they can order or buy them. These patients typically require specific bowel management medications within the first month to protect their anastomosis from hard stool; it is important to review the purpose and importance of those medications.

## 29.4 Bowel management

### 29.4.1 Case 2

A 6-year-old patient with a past surgical history of rectovestibular fistula, and a tethered cord release presents to your bowel management clinic. You've decided to enroll her in a 1-week bowel management program with rectal enemas.

**How do you educate families prior and during the treatment program?**

    **A.** Provide family with information regarding the program prior their clinic visit so they have basic understanding of their expectations during and after the program.

    **B.** Have an informed discussion with family about their child's diagnosis and expectations based on their ARM index continence score.

    **C.** Provide family with handouts and education on how to troubleshoot issues that may arise with the enema.

    **D.** All the above.

*Answer:* E

### 29.4.1.1  Learning points

Patient education regarding bowel management's purpose, strategies for care, and areas of concern are key to long-term success in patients with colorectal anomalies. No matter the program, oral medications versus rectal enemas/antegrade enemas, patients and their caretakers must receive education on the importance of routine bowel management. This education must start early and continue as the child grows with the goals being socially continent and eventually independent in their bowel routine.

A formal bowel management program requires dedication from the medical team, patient, and family (details about the structure of a bowel management program are provided in Chapter 19). Within a program, there are several opportunities to provide education sessions and materials which families can utilize throughout the program and after they are home. Multiple learning formats should be utilized when educating patients and families, which include written materials, hands-on sessions, and visual aids.

## 29.4.2  Program Booklet

A program booklet given to each family with an overview of information about the program and additional education materials provides structure to the program. This booklet serves as a resource throughout the bowel management week, as well as reference guide in the future. In this booklet, it is important to review the basics of bowel management including how continence works, why patients soil, and an outline of what their bowel management day-to-day schedule will look like. In that, include sections on each specific program (oral medication, rectal enema/antegrade enemas) and the goals for each. Including a detailed report sheet for them to fill out after each treatment will allow families to focus on key pieces of the program which are helpful for the medical team to note when determining if a medication change is needed.

## 29.4.3  Hands-on teaching, discussion, and demonstration

For patients and caregivers who are visual or hands-on learners, opportunities for them to hear the basic material in person should be given. This can be done as a formal bowel management talk with the patients and families in attendance. This talk not only can reiterate the basics reviewed in the booklet, but also allow for more open discussion with families and offers an opportunity to ask real-time questions. Keep the content general so that irrespective of the diagnosis, they understand the concept of the program.

For many patients and families, they may be entering a new phase of treatment with rectal enemas. This can be a scary time for them as they may not be familiar with the process of a rectal enema. Create time after the talk to provide group teaching on how to give an enema. In their clinic appointment, one-on-one teaching can also be completed with individuals on how to perform an enema. Consider the importance of the teach-back method in this process. Ensure the family follows your instructions and adequately performs the treatment themselves.

## 29.4.4  Handouts

With several different components of bowel management, it is helpful to have one page handouts with pictures and visual references. For processes like giving an enema, families and patients will likely not be able to remember each step even with hands-on education. A step-by-step visual guide with associated steps written out will allow families the assurance they are doing the treatment correctly. For patients new to laxative therapy, consider a handout with pictures of the types of oral medications used for bowel management. Many of these medications are over the counter and can be confusing which medication to purchase. For those starting on fiber therapy, a chart indicating what types of fiber are recommended and where they can purchase them would help ensure the family gets the right product and can properly tell you what dose they are giving. For programs recommending dietary changes such as following a laxative or constipating diet, a list of foods within that category, or those to avoid would provide a guide for them to reference.

### 29.4.5 Case 3

A 10-year-old patient had a Malone appendicostomy procedure 1 month ago. His Malone catheter is still in place when he arrives to clinic.

**How would you educate families on how to preform Malone catheterization before and during their post-operative clinic appointment?**

- **A.** Have the surgeon or specialized nurse preform the first Malone catheterization. Require the caregiver to return demonstrate their ability to pass the catheter.
- **B.** They will watch a video and will be able to do it on their own at home without the need for education at their clinic appointment.
- **C.** In clinic, provide family with handouts and instruction on what to do if they have trouble with their Malone flush at home.
- **D.** Support to child through the use of medical play to prepare them for what to expect during the Malone catheterization.

*Answers:* A, C, & D

## 29.5 Surgical antegrade options

Patients with colorectal diagnoses may benefit from surgical antegrade enema options including Malone appendicostomy or cecostomy tube. Prior to surgery, these patients benefit from a one-on-one session with the colorectal surgeon discussing surgical options. Written handouts about these surgeries can also be utilized and include information such as the preoperative care, surgical procedure details, and postoperative care. It can also include important details about the care of the surgical site during the postoperative period and step-by-step instructions on how to give an antegrade enema.

### 29.5.1 Hands-on teaching, discussion, and demonstration

When it is identified that the patient can start giving antegrade enemas using the appendicostomy or cecostomy, education should be provided using multiple teaching strategies. This should include hands-on teaching with step-by-step instructions on how to catheterize the Malone appendicostomy channel and how to give the antegrade enema. Written instructions should also be given to the family as a supplement to the verbal instructions provided. Return demonstration is key to identify any pitfalls and improve the patient and family confidence. If available a doll or medical model can be used to help with the return demonstration. It is also important to educate patients and families on care of catheters and enema supplies during this time.

## 29.6 Urology

### 29.6.1 Case 4

**A patient with a history of anorectal malformation- rectoprostatic fistula, tethered cord and neurogenic bladder is asked to start clean intermittent catheterization (CIC)?**

A. The provider discusses with the patient and family the reason for starting CIC and the urological goals
B. The nurse specialized in urology has an appointment with the patient and family and provides verbal instructions on CIC
C. The patient and family are able to practice CIC on a medical model
D. The patient and family watch a video on CIC
E. All of the above

*Answer:* E

Patients with colorectal diagnoses can have associated urological anomalies or complaints. These include patients with anorectal malformation, neurogenic bowel and bladder, and functional constipation. Education on associated urological anomalies should be provided to patients and families early after diagnosis with appropriate follow-up.

## 29.6.2 Clean intermittent catheterization education

Some patients with colorectal diagnoses may also require clean intermittent catheterization (CIC). This can often be scary and challenging for both the patient and the family, especially in patients who have sensation. Appropriate education and follow-up is key to success. When implementing CIC, it is important to provide education about a patient's specific urological plan and how to perform the catheterization, including an opportunity for return demonstration. It is vital the patient and family understand why CIC is being started and the goals of catheterization. A one-on-one discussion about how to perform the catheterization, along with practice using a medical model are included in the education process. Handouts with pictures and step-by-step instructions also supplement this teaching. Return demonstration is key and can help identify any challenges or trouble with catheterization. After a patient/family is taught catheterization, there should be follow-up in place. This can be a clinic visit or telephone call by the nursing team to get an update and help troubleshoot any concerns.

## 29.6.3 Appendicovesicostomy education

In select patients, surgical intervention with urological reconstruction including an appendicovesicostomy may be considered. A one-on-one discussion with the urologist about these surgical procedures is helpful to determine if this procedure would be of benefit. Written handouts can also be utilized and include information including details about the surgical procedure and the typical postoperative course. Other visual aids can also be used such as videos. Often it is helpful for both the patient and the family to see a video of another patient with an appendicovesicostomy showing how the channel is catheterized. When it is time for the patient and/or family to start catheterization, the appendicovesicostomy in the postoperative period education is provided about catheterizations. This information is presented using multiple teaching strategies including verbal discussion, written instructions, and return demonstration with the patient and/or family catheterizing the appendicovesicostomy channel.

# References

1. Friedman AJ, Cosby R, Boyko S, Hatton-Bauer J, Turnbull G. Effective teaching strategies and methods of delivery for patient education: A systematic review and practice guideline recommendations. *J Cancer Educ.* 2011 Mar;26(1):12–21.
2. Langer JC. Hirschsprung disease. *Curr Opin Pediatr.* 2013;25:368–74.

# 30 Resources for families and the burden of therapy

Greg Ryan, Lori Parker, and Sarah Driesbach

## 30.1 Discussion

As the burdens accumulate some patients are overwhelmed, and the consequences are likely to be poor health-care outcomes for individual patients, increasing strain on caregivers, and rising demand and costs of health-care services. In the face of these challenges, we need to better understand the resources that patients draw upon as they respond to the demands of both burdens of illness and burdens of treatment, and the ways that resources interact with health-care utilization.

## 30.2 Summary

Burden of Treatment Theory is oriented to understanding how capacity for action interacts with the work that stems from health care. Burden of Treatment Theory is a structural model that focuses on the work that patients and their networks do. It thus helps us understand variations in health-care utilization and adherence in different health-care settings and clinical contexts.

## 30.3 Case study 1

**As a colorectal surgeon who treats conditions such as anorectal malformations and Hirschsprung disease, what are the main points to discuss with patients and family from a family support point of view?**

A. Quality of life
B. Burden of therapy
C. Support forums
D. Annual family conferences
E. All the above

*Answer:* E

### 30.3.1 Learning points

As an adult or parent of a child affected by ARM, the writers understand the burden of therapy as a concept and a reality. The phrase describes the demands placed on many ill people suffering from chronic health problems. The burden is all aspects of self or child care handled in private and sometimes in secret. The burden is experienced as a complex tapestry of surgery, monitoring, management, emotional self-protection, and consequential social, emotional, and economic effects. For most of the individuals affected with ARM, this burden will last a lifetime.

Research on the topic of burden of treatment is ongoing. There is still a significant need for validated tools to help assess patients' level of burden in order for caregivers to weigh the risks and benefits of the treatment. Consequences of a significant burden of treatment include poor adherence to treatment regimens and poor overall health and well-being in addition to the socioeconomic consequences previously mentioned. Providers for patients who have anorectal malformations and other lifelong colorectal diagnoses should be cognizant of the burden of treatment they are imposing and modify treatment plans so that patients are able to have optimal quality of life. Colorectal diagnoses do not exist in a vacuum, and theoretical "best care" often differs from the care that provides the best overall quality of life for the patient.

Because of historical and cultural perceptions, the anorectal area is viewed as a private domain overlayed with a sense of shame and stigma. Ignorance and fear are attached to the topic of malfunctions, adding an extra layer of anxiety to patients and families. Learning how to deal with physical and mental realities across a lifetime has become the primary task for family and sufferers. Learning how to relate and relay emotional and psychological understandings is even more complex in an area which is seen to be on the dark side of human experience. In contrast, a child born with a congenital heart condition is not treated as a "silent" matter and the awareness, empathy, and understanding in the wider community provide such families with a sense of comfort and support that is not available to ARM families. This difference in perception between a heart defect and an anorectal defect begins the burden of therapy for parents and families. At birth, the parents are faced with the decision of "who to tell" and "what to tell." Many families find it difficult to share information about their child's anorectal and/or urogenital defects with close family, let alone friends. Thus begins the early stages of isolation. In addition, parents, mothers particularly, wonder if they did something to cause this defect to occur, adding to their burden of therapy.

When a child is born with ARM, it is almost always the first time those parents have heard the words "imperforate anus." These parents are told that their child will require surgery, or a series of surgeries, to correct the anorectal malformation. The parents share this information with family and friends, who then incorrectly assume that the child is "fixed" after these surgeries. It's generally after these surgeries that the family learns of "bowel management" and "incontinence" and the therapies required to keep their child "clean." Friends and family don't understand why the child still requires diapers past the "normal" toilet-training years. This is when it is vital for families dealing with the challenges of ARM to find other families living with the same challenges. Pull-thru Network, Inc. (PTN) is a nonprofit family support organization that helps connect these families. PTN has the largest database of families living with ARM from across the United States, in addition to numerous international families. As members, families can request networking lists to connect with other families or individuals either by location, diagnosis, or age.

Pull-thru Network has a close relationship with the leading pediatric colorectal experts in the United States and Canada. They maintain a list of professional members, several of which serve as professional advisors for the organization. PTN publishes a newsletter three times a year including articles written for the organization by its professional advisors. In addition,

Pull-thru Network hosts a 4-day national conference every other summer for its families to attend. The conference includes educational sessions for all family members: parents, affected children and adults, siblings, and grandparents. The speakers are professional members of the organization. During the conference, family members are able to find and meet others living with the same challenges. It's often a life-changing event for all who attend and the formation of many lifelong friendships.

Similar organizational structures, inspired by Pull-thru Network, such as Australia's "ONE in 5000 Foundation" are now emerging. These agencies offer worldwide emotional sustenance to survivors of ARM as does the beginning of an IA/ARM literature written both online and in print.

The advent of online social media (Facebook, Twitter, Instagram, etc.) has changed the lives of ARM patients and families in an overwhelmingly positive way. We have been able to reach out across the globe to the few individuals who share our physical symptoms and emotional needs. These informal networks have enabled us to undertake a level of collective emotional and practical self-care that previously did not exist. For example, almost universally the daily task of performing anal dilatations by parents is an incredibly emotional responsibility, both from the thought of causing pain to the child and the pervasive fear of the moral cloud that hangs over such an intrusive procedure. Being able to make human contact with someone else undergoing the same isolating experience has been hugely important. Connecting with other patients and families who are living with a colorectal diagnosis often provides an immediate sense of relief. Simply connecting with a community who has had similar experiences and struggles helps normalize the diagnosis and helps alleviate the sense of extreme isolation associated with these complex problems.

However, not all online information is accurate or suitably general and, in some cases, may be detrimental to individuals and families. There is much anecdotal evidence of increased anxiety and stress being caused by a bombardment of information, especially at the early stages of treatment. Furthermore, the subtle differences in each person's needs may not be examined and another person's anecdotal examples may be useless or in fact harmful.

From a provider's perspective, incorrect information presented in the social media platform presents a unique challenge to patient care. Considering that many patients and families with colorectal diagnoses have sought care from multiple providers and may have had unpleasant or traumatic relationships with past providers, it is understandably difficult to gain trust and "debunk" some of the misconceptions presented in online communities. Patients often have a strong sense of trust in information they are getting from within their own community, and providers should be aware of this and provide empathetic guidance toward evidence-based treatment while still respecting the patient's past experiences and feelings of trepidation.

Navigating across social media is notoriously difficult and when this comes to health management the stakes are very high. The caregiver ideally needs to be able to provide a direct or online pathway which is sensitive to the individuals' specific diagnosis. Additional resources aimed at providing emotional support must directly help deal with the burden of therapy that families and individuals undertake across their lifetime.

Across the world the perception is that surgery "fixes" the medical issue and ongoing self-care defines the emotional outcome. In truth, for most ARM-related problems the issues will be life long and the surgery is a maintenance rather than curative activity. The advent of social media support groups has created support and also a different dialogue. Both the surgical profession and the ARM community of families and individuals are now looking at a four-strand strategy that ties continually improving medical intervention with greater community awareness, clear and accurate information provision, and social/emotional support services. The innovative partnership arrangements between major hospitals and family support networks in both the United States and Australia are particularly encouraging in this regard.

An interesting dyad in the treatment of children and adults has been obvious for many years but is rarely discussed. Pediatric surgical care has made huge advances and many young lives have been saved and improved as techniques advanced. Sadly, once adulthood is reached it has been expected that the individual must find his or her own way. Due to the lack of transitional care into adulthood, if someone had not made a connection with another ARM patient or family during their time under pediatric care, there is only an extremely slim chance of meeting a supportive other. Adding the ARM issues into the mix of finding a supportive workplace environment, building and maintaining an understanding intimate relationship while maybe dealing with sexual function issues and incontinence has been a massive mental health challenge for these affected adults.

It is widely acknowledged now by the medical profession that the mental health well-being of ARM children in the past has been inadequately serviced. With the incredibly invasive procedures and intrusive examinations a child must endure, and the stigma attached to having "bowel accidents," be it at home, school, or in sporting endeavors, the burden this imparts on a patient's quality of life from a mental health perspective is highly significant. Lack of resources for our relatively rare congenital issues means that there is no blame that can be apportioned to the medical profession for these omissions. However, the gap has now become obvious to most professionals and others from the ARM community. Later as that child moves to adulthood, the patient logically must leave the pediatric care system. Due to the absence of adult or transitional care programs for the overwhelming majority of ARM patients worldwide until very recently, there has been no real quantifiable information which has highlighted this crisis in the broad community. Mental and financial costs arising from this gap are huge. The coalitions that are forming across the globe to address this are demanding a more integrated and systematic approach to all aspects of the care. The gulf between medical intervention and social/emotional/psychological support is beginning to be addressed. Nevertheless, we see many holes yet to be filled.

One of the most momentous and life-changing issues faced by ARM adults is the lack of understanding of the implications of being able to have children. In most cases it wasn't addressed satisfactorily (if at all) whilst in pediatric care. This is understandable in one sense, but nonetheless an important issue that must be tackled during adolescence by medical professionals and our support community. There are numerous examples of female ARM adults who have endured great pain and heartache in their endeavors of becoming pregnant and sustaining that pregnancy due to the complexity of their ARM. The lack of knowledge of ARM in the adult gynecological profession continues to exacerbate the already difficult situation.

There have been cases where the female has been told that ARM plays no part on childbirth which has resulted in extremely painful births and major ramifications for the person's ARM issues. These issues could have been avoided with a basic understanding of an ARM female patient. Similarly it has often been found that the female ARM patient was unable to have children due to the complexity of their ARM but had not been made aware of this devastating news until later in their adult life. For male patients there have been analogous issues regarding those who have associated urological and genital issues which are no less distressing. The need for reproductive health to be discussed in adolescence must become mandatory in the ARM medical community.

For practically every ARM patient in the past, once they are old enough to be ineligible for the care of the pediatric system, they feel abandoned by the medical profession. The main problem is that ARM is viewed primarily as a "pediatric condition" by the adult medical profession. This means that the expertise or experience to deal with such a complex condition is simply not available in the adult health-care system. We have many anecdotal tales of ARM community members presenting at medical clinics or hospitals and finding that the doctors had no knowledge of the issue. Even more disturbing has been the misdiagnoses and inappropriate medical service as a result of this ignorance.

When there is little general awareness and no transition to an adult colorectal specialist available, the patients must rely on their local general practitioners for "maintenance." When those doctors aren't able to cater to the needs of the ARM patient due to its complexity and rarity, the feeling of abandonment and isolation is emphasized.

It is now widely acknowledged that the result of this lack of transitional care has manifested itself into a major crisis regarding the mental health of many ARM patients. The only salvation some have been able to receive is by finding solidarity and information from others with similar issues. For adult ARM community members that informal help has most often emerged through social media communication. The growth of support networks worldwide over the last 4 years, especially a private social media support group on Facebook called "Adults living with IA/ARM," is providing this salvation. This is a "secret" group which ensures people's privacy because of the continued immense shame and embarrassment the majority of adults feel who have to live with the condition.

The feeling people have when they "find" others and become a part of this support group can be incredibly overwhelming. Because most have never met anyone else with the condition in their lifetime, the emotional effect can be substantial. The overriding feeling is that of relief that "I'm not alone anymore." There is also an immense sense of validation when members are able to share experiences openly in a totally safe environment where others automatically understand context and detail. There are countless examples of people expressing that the day they found this group was "the day my life changed." We have made empathetic friends; instigated and supported each other's projects, and begun to feel that the burden of this therapy can be shared and made lighter.

The positive effect has been twofold. First, it has provided much needed clinical information to adults who had not been exposed to new medical advancements such as the Malone Procedure and other bowel management regimes. In addition, the shared advice on new colorectal centers that will care for adult patients has given the opportunity for ARM adults to seek life-changing medical procedures. Second, the groups have provided adults with new levels of support for the mental health issues with great consequence to their quality of life. It has become undeniable due to the overriding evidence of adults' shared experiences that depression, anxiety, panic attacks, and body image issues have been evident in the overwhelming majority of the adult ARM community. The collective experience is beginning to mitigate some of the worst aspects of this alienation.

Over the years, the surgical options for ARM have greatly advanced in both technique and success rates. In addition, the ARM Continence Index has been a wonderful initiative for ARM children and families that provide a good indicator of future continence. Despite these medical advances, the greatest issue for adolescents and adults born with ARM continues to be the mental health consequences of what they experienced physically in childhood. There is a lack of mental health support in the formative years and a lack of transitional care programs to adulthood which contribute largely to this mental health issue.

Fortunately, we live in a newly enlightened era in which this burden is better understood by the medical fraternity. Consequently, we see this burden as being shared in a mutually interactive way between anorectal medical specialists and the families and informal caregivers who make up the ARM community. The isolation previously felt by many sufferers in managing their own therapies for both physical and mental problems is being acknowledged and recent innovations, studies, and activities have thankfully begun to see the tide turn.

In summary the burden of therapy needs to be shared better. The good news is that many of us in the ARM community have begun to step away from our embarrassment and shame and speak up for ourselves and our children. We are offering services to each other. We are talking more clearly with our medical professionals. Our words are being heard and changes are occurring. Our call is for the burden to be identified and for a partnership of the medical fraternity and the ARM community to be reinforced and financially supported. We must ensure that the congenital issues are identified and discussed. Privacy must be protected but medical services need to be enhanced, communities must be encouraged, and better information should be provided by respectable and authenticated sources. Much has been learned by the ARM community over the past 50 years, yet there is much still to be done. It is necessary for the entire colorectal medical system, both pediatric and adult care, to acknowledge and integrate the distinct information for these therapies for the benefit of the current and future generations.

# Creating a collaborative program

Jeffrey Avansino, Robert Dyckes,
Dennis Minzler, and Julie Choueiki

## 31.1  Case 1: Starting a program

You are seeing an 8-year-old female in your clinic with a history of an anorectal malformation. She was managed at a referring facility and the records are not available. She appears socially withdrawn, hiding behind her parents. During the visit, you learn she is fecally incontinent, wears a diaper, and takes a back pack to school with cleaning supplies, diapers, and a change of clothes. You have seen similar patients in your practice and are inspired to start a multidisciplinary colorectal and pelvic reconstruction program.

**Which of the following qualities are most important for ensuring success?**

A. Focus
B. Passion and interest
C. Strong work ethic
D. Deep knowledge about colorectal and pelvic anomalies
E. All of the above

*Answer:* E

### 31.1.1 Learning points

- Our experience has been that having all of these qualities are the key ingredients to creating a successful program. Passion and interest are the most important when initiating a program. To get the program started, the team requires focus, patience, and strong work ethic. A deep knowledge about colorectal and pelvic anomalies will come with time. It is valuable to visit other colorectal centers to develop knowledge about both program development and caring for patients with colorectal disorders.
- It is important to have a physician champion to move the work forward.
  - This individual must have a genuine interest in caring for this patient population.
  - The provider must be committed to the patient before, during, and long after the operation.
- First, find people with passion and interest. They will eventually develop the knowledge, focus, and will work hard to make the program a success.

## 31.2 Case 2: Building the team

You are sitting down to plan for the creation of your program. You begin to plan what specialties should be a part of the initial multidisciplinary conference and clinic.

**Which of the following combination of specialties would be most appropriate to begin building your reconstructive pelvic medicine program?**

- A. General surgery, urology, pathology, and radiology
- B. General surgery, urology, gynecology, and motility
- C. General surgery, motility, gynecology, and radiology
- D. Urology, motility, gynecology, and radiology

*Answer:* B

### 31.2.1 Learning points

- From a reconstructive perspective, starting with the teams that will be partnering in the operating room is the ideal initial team. Often reconstructive cases require urology, gynecology, and general surgery.
  - A patient's reconstructive needs are ideally reviewed in a multidisciplinary conference.
  - These specialties can participate in the OR together. This is especially helpful during cystoscopy, vaginoscopy, and exams under anesthesia.
  - Motility specialists are an excellent adjunct to any pelvic reconstruction program especially one that has a bowel management program.
  - Excellent pathology and radiology are essential to provide optimal care for this patient population.
  - The program can be expanded to include specialties such as neurosurgery, cardiology, psychiatry/psychology, orthopedics, nephrology, genetics, social work, nutrition, and interventional radiology.

## 31.3 Case 3: Building expertise

After planning your approach to starting the program, you realize that you do not have all the expertise to be an "expert" in this field. You also recognize that you do not have experience in starting or running a multidisciplinary program. You conceptualize a list of possibilities to enhance your knowledge surrounding both colorectal and reconstructive surgery as well as operating a multidisciplinary program.

**Which of the possibilities from the following list will give you the most value for your effort?**

A. Reading
B. Watching videos
C. Visiting other multidisciplinary programs in your hospital
D. Visiting colorectal centers of excellence

*Answer:* D

## 31.3.1  Learning points

- Learning from the experts is the quickest way to gain personal knowledge. There is no reason to reinvent the wheel. Respectfully ask for materials (e.g., intake forms) and modify and improve them for your program. Share any improvements you make with the facility who shared the documents. They will also benefit from your team's perspective.
- Spend time learning the clinical medicine. This can be achieved via a number of means:
  - Do a yearlong colorectal fellowship.
  - Spend 1–2 weeks per year visiting the institution.
  - Travel internationally with groups of experts.
  - Attend conferences with other experts.
  - Look beyond your role as a surgeon and observe the nursing component of care along with the other disciplines involved in patient care. Their care will be integral to best long-term outcomes for your patients.

## 31.4  Case 4: Advancing the program (iterative improvement)

You have recently returned home from a 2-week visit at a top tier reconstructive colorectal and pelvic medicine program. The program is much larger and more developed than your new program. You have a lot of new ideas for your program, but it is hard to know where to start. You also feel somewhat overwhelmed with everything that you would need to create a program like the one you just visited.

The most productive way to responsibly grow your program:

A. Write a detailed business plan and demand money for your program
B. Plan a conference similar to the conference hosted by the program you visited
C. Start small and iteratively improve
D. Continue seeing these patients in your general surgery clinic without other specialties

*Answer:* C

## 31.4.1  Learning points

- Starting a successful multidisciplinary program is hard work and takes time. You will not be able to achieve overnight what other mature programs have created over many years.
- Start small and iteratively make small improvements to your program:
  - Continuous rapid cycle improvements are key to responsibly growing your program. Start your first multidisciplinary clinic with two specialties. After a couple of months, add a third.
  - Each phase of change should follow the Demming cycle (plan, do, check, act). The team should not strive for perfection the first time around. Get started and make modifications as you go. Any failures are opportunities to learn and get better.
  - Recognize that constant change and rapid cycle improvements can be stressful to your team and lead to change-related burnout. Critical to success is empowering all team

members to be involved in designing changes and process improvement. Give your team a platform to voice their ideas, suggestions, concerns, and feedback.
- Once the program has started, creating a robust business plan is a good step toward attaining additional resource for the program.
  - Starting the clinic first establishes a proof of concept and demonstrates the commitment of the team to caring for the patient population.
  - Also having the program running helps the team to understand its most pressing needs. This is important to prioritize the team's needs when requesting resources from the administration.
  - Have your administration document the impact your patients have on downstream revenue of the hospital.
- Planning a conference is a great idea for a more mature program. Doing such a task early could be a good boost for the program but would distract the team from building a strong foundation for the program.
- While it is critical to visit well-established programs, it should be recognized that it can be overwhelming and could potentially deter the team from pursing multidisciplinary care. Persistence is a key to starting a successful program. Involve your team in a brainstorming session to allow them to tell you where they think they could improve or develop and what you can do to facilitate their growth.

## 31.5  Case 5: Data

Your multidisciplinary clinic has been operating for about 1 year. You feel it is time to create a business plan for your program to get additional resources you feel are critical for your continued growth.

**Which of the following items will give you the greatest opportunity for success?**

A. A highly efficient clinic
B. A regional reputation
C. A newly developed technique
D. A robust data library

*Answer:* D

### 31.5.1  Learning points

- All of the above are important for making a strong business development plan to ask for additional resource. Data are required to demonstrate you have an efficient clinic, a regional reputation, or the efficacy of your new technique.
- If you cannot measure it, you cannot improve.
- Many data variables can go into a business development plan. Examples of data a program may consider including the following: number of referrals, total visits, new visits, out of region visits, number of OR cases (inpatient vs. outpatient), average daily census, average length of stay, revenues, expenses, safety/quality improvement measures (complication rates, value-added time for patients in clinic).
- Telephone encounters will help support the utilization of your nursing team in providing long distance care to your patients. Make sure your team is accurately reflecting these encounters in the patient's electronic medical record (EMR) so that the data can be extracted later to support your case for staffing. Then patients require a great deal of

"tinkering." Small incremental changes lead to best outcomes. These patients do not follow a traditional surgical model. They do not "drop off the radar" as most surgical patients do. They instead require modifications in their care even years after their surgery."

- Developing a mechanism to track wRVU production is crucial when developing a business plan. The multidisciplinary care model presents challenges with accurately tracking and reporting production metrics but every effort should be made to capture the work effort of each surgeon/physician providing care for the patients in the program. Ultimately this will help illustrate the total physician FTE required to support the program.
- Continuous improvement means tracking in full transparency. Record everything: how many patients call inquiring to your center; how many actually walk through the door for a clinic visit or surgery. What are the reasons why they didn't matriculate after calling? You can't fix what you don't know! Ask the hard questions.
- Data are also critical for performing research, and publishing of outcomes data can be a draw for more physicians and patients to refer to your program.
  - A program should look for opportunities to align data collected for clinical purposes with data needed for research. Sometimes routine clinical data collection in the EMR can be tagged and simultaneously collected for research purposes.

# 31.6  Case 6: Infrastructure

Your multidisciplinary team consists of a general surgeon, an urologist, a gynecologist, a motility expert, and a nurse. Your nurse seems to spend a majority of the time on the phone with the scheduling center to help arrange patient visits. As your team is preparing the business development plan, you are also prioritizing the resources you need.

**Which of the following would be at the top of your list?**

   **A.** Care coordinator/scheduler
   **B.** Another nurse
   **C.** A nurse practitioner
   **D.** A gynecologist
   **E.** A social worker

*Answer:* A

## 31.6.1  Learning points

- While all the positions listed are important, a care coordinator or designated scheduler would be the best position to help your program based on the scenario. A care coordinator/scheduler will be able to schedule all of your patient's visits including clinic, procedures, and radiology exams. They are the one point of contact.
  - Working through centralized scheduling can be demanding on the clinical team, thus imbedding this member on the team will be critical.
- A concept important to a successful multidisciplinary team is building bench strength.
  - Building bench strength can be done by pulling positions from a shared resource. For example, if there is a pool of general surgery nurses, then one nurse could allocate 0.2 FTE to the program. That is more cost effective than hiring an entire nurse when the clinical volumes may not warrant such a hire. This same thought process can be applied to social workers, child life specialists, nutrition, and psychology. Talk with those departments about sharing resources and costs.
  - Asking for FTE then allocating it to portions of different roles helps to expand your team's membership. With time, these part-time team members will develop expertise

and interest in the program, ultimately resulting in an increased role in the program. Ideally the administration links the activity of the program with the budget needed to be adequately staffed.

A collaborative, multidisciplinary colorectal center may theoretically benefit patients, but logistical hurdles—sharing resources among divisions or routinely scheduling several surgical disciplines for a single case—often dissuade institutions from creating such a program.

A recent study in *Frontiers in Surgery* [1] demonstrated that the benefits are not theoretical at all; in fact, children who undergo combined procedures in this setting have fewer overall surgical interventions, reduced anesthetic procedures, fewer intubations, and a shorter length of stay.

The great majority of procedures were combined specifically to save an anesthetic, visits to the hospital, or for another practical advantage. In some cases, though, the procedures were combined to allow for a single entrance to the pelvis when correcting complex malformations. Combined procedures also allowed for tissue sharing, such as using a resected sigmoid colon for bladder augmentation or sharing the appendix for both Malone and Mitrofanoff. The median number of anesthetic events per patient was 1 versus 3 if procedures had been performed individually. The median length of stay in days for patients who required hospitalization was 8 versus 10. The median number of intubations was 1 versus 2. This study demonstrates how vitally important it is for patient care to create multidisciplinary programs.

## 31.7 Components of a multidisciplinary pediatric colorectal and pelvic reconstruction program

This is an extensive list the authors feel creates a full complement of individuals that makes up a team that cares for children with disorders of the pelvic organs. We recognize that all programs will not be able to assemble all recommended members. The needs of each program will differ and may necessitate additional personnel not listed here or negate other specialists who are listed. It is important to remember that successfully building a program is a slow iterative process.

### 31.7.1 Physician providers

- General surgery*
- Urology*
- Gynecology*
- Motility
- Neurosurgery
- Orthopedics
- Cardiology
- Genetics
- Nephrology
- Pathology
- Radiology
- Interventional radiology
- Psychiatry/psychology

### 31.7.2 Other providers

- Nursing*
- Advance practice providers (nurse practitioners and physician assistants)*

---

* Notes positions that are necessary for starting a multidisciplinary program.

- Wound/stoma therapist
- Nutritionist
- Social workers
- Child life specialist
- Care coordinators (scheduling)*
- Medical assistants
- Program manager/program administrator
- Research coordinator
- Research assistants
- Quality and safety manager

## 31.8  Steps for making the business case to the hospital

Most hospitals have planning and data analysis staff who can assist with formulating a business case for a multidisciplinary center [2]. Engage those resources to create a document in whatever format hospital leadership typically requires for business cases or budget decisions. Many hospitals will use a SWOT (strengths, weaknesses, opportunities, and threats) analysis as part of this process. Regardless of the format, you will need to answer the following questions for your hospital:

- What patient population are you seeking to serve?
- What is the normal activity of these patients in your hospital?
- What gaps in service are you addressing for that population?
- Will you be providing additional and/or enhanced services to an existing patient population?
- Will you be treating new patients who are not currently part of the hospital's service area?
- Will patients already cared for in your system come back to take advantage of this new program?
- What resources are needed over time to provide these services?
- What barriers are there to moving forward?
- What will happen if you do not build the program?
- How does the program help fulfill the hospital's mission, vision, and strategic plan?

Given that building a center of excellence takes years, you will need to lay out a plan over several years with milestones for resources and results along the way.

Ultimately the hospital will need projections for the clinical services to be provided: office visits, diagnostic studies, diagnostic OR cases, treatment operating room cases, inpatient stays, and involvement of collaborating services. It may be acceptable to develop multiple projections that represent best-case to worst-case scenarios.

## 31.9  Components of a typical week in a current program

Your multidisciplinary team has been up and running and your patient list is expanding. You are moving toward your goal of becoming a center of excellence (COE). Key components that allow you to care for you patients at this level include weekly meetings with identified team members focused on new and returning patients [2], as follows.

### 31.9.1  New intake meetings

You recognize that processing new patients into your center is critical to capturing potential business. Wishing to streamline this to be done expeditiously, thoroughly, and

---

* Notes positions that are necessary for starting a multidisciplinary program.

in a cost-controlled method you utilize your nursing team to gather and analyze relevant information in a succinct manner. Families are asked to send relevant previous health records, including previous imaging with reports, procedures, pathology, and operative reports. Your nursing team can review the available records and prepare a multidisciplinary care plan. The plan should include a detailed history of present illness along with the reasons for the referral. Any psychosocial, nutritional, or aesthetic concerns should be noted. Next, the nurse communicates with the family to verify the accuracy of the information. The nurse will create a tentative plan, including performing any additional necessary imaging or testing. Precertification and billing concerns are assessed by appropriate teams at this time.

The next step in processing these new patients for your team is to review the nurse's multidisciplinary care plan for each patient at your new Intake Meeting. Here, colorectal surgery, urology, gynecology, GI/motility, nursing team (APN and RN), and social work team members will all join together to discuss each case. If gynecologists, urologists, and/or GI motility surgeons are unable to attend you can include them in the conversation via an email summary of new inquiries each week. At this time any other specialty consultations needed are identified such as anesthesia, nutrition, neurosurgery, psychology, or orthopedics. Discussing patients prior to their arrival with the entire clinical team allows you to gain various perspectives, build a comprehensive plan for your patients, and maximize their time at your center, even before you have met the patient in clinic. This process further facilitates your ability to decrease the number of hospital or clinic visits, along with testing that the patient will experience. It also sends a sharing message to the entire team that is a collaborative process. Consolidating the patient's visit into a few days in succession allows families from outside your area to minimize travel time away from home, thus allowing you to see those patients living a substantial distance from your center. The nurse will then edit the plan if any changes are made and communicate the final plan with the family. Following this meeting the patient's chart will be passed to the scheduling team who work with the family and finalize the itinerary.

## 31.9.2 Weekly collaborative meeting

Your team recognizes that spending time preparing for patients arriving to your center, either in the clinic or in the operating room, is necessary for best outcomes. Reviewing the status of patients set to arrive the upcoming week is done each week in the collaborative meeting. Here, the multidisciplinary team of colorectal surgeons, gynecologists, urologists, anesthetists, GI specialists, inpatient care nursing, ambulatory center nursing, schedulers, social work, and child life specialists join together to discuss updates to the patient's status since the time that they were originally processed as a new intake. The need for any new colorectal/urologic/gynecologic/motility testing is determined as well as if a surgical intervention is needed. Pre- and postoperative considerations are discussed. Weekly multidisciplinary outpatient clinic patients are reviewed, including the reason for the clinic visit, which specialists will need to see the patient, and how much time they will need. This meeting also allows your team to discuss any "updates to plans" when older patients resurface for planned surgeries or interventions previously discussed but not yet acted upon. The final plan for your patient's clinic or operating room upcoming visit is now confirmed.

In addition to the weekly meetings described previously, your center's typical week will include collaboration at the following key components of care each week:

- Weekly outpatient multidisciplinary clinic:
  - *Participants*: Colorectal surgery, urology, gynecology, GI motility, nursing (APN and RN), social work, psychology, and child life specialists
- Operating room:
  - *Participants*: Colorectal surgery, urology, gynecology, GI motility, surgical nursing, and child life specialists

- Inpatient care:
  - *Participants*: Colorectal surgery, urology, gynecology, GI motility, inpatient nursing supplemented with ambulatory bowel management nursing educators (RN and APN), social work, psychology, and child life specialists
- Bowel management program
  - *Participants*: Colorectal advance practice nursing consulting with colorectal surgery, social work, psychology, and child life specialists
- Long-term follow-up clinic visits or phone consultations:
  - *Participants*: Colorectal surgery, urology, gynecology, GI motility, colorectal nursing (APN and RN), social work, psychology, and child life specialists

Incorporating these collaborative experiences each week with your team will allow your center to move beyond basic care for your patient and provide exceptional care patients deserve and expect at a center of excellence.

# References

1. Vilanova-Sánchez A, Reck CA, Wood RJ et al. Impact on patient care of a multidisciplinary center specializing in colorectal and pelvic reconstruction. *Front Surg*. 2018 Nov 19;5:68.
2. Vilanova-Sanchez A, Halleran DR, Reck-Burneo CA et al. A descriptive model for a multidisciplinary unit for colorectal and pelvic malformations. *J Pediatr Surg*. 2019 Apr;54(3):479–485.

# Index

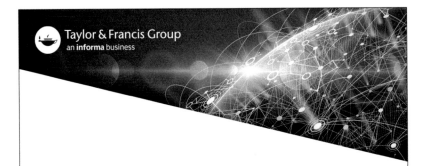